Nurses' Handbook of Health Assessment

Janet R. Weber, RN, EdD
Professor
Director RN-BSN Program
Department of Nursing
Southeast Missouri State University
Cape Girardeau, Missouri

 Wolters Kluwer | Lippincott Williams & Wilkins
Health
Philadelphia · Baltimore · New York · London
Buenos Aires · Hong Kong · Sydney · Tokyo

9 8 7 6 5 4 3 2 1

Printed in China

Care has been taken to confirm the accuracy of the information presented and to describe generally accepted practices. However, the author(s), editors, and publisher are not responsible for errors or omissions or for any consequences from application of the information in this book and make no warranty, expressed or implied, with respect to the currency, completeness, or accuracy of the contents of the publication. Application of this information in a particular situation remains the professional responsibility of the practitioner; the clinical treatments described and recommended may not be considered absolute and universal recommendations.

The author(s), editors, and publisher have exerted every effort to ensure that drug selection and dosage set forth in this text are in accordance with the current recommendations and practice at the time of publication. However, in view of ongoing research, changes in government regulations, and the constant flow of information relating to drug therapy and drug reactions, the reader is urged to check the package insert for each drug for any change in indications and dosage and for added warnings and precautions. This is particularly important when the recommended agent is a new or infrequently employed drug.

Some drugs and medical devices presented in this publication have Food and Drug Administration (FDA) clearance for limited use in restricted research settings. It is the responsibility of the health care provider to ascertain the FDA status of each drug or device planned for use in his or her clinical practice.

Library of Congress Cataloging-in-Publication Data

Nurses' handbook of health assessment / [edited by] Janet R. Weber. — Eighth edition.
      p. ; cm.
  Includes bibliographical references and index.
  ISBN 978-1-4511-4282-2 (alk. paper)
  I. Weber, Janet, editor.
  [DNLM: 1. Nursing Assessment—methods—Handbooks. 2. Medical History Taking—methods—Handbooks. 3. Physical Examination—methods—Handbooks.
WY 49]
  RT48
  616.07′5—dc23

201302419O

To my loving husband, Bill,
for your wise encouragement, patience, and confidence

To my sons:
Joe, *for reviewing the book and providing insights*
to make the content clearer for students;
Wes, *for the book cover graphic illustrating the ongoing*
and complex nature of nursing assessment

To my grandson, Eli,
for reminding me to giggle and have fun

To Ian,
for your caring energy and reminding me what is important in life

To my Mom,
for showing me how to grow old wisely

To my colleagues:
Jane Kelley, RN, PhD, *for your numerous cultural, health promotion,*
and chapter contributions throughout the book
Ann Sprengel, RN, EdD, *for your chapter contributions*
and work as permissions editor
Kathy Casteel, RN, MSN, NP, *for reference contributions*
and your shared Nurse Practitioner expertise

To all my undergraduate and graduate students
who teach me how to teach

To all the practicing nurses
who inspire me to continue to write

Contributors

Jill Cash, MSN, APN
Family Nurse Practitioner
University of Southern Indiana
Evansville, Indiana
CHAPTER 24: ASSESSING CHILDBEARING WOMEN
CHAPTER 25: ASSESSING NEWBORNS AND INFANTS

Brenda Johnson, RN, PHD
Professor
Southeast Missouri State University
Cape Girardeau, Missouri
CHAPTER 26: ASSESSING OLDER ADULTS

Jane H. Kelley, RN, PhD
Adjunct Professor
School of Nursing
Indiana Wesleyan University
Louisville, Kentucky
CHAPTER 7: ASSESSING PAIN: THE 5TH VITAL SIGN
CHAPTER 8: ASSESSING FOR VIOLENCE
NURSING DIAGNOSES, HEALTH PROMOTION TEACHING TIPS, AND REFERENCES

Ann D. Sprengel, RN, EdD
Professor
Director of Undergraduate Studies
Department of Nursing
Southeast Missouri State University
Cape Girardeau, Missouri
CHAPTER 9: ASSESSING NUTRITIONAL STATUS
CHAPTER 18: ASSESSING PERIPHERAL VASCULAR SYSTEM
PERMISSIONS EDITOR

Reviewers

Cherry K. Beckworth, RN, PhD, CNE
Track Administrator—BSN Program
The University of Texas Medical Branch
Galveston, Texas

Celeste Carter, DNS
Assistant Professor
Louisiana State University Health Sciences Center New Orleans
New Orleans, Louisiana

Shelly Daily, MNSc, BSN
Associate Professor of Nursing
Arkansas Tech University
Russellville, Arkansas

Carmela Theresa de Leon, RN-BC, PhD (c), MAN, BSN
Nursing Faculty
Pima Medical Institute
Mesa, Arizona

Cathy R. Kessenich, DSN, ARNP, FAANP
Professor of Nursing
The University of Tampa
Tampa, Florida

Ruth Ann Kiefer, RN, DrNP, CRRN, CNE
Nursing Instructor
Abington Memorial Hospital
Willow Grove, Pennsylvania

Rosemary Macy, RN, PhD, CNE
Associate Professor
Boise State University
Boise, Idaho

Frances Mai, RN-BC, MA, LNC
Director Nursing Resource and Simulation Center
Felician College
Lodi, New Jersey

Juanita Manning-Walsh, PhD
Associate Professor
Western Michigan University
Kalamazoo, Michigan

Kimberly J. Oosterhouse, RN, PhD, CCRN
Associate Professor of Nursing
College of DuPage
Glen Ellyn, Illinois

Julie Slack, RN, MSN
Assistant Professor
Eastern Michigan University
Ypsilanti, Michigan

Debbie Sleik, RN, MSN
Nursing Faculty
Bay College
Escanaba, Michigan

Margaret P. Spain, MSN, APRN, CDE
Assistant Professor
Medical University of South Carolina School of Nursing
Charleston, South Carolina

Terri W. Summers, RN, DNP
Assistant Professor
Clayton State University
Morrow, Georgia

Annette Wounded Arrow, RN, MSN, CEN, CNE
Associate Professor
Illinois Central College
Peoria, Illinois

Preface

Purpose

The eighth edition of the *Nurses' Handbook of Health Assessment* continues to provide students and practicing nurses with an up-to-date reference and guide to assist with interviewing clients and performing a physical assessment.

This 26-chapter guide reminds the reader of questions to ask and assessment procedures to carry out when assessing the client. In addition, it clearly illustrates normal versus abnormal findings and provides examples of precise descriptions of these findings to assist the nurse with accurate documentation.

It may be used as a stand-alone textbook or as a convenient handbook to accompany *Health Assessment in Nursing, 5e,* which contains more comprehensive assessment theory. The small size and spiral binding of this Handbook promote its use at the bedside as a step-by-step guide while performing the exam. A colored tab at the bottom of the page allows for quick referencing of Abnormal Findings.

Because this Handbook can also be used as a freestanding text, more content and illustrative assessment photos have been added. This includes additional content on anatomy and physiology, client preparation for each exam, and more photos of nurses performing the examinations as well as photos of pathologic findings.

Key Features

The key features of this Handbook include **full-color anatomy and physiology** images, illustrations of **normal and abnormal** physiologic findings, highlighted **risk factors**, the **three-column format** of assessment procedures, and the **spiral binding** that allows the Handbook to stay open on any flat surface. This edition includes **additional new photos of nurses performing** each **examination** and new photos of **abnormal findings** throughout the text.

Along with a chapter on older adults, the more common **geriatric variations** that occur with advancing age are located at the end of each of the physical assessment chapters and are easily identified by 🌐 **Pediatric variations** are summarized at the end of each body system assessment chapter and are identified by 🌐 **Cultural variations** are also highlighted, when applicable, with 🌐.

New Chapters in This Edition

The eighth edition includes two new chapters. Chapter 4, "Assessing Psychosocial, Cognitive, and Moral Development," has been added to Unit 2 as the first integrative assessment chapter to help ensure a holistic client assessment. Assessing risk for substance abuse has been added to Chapter 5, "Assessing Mental Status and Substance Abuse."

Organization

This eighth edition has been organized into four units to correlate with the fifth edition of *Health Assessment in Nursing. Unit 1* contains three chapters that focus on nursing data collection and analysis. *Chapter 1* explains the purpose of obtaining a nursing health history and describes basic guidelines for an effective interview. *Chapter 2* describes questions to ask to elicit a client's profile, developmental history, and functional health patterns (Gordon, 1994). The reader is referred to specific physical assessment chapters for related objective data. A list of associated nursing diagnoses, based on the currently accepted North American Nursing Diagnosis Association (NANDA) taxonomy of diagnostic categories, follows each section. *Chapter 3* consists of skills and techniques for performing the physical assessment.

Unit 2 contains *Chapters 4 to 9* and focuses on Integrative Holistic Nursing Assessment. These chapters describe assessment of the client's developmental level; mental status; risk for substance abuse; general overall health status, vital signs, including pain assessment; potential for being a victim of violence; and nutritional status. This unit precedes the *Nursing Assessment of Physical Systems* located in *Unit 3* because these integrative assessments may affect physical assessment findings and vice versa.

Unit 3 contains *Chapters 10 to 23*, covering all the physical body systems. Each chapter consists of the following:

• Illustrations of relevant anatomy or physiologic processes
• Written description of anatomy and physiology

- Equipment needed for the examination
- Focus questions specific to the body system being assessed
- Preparations of the client for each exam
- Risk factors
- Overview of exam
- Physical assessment procedure (three-column format: procedure, normal findings, and abnormal findings)
- Pediatric variations
- Geriatric variations
- Cultural variations
- Teaching tips for selected nursing diagnoses

Unit 4 focuses on nursing assessment of special groups: childbearing women, newborns and infants, and older adults.

Appendices

The appendices at the end of the Handbook contain useful tools to complete a holistic assessment. The first two appendices contain an interview guide based on functional health patterns followed by a physical assessment guide to pull it all together. These are followed by an example of how to document the entire adult assessment. Other reference tools needed for health assessment include:

assessment of family functional health patterns, developmental information, immunization schedule, growth charts, nursing diagnoses and collaborative problem lists, a convenient Spanish Translation Guide to conduct an interview and explain the physical assessment, and an example of Canada's Food Guide.

Student Resources Available on thePoint

- Assessment Tool: Nursing History Guide
- Assessment Tool: Physical Assessment Guide
- Full Text Online
- Concepts in Action Animations
- Watch and Learn Video Clips
- Heart and Breath Sounds
- Nursing Professional Roles and Responsibilities

Instructor Resources Available on thePoint

- Image Bank
- Strategies for Effective Teaching

Janet R. Weber, RN, EdD

Contents

UNIT 4 : NURSING ASSESSMENT OF SPECIAL GROUPS

APPENDICES

CHAPTER **1**

Obtaining a Nursing Health History

A nursing health assessment can be defined as the systematic collection of subjective data (stated by the client) and objective data (observed by the nurse) used to determine a client's functional health pattern status (Table 1-1). The nurse collects physiologic, psychological, sociocultural, developmental, and spiritual client data.

Guidelines for a nursing health history and the difference between nursing diagnoses, collaborative problems, and medical diagnoses are discussed in this chapter. Chapter 2 focuses on collecting subjective and objective data using functional health patterns and Chapter 3 focuses on performing physical assessment skills.

Guidelines for Obtaining a Nursing Health History

A nursing health history usually precedes the physical assessment and guides the nurse as to which body systems must be assessed.

TABLE 1-1   Comparing Subjective and Objective Data

	Subjective	Objective
Description	Data elicited and verified by the client	Data directly or indirectly observed through measurement
Sources	Client Family and significant others Client record Other health-care professionals	Observations and physical assessment findings of the nurse or other health-care professionals Documentation of assessments made in client record Observations made by the client's family or significant others
Methods used to obtain data	Client interview	Observation and physical examination
Skills needed to obtain data	Interview and therapeutic communication skills Caring ability and empathy Listening skills	Inspection Palpation Percussion Auscultation
Examples	"I have a headache." "It frightens me." "I am not hungry."	Respirations 16 per minute BP 180/100, apical pulse 80 and irregular X-ray film reveals fractured pelvis

It also assists the nurse in establishing a nurse–client relationship and allows client participation in identifying problems and goals. The primary source of data is the client; valuable information may also be obtained from the family, other health team members, and the client record.

PHASES OF THE NURSING INTERVIEW

Professional interpersonal and interviewing skills are necessary to obtain a valid nursing health history. The nursing interview is a communication process that focuses on the client's developmental, psychological, physiologic, sociocultural, and spiritual responses that can be treated with nursing and collaborative interventions. The nursing interview has three basic phases: Introductory phase, working phase, and summary and closure phase.

Introductory Phase

Introduce yourself and describe your role (i.e., RN, student, etc.). Address the client with surname. Next, explain the purpose of the interview to the client (i.e., to collect data, to understand the client's needs, and to plan nursing care). Explain the purpose of note taking, confidentiality, and the type of questions to be asked. Provide comfort, privacy, and confidentiality.

Working Phase

Facilitate the client's comments about major biographical data, reason for seeking health care and functional health pattern responses. Use critical thinking skills to listen for and observe cues and to interpret and validate the information received from the client. Collaborate with the client to identify problems and goals. The approach used for facilitation may be either free-flowing or more structured with specific questions, depending on available time and type of data needed.

Summary and Closure Phase

Summarize the information obtained during the working phase and validate the problems and goals with the client. You may begin to discuss possible plans to resolve the problems (nursing diagnoses and collaborative problems). Allow the client time to express feelings, concerns, and questions.

SPECIFIC COMMUNICATION TECHNIQUES

Specific communication techniques are used to facilitate the interview. The following sections include specific guidelines for phrasing questions and statements to promote an effective and productive interview.

Types of Questions to Use

- Use open-ended questions to elicit the client's feelings and perceptions. These questions begin with "What," "How," or "Which," and require more than a one-word response.

- Use closed-ended questions to obtain facts and zero in on specific information. The client can respond with one or two words. These questions begin with "Is," "Are," "Will," "When," or "Did," and help avoid rambling by the client.

- Use a laundry list (scrambled words) approach to obtain specific answers. For example, "Is the pain severe, dull, sharp, mild, cutting, piercing?" "Does the pain occur once every year, day, month, hour?" This reduces the likelihood of the client's perceiving and providing an expected answer.

- Explore all data that deviate from normal with the following questions: "What alleviates or aggravates the problem?" "How long has it occurred?" "How severe is it?" "Does it radiate?" "When does it occur?" "Is its onset gradual or sudden?" The mnemonic COLDSPA may be used to further explore the client's symptoms (see Box 1-1).

Types of Statements to Use

- Rephrase or repeat your perception of the client's response to reflect or clarify the information shared. For example, "You feel you have a serious illness?"

- Encourage verbalization of client by saying "Um hum," "Yes," or "I agree," or nodding.

- Describe what you observe in the client. For example, "It seems you have difficulty on the right side."

Additional Helpful Hints

- Accept the client; display a nonjudgmental attitude.

- Use silence to help the client and yourself reflect and reorganize thoughts.

- Provide the client with information during the interview as questions and concerns arise.

- Note that not all clients can read. Basic care terms can be communicated best by using pictures.

Communication Styles to Avoid

- Excessive or insufficient eye contact (varies with cultures).

- Doing other things while taking the history, and being mentally distant or physically far away from the client (more than 60.9 to 91.4 cm [2 to 3 ft]).

BOX 1-1	SAMPLE APPLICATION OF COLDSPA: EXPLORING THE SYMPTOMS OF BACK PAIN	
Mnemonic	**General Question**	**Adapted Question**
Character	Describe the sign or symptom (feeling, appearance, sound, smell, or taste if applicable).	"What does the pain feel like?"
Onset	When did it begin?	"When did this pain start?"
Location	Where is it? Does it radiate? Does it occur anywhere else?	"Where does it hurt the most? Does it radiate or go to any other part of your body?"
Duration	How long does it last? Does it recur?	"How long does the pain last? Does it come and go or is it constant?"
Severity	How bad is it? How much does it bother you?	"How intense is the pain? Rate it on a scale of 1 to 10."
Pattern	What makes it better or worse?	"What makes your back pain worse or better? Are there any treatments you've tried that relieve the pain?"
Associated factors/ How it Affects the client	What other symptoms occur with it? How does it affect you?	"What do you think caused it to start? Do you have any other problems that seem related to your back pain? How does this pain affect your life and daily activities?"

- Biased or leading questions—for example, "You don't feel bad, do you?"
- Relying on memory to recall all the information or recording all the details.
- Rushing the client.
- Reading questions from the history form, distracting attention from the client.

Specific Age Variations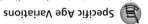

When interviewing the pediatric client from birth to early ado-lescence (through age 14 years), validate information from the history for reliability with the responsible significant others (e.g., parent, grandparent). Use the following guidelines when inter-viewing the pediatric client:

- Use language that is familiar for the appropriate age.
- Involve the parent and/or significant other when interviewing the child to achieve accurate information.
- Allow the child to sit with parent, or in parent's lap, if desired.

When interviewing the older adult client, remember that age affects and often slows all body systems within a person to vary-ing degrees.

Use the following guidelines when interviewing the older adult client.

- Use a gentle, genuine approach.
- Use simple, straightforward questions in lay terms. Let the client set the pace of the conversation. Be patient and listen well. Allow ample time.
- Introduce yourself, but remember that an older client may forget your name—you may have to write it for the client later in the interview.
- Use direct eye contact and sit at client's eye level. Establish and maintain privacy (especially important).
- Assess hearing acuity; with hearing loss, speak the client, and speak on the side on which hearing is more adequate. Speak louder only if you confirm the client has a hearing defi-cit. Turn off any background noises.
- Wear a nametag and provide written notes for the client to refer to in the future.

Emotional Variations

Not all clients are calm and friendly. It is important to assess the client's mood in order to adapt your approach to promote an effective interaction with the client.

- *Angry client:* Approach in a calm, reassuring, in-control man-ner. Allow ventilation of client's feelings. Avoid arguing and provide personal space.
- *Anxious client:* Approach with simple, organized information. Explain your role and purpose.
- *Manipulative client:* Provide structure and set limits.
- *Depressed client:* Express interest and understanding in a neu-tral manner.
- *Sensitive issues* (e.g., sexuality, dying, spirituality): Be aware of your own thoughts and feelings. These factors may affect the

client's health and need to be discussed with someone. Such personal, sensitive topics may be referred when you do not feel comfortable discussing these topics.

 Cultural Variations

Cultural variations in communication and self-disclosure styles may seriously affect the information obtained. Be aware of possible variations in the communication styles of yourself and client. If misunderstanding or difficulty in communicating is evident, seek help from a "culture broker" who is skilled at cross-cultural communication. See Box 1-2 for observations and questions to ask clients from another culture.

BOX 1-2 EXAMPLE OF OBSERVATIONS AND QUESTIONS TO ASK A CLIENT FROM ANOTHER CULTURE

1. What is your full name?
2. What is your legal name?
3. By what name do you wish to be called?
4. What is your primary language?
5. Do you speak a specific dialect?
6. What other languages do you speak?
7. Do you find it difficult to share your thoughts, feelings, and ideas with family? Friends? Health-care providers?
8. Do you mind being touched by friends? Strangers? Health-care workers?
9. How do you wish to be greeted? Handshake? Nod of the head, etc.?
10. Are you usually on time for appointments?
11. Are you usually on time for social engagements?
12. Observe the client's speech pattern. Is the speech pattern low- or high-context? Remember, clients from highly contexted cultures place greater value on silence.
13. Observe the client when physical contact is made. Does he or she withdraw from the touch or become tense?
14. How close does the client stand when talking with family members? With health-care providers?
15. Does the client maintain eye contact when talking with the nurse/physician, etc.?

Frequently noted cultural variations include the following:

• Reluctance to reveal personal information to strangers for various culturally based reasons.
• Variation in willingness to express emotional distress or pain openly.
• Variation in ability to receive information and/or listen.
• Variation in meaning conveyed by use of language (e.g., by nonnative speakers, by use of slang).
• Variation in use and meaning of nonverbal communication: Eye contact, stance, gestures, demeanor (e.g., eye contact may be perceived as rude, aggressive, or immodest by some cultures, but lack of eye contact may be perceived as evasive, insecure, or inattentive by other cultures; slightly bowed stance may indicate respect in some groups; size of personal space affects one's comfortable interpersonal distance; touch may be perceived as comforting or threatening).
• Variation in disease/illness perception; culture-specific syndromes or disorders are accepted by some groups (e.g., *susto* in Latin America). *Susto* (fright, emotional shock, soul loss) is perceived to have either a physical or supernatural cause resulting in loss of appetite, weight, strength, and motivation to carry out even simple tasks (From culture bound syndrome "Susto," 2011; Guarnero, 2005).

• Variation in past, present, or future time orientation (e.g., United States' dominant culture is future-oriented; other cultures vary).
• Variation in family decision-making process: Person other than the client or the client's parent may be the major decision maker re: appointments, treatments, or follow-up care for client.

Assessing Non–English-Speaking Clients

• Use a bilingual interpreter familiar with the client's culture and with health care, when possible (e.g., a nurse culture broker).
• Consider the relationship of the interpreter to the client. If the interpreter is a child or is of the opposite sex, different age, or different social status, interpretation may be impaired.

Nursing Diagnoses, Collaborative Problems, and Medical Diagnoses

The subjective and objective data that are collected during a nursing health assessment assist the nurse in identifying nursing diagnoses and/or collaborative problems.

As outlined by NANDA (2012a, b), nursing diagnoses may fall into one of four categories: Health promotion, risk, actual, or syndrome. A "health promotion" nursing diagnosis describes human responses of a person, family, or community that have a readiness for enhancing a healthy state. A "risk" diagnosis describes human responses of an individual, family, or community and is supported by risk factors that contribute to increased vulnerability. An "actual" nursing diagnosis is a human response to health conditions/life processes that currently exist in a person, family, or community that can be validated by the defining characteristics of that diagnostic category. A syndrome nursing diagnosis involves clusters of nursing diagnoses that comprise a single syndrome.

An actual nursing diagnosis is a human response to health conditions or life processes that currently exist at the present time in an individual, family, or community that can be validated by the defining characteristics of that diagnostic category. NANDA (2012) defines a health promotion diagnosis as "a clinical judgment about a person's, family's, or community's motivation and desire to increase well-being and actualize human health potential as expressed in the readiness to enhance specific health behaviors, and can be used in any health state." Wording may include "readiness for enhanced" (e.g., readiness for enhanced self-health management) or as a problem to be addressed that will enhance health status (e.g., ineffective protection). A risk diagnosis describes vulnerability, especially as a result of exposure to factors that increase the chance of injury or loss. A newer category of "syndrome" nursing diagnosis is defined as "a clinical judgment describing a specific cluster of nursing diagnoses that occur together and are best addressed together and through similar interventions" (NANDA, 2012a). Syndromes such as rape trauma syndrome, post trauma syndrome, risk for disuse syndrome are included in this category. See Table 1-2 for an example of the four nursing diagnosis categories and the directions for stating each type of diagnosis.

In addition to nursing diagnoses, Carpenito-Moyet (2012) defines collaborative problems as "certain physiologic complications that nurses monitor to detect their onset or changes in status. Nurses manage collaborative problems using both physician-prescribed and nursing-prescribed interventions to minimize the complications of the events" (p. 841). The definitive treatment for a nursing diagnosis is developed by the nurse; the definitive treatment for a collaborative problem

TABLE 1-2 Comparison of Health Promotion, Risk, Actual, and Syndrome Nursing Diagnoses

	Health Promotion Diagnoses	Risk Diagnoses	Actual Nursing Diagnoses	Syndrome Nursing Diagnoses
Client Status	A clinical judgment about an individual, family, or community's motivation to increase well-being and actualize human health potential (NANDA, 2012)	Human responses that may develop in a vulnerable individual, family, or community especially as a result of exposure to factors that increase the chance of injury or loss (NANDA, 2012)	Human experiences/responses to health conditions/life processes that exist in reality or at the present time (NANDA, 2012).	A clinical judgment describing a specific cluster of nursing diagnoses that occur together and are best addressed together and through similar interventions (NANDA, 2012).
Format for Stating	"Readiness for Enhanced . . ." Or a possible problem area that can be addressed to enhance well-being	"Risk for . . ."	"Nursing diagnoses and related to clause"	Includes a "syndrome" in the nursing diagnosis along with a "related to" clause.
Examples	Readiness for Enhanced Body Image Readiness for Enhanced Family Processes Readiness for Enhanced Effective Breast-feeding Readiness for Enhanced Skin Integrity	Risk for Disturbed Body Image Risk for Interrupted Family Processes Risk for Ineffective Breast-feeding Risk for Impaired Skin Integrity	Dysfunctional Family Processes: Alcoholism Ineffective Breast-feeding related to poor infant-mother attachment Impaired Skin Integrity related to immobility	Syndrome diagnoses can be risk or actual: Risk for Relocation Stress Syndrome related to change of school, house, city of residence and moving far from grandparents. Rape Trauma Syndrome related to experience of violent rape. Post Trauma Syndrome related to presence in riot conditions.

is developed by both the nurse and the physician. Not all physiologic complications are collaborative problems. If the nurse can prevent the complication or provide the primary treatment, then the problem may very well be a nursing diagnosis. For example, nurses can prevent and treat pressure ulcers. The NANDA nursing diagnosis to use, therefore, is Risk for Impaired Skin Integrity. Nursing diagnoses, risk nursing diagnoses, health promotion nursing diagnoses, syndrome nursing diagnoses, and collaborative problems are listed in Appendices 9 and 10.

Collaborative problems are equivalent in importance to nursing diagnoses but represent the interdependent or collaborative role of nursing, whereas nursing diagnoses represent the independent role of the nurse (Carpenito-Moyet, 2012). Figure 1-1 illustrates the decision-making process involved in distinguishing a nursing diagnosis from a collaborative health problem. The nurse can use this model to decide whether the identified problem can be treated independently as a nursing diagnosis or whether the nurse will monitor and use both medical and nursing interventions to treat or prevent the problem. Table 1-3 provides guidelines for formulating nursing diagnoses and collaborative problems.

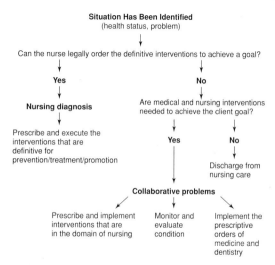

FIGURE 1-1 Differentiation of nursing diagnoses from collaborative problems. (From: Carpenito-Moyet, L.J. (2012). *Nursing diagnoses: Application to clinical practice* (13th ed.). Philadelphia: Lippincott Williams & Wilkins, pp. 28. © 1990 Lynda Juall Carpenito.)

TABLE 1-3 Comparison of Nursing Diagnoses and Collaborative Problems

Identifying Criteria of a Nursing Diagnosis	Identifying Criteria of a Collaborative Problem
1. The client problem is physiologic, psychosocial, or spiritual.	1. The client problem is a physiologic complication.
2. The nurse monitors and treats.	2. The nurse monitors for signs and symptoms of the complication and notifies the physician if a change occurs. (In some cases the nurse may initiate interventions.)
3. The nurse independently orders and implements the primary nursing interventions.	3. The physician orders the primary treatment, and the nurse collaborates to implement additional treatments that are licensed to be implemented and monitors for responses to and effectiveness of treatments.

Format and Follow-up for Nursing Diagnoses	Format and Follow-up for Collaborative Problems
1. Use diagnostic category + "related to" + etiology.	1. Use "Risk for complication: _____."
2. Write specific client goals.	2. Write nursing goals.
3. Write specific nursing orders (interventions) including assessments, teaching, counseling, referrals, and direct client care.	3. Write which parameters the nurse must monitor, including how often. Indicate when the physician should be notified. Identify the nursing interventions to prevent the complication and those to be initiated if a change occurs.

If collaborative medical and nursing interventions are not needed, the problem is a medical diagnosis. A medical diagnosis is the identification of a disease or a disorder. The nurse should refer all medical diagnoses to medicine and/or dentistry. Table 1-4 highlights the differences between nursing diagnoses, collaborative problems, and medical diagnoses.

TABLE 1-4   **Examples of Nursing Diagnoses, Collaborative Problems, and Medical Diagnoses**

Nursing Diagnoses	Collaborative Problems	Medical Diagnoses
Altered Oral Mucous Membrane related to difficulty with hygiene secondary to fixation devices Acute Pain related to tissue trauma	Risk for complication: Aspiration	Fractured jaw
Impaired Skin Integrity related to poor circulation to lower extremities Deficient Knowledge (effects of exercise on need for insulin)	Risk for complication: Hyperglycemia	Diabetes mellitus
Ineffective Airway Clearance related to the presence of excessive mucus production Deficient Fluid Volume related to poor fluid intake	Risk for complication: Hypoglycemia Risk for complication: Hypoxemia	Pneumonia

CHAPTER 2

Collecting Subjective and Objective Data

This chapter will focus on how a nursing model or framework is needed to correctly collect objective and subjective data from a client. The differences between a medical model and a nursing model will be described. Finally, a Functional Health Patterns nursing framework by Gordon (2010) will be used to describe the parts of a holistic nursing assessment.

Nursing Model Versus Medical Model for Data Collection

Several models of nursing may be used to guide the nurse in data collection. However, Marjory Gordon's Functional Health Pattern assessment framework (2010) is particularly useful in collecting health data to formulate nursing diagnoses. Gordon has defined 11 functional health patterns that provide for a holistic client database. A pattern is a sequence of related behaviors that assists the nurse in collecting and categorizing data. These 11 functional health patterns can be used for nursing assessment in any practice areas for clients of all ages and in the assessment of families and communities. For the purpose of this handbook, assessment is focused on the individual. However, guideline questions for families organized according to functional health patterns are included in Appendix 1 (p. 664). The NANDA list of accepted nursing diagnoses has been grouped according to the appropriate functional health patterns. These diagnoses are listed at the end of each functional health pattern section in this chapter. In addition, Box 2-1 presents a brief overview of the subjective and objective assessment focus data needed for each functional health pattern.*

Using a functional health pattern framework assists the nurse with collecting data necessary to identify and validate nursing diagnoses. This approach eliminates repetition of medical data

---

*Adapted from: Gordon, M. (2010). *Manual of nursing diagnosis* (12th ed.). St. Louis, MO: Mosby.

already obtained by physicians and other members of the healthcare team. The medical systems model (biographical data, reason for seeking care, personal history, past medical history, family history, psychosocial history, and review of systems) is more useful for the physician in making medical diagnoses. Clients often complain that the same information is requested by both nurses and physicians. A nursing history based on functional health patterns, however, will help eliminate this problem by assisting the nurse to assess client responses associated with nursing diagnoses and collaborative problems.

It is important for the nurse to assess each functional health pattern with clients because alterations in health can affect functioning in any of these areas, and alterations in functional health patterns can, in turn, affect health. See Appendix 1 for a sample nursing assessment form based on functional health patterns.

Nursing Assessment by Functional Health Patterns

The components of a nursing health assessment incorporating a functional health pattern approach (Gordon, 2010) are listed below. Prior to data collection for each functional health pattern,

Continued on page 17

BOX 2-1 SUBJECTIVE AND OBJECTIVE ASSESSMENT FOCUS FOR FUNCTIONAL HEALTH PATTERNS

1. Health Perception–Health Management Pattern

   Subjective data: Perception of health status and health practices used by client to maintain health

   Objective data: Appearance, grooming, posture, expression, vital signs, height, weight

2. Nutritional–Metabolic Pattern

   Subjective data: Dietary habits, including food and fluid intake

   Objective data: General physical survey, including examination of skin, mouth, abdomen, and cranial nerves (CN) V, IX, X, and XII

3. Elimination Pattern

   Subjective data: Regularity and control of bowel and bladder habits

   Objective data: Skin examination, rectal examination

4. Activity–Exercise Pattern

   Subjective data: Activities of daily living that require energy expenditure

   Objective data: Examination of musculoskeletal system, including gait, posture, range of motion (ROM) of joints, muscle tone, and strength; cardiovascular examination; peripheral vascular examination; thoracic examination

5. Sexuality–Reproduction Pattern

   Subjective data: Sexual identity, activities, and relationships; expression of sexuality and level of satisfaction with sexual patterns; reproduction patterns

   Objective data: Genitalia examination, breast examination

6. Sleep–Rest Pattern

   Subjective data: Perception of effectiveness of sleep and rest habits

   Objective data: Appearance and attention span

7. Cognitive–Perceptual Pattern

   For the purposes of this handbook, the cognitive pattern has been divided into two parts: (1) The sensory–perceptual pattern, to include the senses of hearing, vision, smell, taste, and touch, and (2) the cognitive pattern, to include knowledge, thought, perception, and language.

   a. Sensory–Perceptual Pattern

   Subjective data: Perception of ability to hear, see, smell, taste, and feel (including light touch, pain, and vibratory sensation)

   Objective data: Visual and hearing examinations, pain perception, cranial nerve examination; testing for taste, smell, and touch

b. Cognitive Pattern
   Subjective data: Perception of messages, decision making, thought processes
   Objective data: Mental status examination
8. Role–Relationship Pattern
   Subjective data: Perception of and level of satisfaction with family, work, and social roles
   Objective data: Communication with significant others, visits from significant others and family, family genogram
9. Self-Perception–Self-Concept Pattern
   Subjective data: Perception of self-worth, personal identity, feelings

   Objective data: Body posture, movement, eye contact, voice and speech pattern, emotions, moods, and thought content
10. Coping–Stress Tolerance Pattern
    Subjective data: Perception of stressful life events and ability to cope
    Objective data: Behavior, thought processes
11. Value–Belief Pattern
    Subjective data: Perception of what is good, correct, proper, and meaningful; philosophical beliefs; values and beliefs that guide choices
    Objective data: Presence of religious articles, religious actions and routines, and visits from clergy

it is important to obtain a client profile and developmental history.

1. Client Profile
2. Developmental History
3. Health Perception–Health Management Pattern
4. Nutritional–Metabolic Pattern
5. Elimination Pattern
6. Activity–Exercise Pattern
7. Sexuality–Reproduction Pattern
8. Sleep–Rest Pattern
9. Sensory–Perceptual Pattern
10. Cognitive Pattern
11. Role–Relationship Pattern
12. Self-Perception–Self-Concept Pattern

13. Coping–Stress Tolerance Pattern
14. Value–Belief Pattern

In the following sections, the purpose of each nursing health assessment functional health pattern component is explained, followed by guideline statements and questions to elicit subjective data from the client, objective data information and referral, and a list of nursing diagnostic categories for the specific nursing health assessment functional health pattern component.

For subjective data collection, ask open-ended questions first to encourage the client to verbalize freely. Then ask specific questions to obtain specific information. It is important to remember that not every question will apply to every client. Use common sense and professional judgment to determine which questions are a priority and appropriate for each individual client. Consider certain factors, such as comfort level, anxiety level, age, and current health status, because they influence the client's ability to participate fully in the interview.

When appropriate, an objective data outline follows the subjective data questions and refers the examiner to the section where the specific examination technique, normal findings, and deviations from normal are located. At the end of each section is a list of corresponding nursing diagnostic categories for that specific nursing health assessment component. This list is divided into wellness, risk, and actual (problem) nursing diagnoses. Although clients can be at risk for most problem diagnoses, only NANDA-approved and a few selected other risk diagnoses are listed. Appendix 1 (p. 664) provides a documentation form for the collection of subjective and objective data for each of the functional health patterns.

CLIENT PROFILE

Purpose

The purpose of the client profile is to determine biographical client data and to obtain an overview of past and present medical diagnoses and treatment that may alter a client's response. This section also helps the interviewer elicit collaborative health problems.

Subjective Data: Guideline Questions

Biographical Data

- What is your name?
- Tell me about your background.
- When were you born?
- What is your ethnic origin?

- How old are you?
- What level of education have you completed?
- Have you ever served in the military?
- Do you have a religious preference? Specify.
- Where do you live?
- What form of transportation do you use?
- Where is the closest health-care facility to you that you would go to if ill or in an emergency?

Reason for Seeking Health Care and Current Understanding of Health

- Explain your major reason for seeking health care.
- What has the doctor told you regarding your health?
- Do you understand your medical diagnosis? Explain.
- Use the following mnemonic—**COLDSPA**—to explore any abnormal signs, symptoms, or problems the client reports.
  - **C**haracter: Describe the sign or symptom.
  - **O**nset: When did it begin?
  - **L**ocation: Where is it? Does it radiate?
  - **D**uration: How long does it last? Does it recur?
  - **S**everity: How bad is it (on a scale of 1 to 10, 1 being mild and 10 being severe)?
  - **P**attern: What makes it better? What makes it worse?
  - **A**ssociated factors: What other symptoms occur with it?

Treatments/Medications

- Describe the treatments and medications you have received.
- How has your illness been treated in the past?
- What is being planned for your treatment now?
- Do you understand the purpose of your treatment?
- Have you been satisfied with past treatments? Explain.
- What prescribed medications are you taking?
- What over-the-counter medications are you taking?
- Do you take any supplements, alternative, or complementary medications?
- Do you have any difficulties with these medications?
- How do they make you feel?
- What is the purpose of these medications?

Past Illnesses/Hospitalizations

- Tell me about any past illnesses/surgeries you have had.
- Have you had other illnesses in the past? Specify.
- How were the past illnesses treated?
- Have you been in hospital before? Where? For what purpose?

- How did you feel about your past hospital stays?
- How can we help to improve this hospital stay for you?
- Have you received any home health care? Explain.
- How satisfied were you with this care?

Allergies

- Are you allergic to any drugs, foods, or other environmental substances (e.g., dust, molds, pollens, latex)?
- Describe the reaction you have when exposed to the allergen.
- What do you do for your allergies?

DEVELOPMENTAL HISTORY

Purpose

The purpose of the developmental history is to determine the physical, cognitive, and psychosocial development of the client to assess any developmental delays. Subjective data obtained from assessment of the functional health patterns (Role–Relationship, Cognitive, Value–Belief, and Coping–Stress Tolerance) will assist you in determining cognitive and psychosocial development. Appendix 5 provides a comparison developmental table for the child. Objective data obtained from the physical examination regarding height, weight, and musculoskeletal function provides a basis for determining physical development (see Appendix 8).

Subjective Data: Guideline Questions

- Describe any physical handicaps you have.
- Tell me about your health and growth as a child.
- Tell me about your accomplishments in life.
- What are your lifelong goals?
- Has your illness interfered with these goals?

Objective Data

Appendices 5 and 8 provide normal information and developmental norms based on age to provide a baseline by which to compare your client's physical and cognitive development.

- Does this client have obvious developmental lags that need further assessment?
- Does this client's illness interfere with the ability to accomplish the necessary developmental, physical, psychosocial, and cognitive tasks required at each age level for normal development?
- Does this client have any physical, psychosocial, or cognitive developmental lags that aggravate his or her illness or inhibit self-care?

HEALTH PERCEPTION–HEALTH MANAGEMENT PATTERN

Purpose

The purpose of assessing the client's health perception–health management pattern is to determine how the client perceives and maintains his or her health. Compliance with current and past nursing and medical recommendations is assessed. The client's ability to perceive the relationship between activities of daily living and health is also determined.

Subjective Data: Guideline Questions

Client's Perception of Health

- Describe your health.
- How would you rate your health on a scale of 1 to 10 (10 is excellent) now, 5 years ago, and 5 years ahead?

Client's Perception of Illness

- Describe your illness or current health problem.
- How has this affected your normal daily activities?
- How do you feel your current daily activities have affected your health?
- What do you believe caused your illness?
- What course do you predict your illness will take?

- How do you believe your illness should be treated?
- Do you have or anticipate any difficulties in caring for yourself or others at home? If yes, explain.

Health Management and Habits

- Tell me what you do when you have a health problem.
- When do you seek nursing or medical advice?
- How often do you go for professional exams (dental, Pap smears, breast, blood pressure)?
- What activities do you believe keep you healthy? Contribute to illness?
- Do you perform self-exams (blood pressure, breast, testicular)?
- When were your last immunizations? Are they up-to-date? (See Immunization Schedule, Appendices 6 and 7.)
- Do you use alcohol, tobacco, drugs, caffeine? Describe the amount and length of time used.
- Are you exposed to pollutants or toxins? Describe.

Compliance with Prescribed Medications and Treatments

- Have you been able to take your prescribed medications? If not, what caused your inability to do so?
- Have you been able to follow through with your prescribed nursing and medical treatment (e.g., diet, exercise)? If not, what caused your inability to do so?

Objective Data

Refer to Chapter 6, Assessing General Status and Vital Signs.

Associated Nursing Diagnostic Categories to Consider

Health Promotion Diagnoses

- Deficient diversional activity
- Sedentary lifestyle
- Deficient community health
- Risk-prone health behavior
- Ineffective health maintenance
- Readiness for enhanced immunization status
- Ineffective protection
- Ineffective self-health management
- Readiness for enhanced self-health management
- Ineffective family therapeutic regimen management
- Readiness for enhanced sleep
- Readiness for enhanced self-care

Risk Diagnoses

- Risk for falls
- Risk for activity intolerance
- Risk for disorganized infant behavior
- Risk for autonomic dysreflexia
- Risk for injury
- Risk for suffocation
- Risk for poisoning
- Risk for trauma
- Risk for perioperative positioning injury

Actual Diagnoses

- Adult failure to thrive
- Disturbed energy field
- Delayed surgical recovery
- Ineffective health maintenance
- Ineffective therapeutic regimen: Management (individual, family, community)
- Sedentary lifestyle
- Risk-prone health behavior

NUTRITIONAL–METABOLIC PATTERN

Purpose

The purpose of assessing the client's nutritional–metabolic pattern is to determine the client's dietary habits and metabolic needs. The conditions of hair, skin, nails, teeth, and mucous membranes are assessed.

Subjective Data: Guideline Questions

Dietary and Fluid Intake

- Describe the type and amount of food you eat at breakfast, lunch, and supper on an average day.
- Do you attempt to follow any certain type of diet? Explain.
- What time do you usually eat your meals?
- Do you find it difficult to eat meals on time? Explain.
- What types of snacks do you eat? How often?
- Do you take any vitamin supplements? Describe.
- Do you take herbal supplements? Describe.
- Do you consider your diet high in fat? Sugar? Salt?
- Do you find it difficult to tolerate certain foods? Specify.
- What kind of fluids do you usually drink? How much per day?
- Do you have difficulty chewing or swallowing food?
- When was your last dental exam? What were the results?
- Do you ever experience a sore throat, sore tongue, or sore gums? Describe.
- Do you ever experience nausea and vomiting? Describe.
- Do you ever experience abdominal pains? Describe.
- Do you use antacids? How often? What kind?

Condition of Skin

- Describe the condition of your skin.
- Describe your bathing routine.
- Do you use sunscreens, lotions, oils? Describe.
- How well and how quickly does your skin heal?
- Do you have any skin lesions? Describe.
- Do you have excessively oily or dry skin?
- Do you have any itching? What do you do for relief?

Condition of Hair and Nails

- Describe the condition of your hair and nails.
- Do you use artificial nails? How often? How long? Have you ever had problems with these nails?
- Do you have excessively oily or dry hair?
- Have you had difficulty with scalp itching or sores?
- Do you use any special hair- or scalp-care products (i.e., permanents, coloring, straighteners)?
- Have you noticed any changes in your nails? Color? Cracking? Shape? Lines?

Metabolism

- What would you consider to be your ideal weight?
- Have you had any recent weight gains or losses? Describe.
- Have you used any measures to gain or lose weight? Describe.
- Do you have any intolerances to heat or cold?
- Have you noted any changes in your eating or drinking habits? Explain.
- Have you noticed any voice changes?
- Have you had difficulty with nervousness?

Objective Data

Refer to Chapter 6 to assess the client's temperature, pulse, respirations, and height and weight. Refer to Chapter 10, Assessing Skin, Hair, and Nails; Chapter 11, Assessing Head and Neck; and Chapter 14, Assessing Mouth, Throat, Nose, and Sinuses.

Associated Nursing Diagnostic Categories to Consider

Health Promotion Diagnoses

- Insufficient breast milk
- Readiness for enhanced nutrition
- Readiness for enhanced fluid balance

Risk Diagnoses

- Risk for imbalanced nutrition: More than body requirements
- Risk for Imbalanced Body Temperature
- Hypothermia
- Hyperthermia
- Risk for unstable blood glucose level
- Risk for neonatal jaundice
- Risk for impaired liver function
- Risk for electrolyte imbalance
- Risk for infection
- Risk for aspiration
- Risk for deficient fluid volume
- Risk for imbalanced fluid volume
- Risk for constipation
- Risk for delayed surgical recovery
- Risk for impaired skin integrity

Actual Diagnoses

- Ineffective infant feeding pattern
- Imbalanced nutrition: Less than body requirements
- Imbalanced nutrition: More than body requirements
- Decreased intracranial adaptive capacity

- Ineffective thermoregulation
- Deficient fluid volume
- Excess fluid volume
- Insufficient breast milk
- Impaired swallowing
- Impaired tissue integrity
- Impaired skin integrity

ELIMINATION PATTERN

Purpose

The purpose of assessing the client's elimination pattern is to determine the adequacy of function of the client's bowel and bladder for elimination. The client's bowel and urinary routines and habits are assessed. In addition, any bowel or urinary problems and use of urinary or bowel elimination devices are examined.

Subjective Data: Guideline Questions

Bowel Habits

- Describe your bowel pattern. Have there been any recent changes?
- How frequent are your bowel movements?
- What is the color and consistency of your stools?
- Do you use laxatives? What kind and how often do you use them?
- Do you use enemas? How often and what kind?
- Do you use suppositories? How often and what kind?
- Do you have any discomfort with your bowel movements? Describe.
- Have you ever had bowel surgery? What type? Ileostomy? Colostomy?

Bladder Habits

- Describe your urinary habits.
- How frequently do you urinate (when and number of times)?
- What is the amount and color of your urine?
- Do you have any of the following problems with urinating:
- Pain?
- Blood in urine?
- Difficulty starting a stream?
- Incontinence?
- Voiding frequently at night?
- Voiding frequently during day?
- Bladder infections?

- Have you ever had bladder surgery? Describe.
- Have you ever had a urinary catheter? Describe. When? How long?

Objective Data

Refer to Chapter 19, Assessing Abdomen, and the External Rectal Area Assessment section, in Chapters 22 and 23.

Associated Nursing Diagnostic Categories to Consider

Health Promotion Diagnoses

- Readiness for enhanced urinary elimination

Risk Diagnoses

- Risk for constipation
- Risk for impaired urinary elimination
- Risk for urge urinary incontinence
- Risk for dysfunctional gastrointestinal motility

Actual Diagnoses

- Functional urinary incontinence
- Overflow urinary incontinence
- Reflex urinary incontinence
- Stress urinary incontinence
- Urge urinary incontinence
- Risk for urge urinary incontinence
- Impaired urinary elimination
- Readiness for enhanced urinary elimination
- Urinary retention
- Constipation
- Perceived constipation
- Risk for constipation
- Diarrhea
- Dysfunctional gastrointestinal motility
- Risk for dysfunctional gastrointestinal motility
- Bowel incontinence
- Impaired gas exchange

ACTIVITY–EXERCISE PATTERN

Purpose

The purpose of assessing the client's activity–exercise pattern is to determine the client's activities of daily living, including routines of exercise, leisure, and recreation. This includes activities necessary for personal hygiene, cooking, shopping, eating, maintaining the home, and working. An assessment is made of any factors that affect or interfere with the client's routine activities of daily living. Activities are evaluated in reference to the client's perception of their significance in his or her life.

Subjective Data: Guideline Questions

Activities of Daily Living

- Describe your activities on a normal day (including hygiene activities, cooking activities, shopping activities, eating activities, house and yard activities, other self-care activities).
- How satisfied are you with these activities?
- Do you have difficulty with any of these self-care activities? Explain.
- Does anyone help you with these activities? How?
- Do you use any special devices to help you with your activities?
- Does your current physical health affect any of these activities (e.g., dyspnea, shortness of breath, palpitations, chest pain, pain, stiffness, weakness)? Explain.

Leisure Activities

- Describe the leisure activities you enjoy.
- Has your health affected your ability to enjoy your leisure? Explain.
- Do you have time for leisure activities?
- Describe any hobbies you have.

Exercise Routine

- Describe those activities that you believe give you exercise.
- How often are you able to do this type of exercise?
- Has your health interfered with your exercise routine?

Occupational Activities

- Describe what you do to make a living.
- How satisfied are you with this job?
- Do you believe it has affected your health? If yes, how?
- How has your health affected your ability to work?

Objective Data

Refer to Chapter 15, Assessing Thorax and Lungs; Chapter 17, Assessing Heart and Neck Vessels; Chapter 18, Assessing Peripheral Vascular System; and Chapter 20, Assessing Musculoskeletal System.

Associated Nursing Diagnostic Categories to Consider

Health Promotion Diagnoses

- Readiness for enhanced sleep
- Readiness for enhanced self-care

Risk Diagnoses

- Risk for disuse syndrome
- Risk for activity intolerance
- Risk for ineffective gastrointestinal perfusion
- Risk for ineffective renal perfusion
- Risk for decreased cardiac tissue perfusion
- Risk for ineffective cerebral tissue perfusion
- Risk for ineffective peripheral tissue perfusion
- Risk for ineffective renal perfusion
- Risk for perioperative positioning injury
- Risk for disorganized infant behavior
- Risk for peripheral neurovascular dysfunction

Actual Diagnoses

- Insomnia
- Sleep deprivation
- Disturbed sleep pattern
- Impaired bed mobility
- Impaired physical mobility
- Impaired wheelchair mobility
- Impaired transfer ability
- Impaired walking
- Disturbed energy field
- Fatigue
- Wandering
- Activity intolerance
- Ineffective breathing pattern
- Decreased cardiac output
- Impaired spontaneous ventilation
- Ineffective peripheral tissue perfusion
- Impaired gas exchange
- Ineffective airway clearance
- Dysfunctional ventilatory weaning response
- Impaired home maintenance
- Bathing self-care deficit
- Dressing self-care deficit
- Feeding self-care deficit
- Toileting self-care deficit
- Self-neglect

SEXUALITY–REPRODUCTION PATTERN

Purpose

The purpose of assessing the client's sexuality–reproduction pattern is to determine the client's fulfillment of sexual needs and perceived level of satisfaction. The reproductive pattern and developmental level of the client are determined, and perceived problems related to sexual activities, relationships, or self-concept are elicited. The physical and psychological effects of the client's current health status on his or her sexuality or sexual expression are examined.

Subjective Data: Guideline Questions

Female

- Menstrual history
  - How old were you when you began menstruating?
  - On what date did your last cycle begin?
  - How many days does your cycle normally last?
  - How many days elapse from the beginning of one cycle until the beginning of another?
  - Have you noticed any change in your menstrual cycle?
  - Have you noticed any bleeding between your menstrual cycles?
  - Do you experience episodes of flushing, chilling, or intolerance to temperature changes?
  - Describe any mood changes or discomfort before, during, or after your cycle.
  - What was the date of your last Pap smear? Results?

- Obstetric history
  - How many times have you been pregnant?
  - Describe the outcome of each of your pregnancies.
  - If you have children, what are the ages and sex of each?
  - Describe your feelings with each pregnancy.
  - Explain any health problems or concerns you had with each pregnancy.
  - If pregnant now:
    - Was this a planned or unexpected pregnancy?
    - Describe your feelings about this pregnancy.
    - What changes in your lifestyle do you anticipate with this pregnancy?
    - Describe any difficulties or discomfort you have had with this pregnancy.
    - How can I help you meet your needs during this pregnancy?

Male or Female

- Contraception
  - What do you or your partner do to prevent pregnancy?
  - How acceptable is this method to both of you?
  - Does this means of birth control affect your enjoyment of sexual relations?

- Describe any discomfort or undesirable effects this method produces.
- Have you had any difficulty with fertility? Explain.
- Has infertility affected your relationship with your partner? Explain.
- Perception of sexual activities
  - Describe your sexual feelings. How comfortable are you with your feelings of femininity/masculinity?
  - Describe your level of satisfaction from your sexual relationship(s) on a scale of 1 to 10 (with 10 being very satisfying).
  - Explain any changes in your sexual relationship(s) that you would like to make.
  - Describe any pain or discomfort you have during intercourse.
  - Have you (has your partner) experienced any difficulty achieving an orgasm or maintaining an erection? If so, how has this affected your relationship?
- Concerns related to illness
  - How has your illness affected your sexual relationship(s)?
  - How comfortable are you discussing sexual problems with your partner?
  - From whom would you seek help for sexual concerns?

- Special problems
  - Do you have or have you ever had a sexually transmitted disease? Describe.
  - What method do you use to prevent contracting a sexually transmitted disease?
  - Describe any pain, burning, or discomfort you have while voiding.
  - Describe any discharge or unusual odor you have from your penis/vagina.
- History of sexual abuse
  - Describe the time and place the incident occurred.
  - Explain the type of sexual contact that occurred.
  - Describe the person who assaulted you.
  - Identify any witnesses present.
  - Describe your feelings about this incident.
  - Have you had any difficulty sleeping, eating, or working since the incident occurred?

Objective Data

Refer to Chapter 16, Assessing Breasts and Lymphatic System; Chapter 19, Assessing Abdomen; Chapter 23, Assessing Female Genitalia and Rectum; and Chapter 22, Assessing Male Genitalia and Rectum.

Associated Nursing Diagnostic Categories to Consider

Health Promotion Diagnosis

- Readiness for enhanced childbearing process

Risk Diagnoses

- Risk for ineffective childbearing process
- Risk for disturbed maternal–fetal dyad

Actual Diagnoses

- Sexual dysfunction
- Ineffective sexuality pattern
- Ineffective childbearing process

SLEEP–REST PATTERN

Purpose

The purpose of assessing the client's sleep–rest pattern is to determine the client's perception of the quality of his or her sleep, relaxation, and energy levels. Methods used to promote relaxation and sleep are also assessed.

Subjective Data: Guideline Questions

Sleep Habits

- Describe your usual sleeping time and habits (i.e., reading, warm milk, medications, etc.) at home.
- How long does it take you to fall asleep?
- If you awaken, how long does it take you to fall asleep again?
- Do you use anything to help you fall asleep (i.e., medication, reading, eating)?
- How would you rate the quality of your sleep?

Special Problems

- Do you ever experience difficulty with falling asleep? Remaining asleep?
- Do you ever feel fatigued after a sleep period?
- Has your current health altered your normal sleep habits? Explain.
- Do you feel your sleep habits have contributed to your current illness? Explain.

Sleep Aids

- What helps you fall asleep?
- Medications?

SENSORY-PERCEPTUAL PATTERN

Purpose

The purpose of assessing the client's sensory–perceptual pattern is to determine the functioning status of the five senses: Vision, hearing, touch (including pain perception), taste, and smell. Devices and methods used to assist the client with deficits in any of these five senses are assessed.

Subjective Data: Guideline Questions

Perception of Senses

- Describe your ability to see, hear, feel, taste, and smell.
- Describe any difficulty you have with your vision, hearing, ability to feel (e.g., touch, pain, heat, cold), taste (salty, sweet, bitter, sour), or smell.

Objective Data

Observe Appearance

- Pale
- Puffy eyes with dark circles

Observe Behavior

- Yawning
- Dozing during day
- Irritability
- Short attention span

Associated Nursing Diagnostic Categories to Consider

Health Promotion Diagnosis

- Readiness for enhanced sleep

Risk Diagnoses

- Risk for disturbed sleep pattern
- Risk for sleep deprivation

Actual Diagnoses

- Insomnia
- Disturbed sleep pattern
- Sleep deprivation

- Reading?
- Relaxation technique?
- Watching TV?
- Listening to music?

Pain Assessment

(See Chapter 7 for detailed pain assessment.)

- Describe any pain you have now.
- What brings it on? What relieves it?
- When does it occur? How often? How long does it last?
- What else do you feel when you have this pain?
- Show me on this drawing (of a figure) where you have pain.
- Rate your pain on a scale of 1 to 10, with 10 being the most severe pain. (Have a child use the Oucher Scale, with faces ranging from frowning to crying.)
- How has your pain affected your activities of daily living?

Special Aids

- What devices (e.g., glasses, contact lenses, hearing aids) or methods do you use to help you with any of these problems?
- Describe any medications you take to help you with these problems.

Objective Data

Refer to the section on Nose and Sinus Assessment in Chapter 14 (pp. 295–298); Chapter 12, Assessing Eyes; Chapter 13, Assessing Ears; and the section on Cranial Nerve Assessment in Chapter 21 (pp. 463–469).

Associated Nursing Diagnostic Categories to Consider

Health Promotion Diagnosis

- Readiness for enhanced comfort

Risk Diagnoses

- Risk for pain (acute, chronic)
- Risk for aspiration
- Risk for autonomic dysreflexia

Actual Diagnoses

- Impaired comfort
- Acute pain
- Chronic pain
- Dysreflexia
- Impaired environmental interpretation syndrome
- Nausea
- Unilateral neglect

COGNITIVE PATTERN

Purpose

The purpose of assessing the client's cognitive pattern is to determine the client's ability to understand, communicate, remember, and make decisions.

Subjective Data: Guideline Questions

Ability to Understand
- Explain what your doctor has told you about your health.
- Are you satisfied with your understanding of your illness and prescribed care? Explain.
- What is the best way for you to learn something new (read, watch television, etc.)?

Ability to Communicate
- Can you tell me about how you feel about your current state of health?
- Are you able to ask questions about your treatments, medications, and so forth?
- Do you ever have difficulty expressing yourself or explaining things to others? Explain.

Ability to Remember
- Are you able to remember recent events and events of long ago? Explain.

Ability to Make Decisions
- Describe how you feel when faced with a decision.
- What assists you in making decisions?
- Do you find decision making difficult, fairly easy, or variable? Describe.

Objective Data

Refer to the Mental Status Assessment section of Chapter 5 (pp. 92–100).

Associated Nursing Diagnostic Categories to Consider

Health Promotion Diagnosis
- Readiness for enhanced knowledge
- Readiness for enhanced communication

Risk Diagnosis
- Risk for acute confusion

Actual Diagnoses

- Impaired verbal communication
- Impaired memory
- Unilateral neglect
- Ineffective impulse control
- Acute confusion
- Chronic confusion
- Impaired environmental interpretation syndrome
- Deficient knowledge

ROLE–RELATIONSHIP PATTERN

Purpose

The purpose of assessing the client's role–relationship pattern is to determine the client's perceptions of responsibilities and roles in the family, at work, and in social life. The client's level of satisfaction with these is assessed. In addition, any difficulties in the client's relationships and interactions with others are examined.

Subjective Data: Guideline Questions

Perception of Major Roles and Responsibilities in Family

- Describe your family.
- Do you live with your family? Alone?
- How does your family get along?
- Who makes the major decisions in your family?
- Who is the main financial supporter of your family?
- How do you feel about your family?
- What is your role in your family? Is this an important role?
- What is your major responsibility in your family? How do you feel about this responsibility?
- How does your family deal with problems?
- Are there any major problems now?
- Who is the person you feel closest to in your family? Explain.
- How is your family coping with your current state of health?

Perception of Major Roles and Responsibilities at Work

- Describe your occupation.
- What is your major responsibility at work?
- How do you feel about the people you work with?
- If you could, what would you change about your work?
- Are there any major problems you have at work? If yes, explain.

Perception of Major Social Roles and Responsibilities

- Who is the most important person in your life? Explain.
- Describe your neighborhood and the community in which you live.
- How do you feel about the people in your community?
- Do you participate in any social groups or neighborhood activities? If yes, describe.
- What do you see as your contribution to society?
- What would you change about your community if you could?

Objective Data

- Outline a family genogram for your client. See Figure 2-1 for an example.
- Observe your client's family members.
  - How do they communicate with each other?
  - How do they respond to the client?
  - Do they visit, and how long do they stay with the client?

Associated Nursing Diagnostic Categories to Consider

Health Promotion Diagnoses

- Readiness for enhanced family processes
- Readiness for enhanced relationship

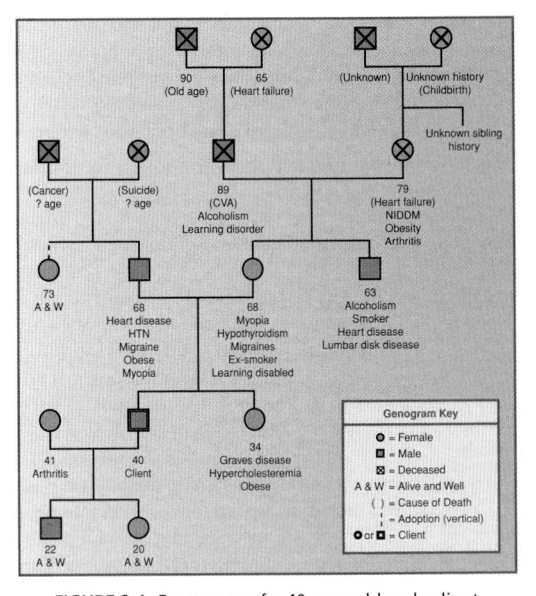

FIGURE 2-1 Genogram of a 40-year-old male client.

- Readiness for enhanced parenting
- Readiness for enhanced breastfeeding

Risk Diagnoses

- Risk for caregiver role strain
- Risk for impaired parenting
- Risk for impaired attachment
- Risk for ineffective relationship
- Risk for dysfunctional grieving
- Risk for loneliness
- Risk for impaired parent/infant/child attachment

Actual Diagnoses

- Impaired verbal communication
- Dysfunctional family processes
- Anticipatory grieving
- Dysfunctional grieving
- Social isolation
- Ineffective breastfeeding
- Interrupted breastfeeding
- Caregiver role strain
- Impaired parenting
- Interrupted family processes

- Ineffective relationship
- Parental role conflict
- Ineffective role performance
- Impaired social interaction

SELF-PERCEPTION–SELF-CONCEPT PATTERN

Purpose

The purpose of assessing the client's self-perception–self-concept pattern is to determine the client's perception of his or her identity, abilities, body image, and self-worth. The client's behavior, attitude, and emotional patterns are also assessed.

Subjective Data: Guideline Questions

Perception of Identity

- Describe yourself.
- Has your illness affected how you describe yourself?

Perception of Abilities and Self-Worth

- What do you consider to be your strengths? Weaknesses?
- How do you feel about yourself?
- How does your family feel about you and your illness?

Body Image

- How do you feel about your appearance?
- Has this changed since your illness? Explain.
- How would you change your appearance if you could?
- How do you feel about other people with disabilities?

Objective Data

Refer to the procedures for observing appearance, behavior, and mood in the Mental Status Assessment section of Chapter 5 (pp. 94–96).

Associated Nursing Diagnostic Categories to Consider

Health Promotion Diagnoses

- Readiness for enhanced self-control
- Readiness for enhanced organized infant behavior

Risk Diagnoses

- Risk for hopelessness
- Risk for compromised human dignity
- Risk for loneliness
- Risk for disturbed personal identity
- Risk for chronic low self-esteem
- Risk for situational low self-esteem
- Risk for disorganized infant behavior
- Risk for autonomic dysreflexia

Actual Diagnoses

- Hopelessness
- Disturbed personal identity
- Chronic low self-esteem
- Situational low self-esteem
- Disturbed body image
- Stress overload
- Autonomic dysreflexia
- Disorganized infant behavior
- Decreased intracranial adaptive capacity
- Anxiety
- Fatigue
- Fear
- Powerlessness
- Disturbed self-esteem
- Death anxiety

COPING–STRESS TOLERANCE PATTERN

Purpose

The purpose of assessing the client's coping–stress tolerance pattern is to determine the areas and amount of stress in a client's life and the effectiveness of coping methods used to deal with it. Availability and use of support systems such as family, friends, and religious beliefs are assessed.

Subjective Data: Guideline Questions

Perception of Stress and Problems in Life

- Describe what you believe to be the most stressful situation in your life.
- How has your illness affected the stress you feel? *or* How do you feel stress has affected your illness?
- Has there been a personal loss or major change in your life over the last year? Explain.
- What has helped you to cope with this change or loss?

Coping Methods and Support Systems

- What do you usually do first when faced with a problem?
- What helps you to relieve stress and tension?
- To whom do you usually turn when you have a problem or feel under pressure?
- How do you usually deal with problems?
- Do you use medication, drugs, or alcohol to help relieve stress? Explain.

Objective Data

Refer to Chapter 5, Assessing Mental Status and Substance Abuse.

Associated Nursing Diagnostic Categories to Consider

Health Promotion Diagnoses

- Readiness for enhanced coping
- Readiness for enhanced family coping
- Readiness for enhanced organized infant behavior
- Readiness for enhanced power
- Readiness for enhanced resilience

Risk Diagnoses

- Risk for self-mutilation
- Risk for Suicide
- Risk for Violence: Self-Directed or Other Directed

- Compromised Family Coping
- Ineffective Community Coping
- Post trauma Response
- Self-Mutilation
- Post trauma syndrome
- Rape trauma syndrome
- Relocation stress syndrome
- Ineffective activity planning
- Anxiety
- Ineffective coping
- Death anxiety
- Adult failure to thrive
- Fear
- Grieving
- Powerlessness
- Impaired individual resilience
- Chronic sorrow
- Stress overload
- Autonomic dysreflexia
- Disorganized infant behavior
- Decreased intracranial adaptive capacity

- Ineffective Denial
- Ineffective Family Coping: Disabling
- Defensive Coping
- Ineffective Individual Coping
- Complicated Grieving
- Disturbed Energy Field
- Disabled Family Coping
- Caregiver Role Strain
- Impaired Adjustment

Actual Diagnoses

- Risk for autonomic dysreflexia
- Risk for disorganized infant behavior
- Risk for compromised resilience
- Risk for powerlessness
- Risk for relocation stress syndrome
- Risk for complicated grieving
- Risk for ineffective activity planning
- Risk for post trauma syndrome
- Risk for Relocation Syndrome
- Risk for Spiritual Distress

VALUE–BELIEF PATTERN

Purpose

The purpose of assessing the client's value–belief pattern is to determine the client's life values and goals, philosophical beliefs, religious beliefs, and spiritual beliefs that influence his or her choices and decisions. Conflicts between these values, goals, beliefs, and expectations that are related to health are assessed.

Subjective Data: Guideline Questions

Values, Goals, and Philosophical Beliefs

- What is most important to you in life?
- What do you hope to accomplish in your life?
- What is the major influencing factor that helps you make decisions?
- What is your major source of hope and strength in life?

Religious and Spiritual Beliefs

- Do you have a religious affiliation?
- Is this important to you?

- Are there certain health practices or restrictions that are important for you to follow while you are ill or hospitalized? Explain.
- Is there a significant person (e.g., minister, priest) from your religious denomination whom you want to be contacted?
- Would you like the hospital chaplain to visit?
- Are there certain practices (e.g., prayer, reading scripture) that are important to you?
- Is a relationship with God an important part of your life? Explain.
- Describe any other sources of strength that are important to you.
- How can I help you continue with this source of spiritual strength while you are ill in the hospital?

Objective Data

- Observe religious practices:
  - Presence of religious articles in room (e.g., Bible, cards, medals, statues)
  - Visits from clergy
  - Religious actions of client: Prayer, visit to chapel, request for clergy, watching of religious TV programs, or listening to religious radio stations

- Observe client's behavior for signs of spiritual distress:
  - Anxiety
  - Anger
  - Depression
  - Doubt
  - Hopelessness
  - Powerlessness

Associated Nursing Diagnostic Categories to Consider

Health Promotion Diagnoses

- Readiness for enhanced spiritual well-being
- Readiness for enhanced hope
- Readiness for enhanced spiritual well-being

- Readiness for enhanced decision making
- Readiness for enhanced religiosity

Risk Diagnoses

- Risk for spiritual distress
- Risk for impaired religiosity

Actual Diagnoses

- Impaired religiosity
- Spiritual distress
- Death anxiety
- Decisional conflict
- Moral distress
- Noncompliance

CHAPTER 3

Performing Physical Assessment Skills

Physical Assessment Skills

Four basic techniques are used in performing a physical assessment: *Inspection, palpation, percussion,* and *auscultation*. The definition and proper technique for each of these are described below. Always use Standard Precautions as recommended by the Hospital Infection Control Practices Advisory Committee (HICPAC) and the Centers for Disease Control and Prevention (CDC).

INSPECTION

Definition

Inspection is using the senses of vision, smell, and hearing to observe the condition of various body parts, including any deviations from normal.

Technique

- Expose body parts being observed while keeping the rest of the client properly draped.
- *Always* look before touching.
- Use good lighting. Tangential sunlight is best. Be alert for the effect of bluish red-tinted or fluorescent lighting that interferes with observing bruises, cyanosis, and erythema.
- Provide a warm room for examination of the client. (An environment that is too cold or hot may alter skin color and appearance.)
- Observe for color, size, location, texture, symmetry, odors, and sounds.

PALPATION

Definition

Palpation is touching and feeling body parts with your hands to determine the following characteristics.

- Texture (roughness/smoothness)
- Temperature (warm/hot/cold)
- Moisture (dry/wet/moist)
- Motion (stillness/vibration)
- Consistency of structures (solid/fluid-filled)

Technique

- Keep your fingernails short.
- Use the most sensitive part of the hand to detect various sensations. See Table 3-1.
- Use four different types of palpation, depending on the purpose of the exam. The purpose and technique for each are described in Table 3-2.
- Perform light palpation before deep palpation.
- Palpate tender areas last.

TABLE 3-1 Sensitivity of Parts of the Hand

Hand Part Used	Type of Sensation Felt
Fingertips	Fine discriminations, pulsations
Palmar/ulnar surface	Vibratory sensations (e.g., thrills, fremitus)
Dorsal surface (back of hand)	Temperature

TABLE 3-2 **Types of Palpation**

Type	Purpose	Technique
Light palpation	To determine surface variations such as pulses, tenderness, surface skin texture, temperature, and moisture.	Place your dominant hand lightly on the surface of the structure. There should be very little or no depression (less than 1 cm). Feel the surface structure using a circular motion.
Moderate palpation	To feel for easily palpable body organs and masses.	Depress the skin surface 1–2 cm (0.5–0.75 in) with your dominant hand, using a circular motion. Note size, consistency, and mobility of structures.

Continued on following page

TABLE 3-2 Types of Palpation (Continued)

Type	Purpose	Technique
Deep palpation	To feel very deep organs or structures that are covered by thick muscle.	Place your dominant hand on the skin surface and your nondominant hand on top of your dominant hand to apply pressure. This should result in a surface depression between 2.5 cm and 5 cm (1 and 2 in).
Bimanual palpation (use with caution as it may provoke internal injury)	To palpate breasts and deep abdominal organs.	Use two hands, placing one on each side of the body part (e.g., uterus, breasts, spleen) being palpated. Use one hand to apply pressure and the other hand to feel the structure. Note the size, shape, consistency, and mobility of the structures you palpate.

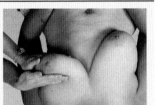

PERCUSSION

Definition

Percussion is tapping a portion of the body to elicit tenderness or sounds that vary with the density of underlying structures. The reliability of this technique is often questioned due to variations in the specificity and sensitivity of percussion.

Technique

Use three types of percussion, depending on the purpose of the examination. The three types of percussion are explained in Table 3-3. Percussion notes elicited through indirect percussion vary with the density of the underlying structures. Five percussion notes are described in Table 3-4, p. 51.

AUSCULTATION

Definition

Auscultation is listening for various breath, heart, vasculature, and bowel sounds using a stethoscope.

Technique

Use a good stethoscope that has the following.

- Snug-fitting earplugs
- Tubing not longer than 38.1 cm (15 in) and internal diameter not greater than 2.5 cm (1 in)
- Diaphragm and bell

The diaphragm and bell are used differently to detect various sounds, as shown in Table 3-5, p. 51.

Basic Guidelines for Physical Assessment

Obtain a nursing history and survey the client's general physical status for an overall impression before performing the physical assessment. This is done to determine which specific body systems should be examined (e.g., if the client complains of chest pain, the nurse should perform a thoracic and cardiac physical examination). A complete examination of all body systems may be done only on admission to the hospital or health-care facility; otherwise, the physical assessment may only include one or a few body systems.

Guidelines for performing a physical assessment include the following.

- Wash hands before beginning the examination; after completing the physical examination; or after removing gloves.

Continued on page 52

TABLE 3-3   Types of Percussion

Type	Purpose	Technique
Direct percussion	To elicit tenderness or pain	Directly tap a body part with one or two fingertips such as over the sinuses.

Direct percussion of sinuses

TABLE 3-3 **Types of Percussion** (Continued)

Type	Purpose	Technique
Blunt percussion (most commonly used method of percussion) Blunt percussion of the kidneys	To detect tenderness over organs (e.g., kidneys)	Place one hand flat on the body surface and use the fist of the other hand to strike the back of the hand flat on the body surface.

Continued on following page

TABLE 3-3 Types of Percussion (Continued)

Type	Purpose	Technique
Indirect percussion (least used method of percussion because of its low reliability) 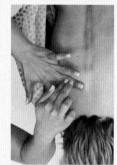 Indirect or mediate percussion of lungs	To elicit one of the following sounds over the chest or abdomen: Tympany, resonance, hyperresonance, dullness, and flatness. As density increases, the sound of the tone becomes quieter. Solid tissue produces a soft tone, fluid produces a louder tone, and air produces an even louder tone (see Table 3-4)	Press middle finger of nondominant hand firmly on body part. Keep other fingers off body part to avoid dampening of the sound elicited. Strike the finger on the body part with the middle finger (with short fingernail) with two quick taps of the dominant hand. Flex dominant wrist (not forearm) quickly. Listen to sound (Use quick wrist movement, not forearm.)

TABLE 3-4 Sounds (Tones) Elicited by Percussion

Sound	Intensity	Pitch	Length	Quality	Example of Origin
Resonance (heard over part air and part solid)	Loud	Low	Long	Hollow	Normal lung
Hyperresonance (heard mostly over air)	Very loud	Low	Long	Booming	Lung with emphysema
Tympany (heard over air)	Loud	High	Moderate	Drum-like	Puffed-out cheek, gastric bubble
Dullness (heard over more solid tissue)	Medium	Medium	Moderate	Thud-like	Diaphragm, pleural effusion, liver
Flatness (heard over very dense tissue)	Soft	High	Short	Flat	Muscle, bone, sternum, thigh

TABLE 3-5 Uses for Diaphragm and Bell of Stethoscope

		Purpose	Technique
	Diaphragm	To detect high-pitched sounds (e.g., breath sounds, normal heart sounds, bowel sounds)	Press firmly on body part.
	Bell	To detect low-pitched sounds (e.g., abnormal extra heart sounds, heart murmurs, carotid bruits)	Press lightly over body part.

- Use each technique to compare symmetrical sides of the body and organs.
- Assess both structure *and* function of each body part and organ (e.g., the appearance and condition of the ear, as well as its hearing function).
- When you identify an abnormality, assess for further data on the extent of the abnormality and the client's responses to the abnormality. Is there radiation of pain to other areas? Is there an effect on eating? Bowels? Activities of daily living? (e.g., with left upper quadrant abdominal pain: is there radiation of the pain?)
- Integrate client education with the physical assessment (e.g., breast self-exam, testicular self-exam, foot care for the client with diabetes).
- Allow time for client questions.

Variations in Physical Assessment of the Pediatric Client

Note: *The physical assessment sequence is dependent upon the development level of the client. (For a detailed discussion, see Appendix 5, Developmental Information—Age 1 Month to 18 Years.)*

- Wear gloves if you will have direct contact with blood or other body fluids, if you have an open wound, when collecting body fluids (e.g., blood, sputum, urine, or wound drainage, when handling contaminated surfaces (e.g., linen, tongue blades, vaginal speculum), and when performing an examination of the mouth, an open wound, genitalia, vagina, or rectum.
- Maintain privacy and proper draping; make sure the examination area has adequate lighting and a comfortable temperature (provide blanket if necessary).
- Explain the procedure and purpose of each part of the examination to the client.
- Follow a planned examination order for each body system, using the four techniques described earlier. Specific history questions related to each body part being examined may be integrated with the physical examination (e.g., when examining vision, ask the date of the client's last eye examination, if he or she has a history of blurring or double vision).
- First inspect, palpate, percuss, and then auscultate, except in the abdominal examination. To avoid alterations in bowel sounds: First auscultate and then percuss the abdomen, palpating the abdomen.

- Establishing rapport with the child and caregiver is the most essential step in obtaining meaningful physical assessment data.
- Allowing time for interaction with the child before beginning the examination helps to reduce fears.
- Allowing the child to use play medical instruments and/or allowing the child to touch and see instruments used, such as the stethoscope, otoscope, and ophthalmoscope may reduce anxiety and fear in the child, making use of instruments on the child more accepting by the child.
- In certain age groups, portions of the assessment will require physical restraint of the client with the help of another adult.
- Intermingling distraction and play throughout the examination assists in maintaining rapport with the pediatric client.
- Involving assistance from the child's parent or guardian may facilitate a more meaningful examination of the younger client.
- Based on the child's responses, prepare to alter the order of the assessment and your approach to the child.
- For infants and small children, the examiner should use a pediatric stethoscope to auscultate the heart and the lungs. If a pediatric stethoscope is not available, use of the bell of the adult scope may be used.
- Protest or an uncooperative attitude toward the examiner is a normal finding in children from birth to early adolescence, throughout parts or even all of the assessment process. Appendix 5 describes normal behavior at various developmental levels for the pediatric client.
- If another member of the health-care team is needed to help restrain the child, allow the parent to comfort the child *after* the procedure.

Variations in Physical Assessment of the Geriatric Client

Note: Normal variations related to aging may be observed in all parts of the physical examination.

- To avoid fatiguing the older client, allow rest periods between parts of the physical assessment. Provide a room with a comfortable temperature setting and no drafts, close to the restroom.
- Allow sufficient time for client to respond to directions and to change positions. Use silence to provide more time for the client to process thoughts and respond.
- If possible, assess geriatric clients in a setting where they have an opportunity to perform normal activities of daily living to determine their optimum potential.
- Conduct the examination in an area with ample space to accommodate wheelchairs and other supportive devices.

Assessing Psychosocial, Cognitive, and Moral Development

Growth and Development Overview

The developmental theories presented in this chapter focus on the psychosocial, cognitive, and moral *growth* (addition of new skills) and *development* (improvement of existing skills) of an individual throughout the lifespan. Psychosocial growth and development is explained using the works of Freud and Erikson. Cognitive development is explained using Piaget's theory and moral development is described using Kohlberg's theory.

FREUD'S THEORY OF PSYCHOSEXUAL DEVELOPMENT

Sigmund Freud's revised theory of personality included three basic personality structures: The *id, ego,* and *superego* (Freud, 1949). He believed they could operate within any of the levels of awareness. However, he declared the *id* to be completely *unconscious,* which is the inherited system. Containing the basic motivational drives for such entities as air, water, warmth, and sex, the *id* seeks instant gratification and supplies the psychic energy for the *ego* and the *superego.* Freud defined sex as the most important drive that included all pleasurable thoughts and beliefs. He added that the *id* knows no perception of reality or morality (what is right and wrong). Until the *ego* begins to develop in late infancy, the infant performs only at the level of the *id.* The *ego* plays an important role in behavior, but does not possess a concept of morality. The *superego,* often referred to as the moral component ("conscience"), provides feedback to the person regarding how closely his behavior conforms to the external value system. Adult behavior is described as the result of the interactions among the *id, ego,* and *superego.* The *id* seeks pleasure, avoiding pain, while the *superego* tries to reconcile the instincts of the *id* while discouraging the expression of undesirable behavior. The *ego*

must decide whether the *id* or the *superego* prevails to compromise the two opposing forces. He postulated that one's psychological nature is determined by the outcome of conflict between one's instincts and social expectations. Freud explained that how a child's sexual and aggressive drives are managed and affect personality development. He believed people may go through five psychosexual stages of development that could overlap or exist simultaneously. He postulated that as the child matures, he invests instinctual, sexual–sensual energy (*libido*) in one biophysical area of the body (*pleasure-seeking* or *erogenous zone*) during each stage. He also posited that if an individual became either *undergratified* or *overgratified* during any of these stages, he could become *fixated. See Table 4-1* for a summary of Freud's psychosexual stages of development.

ERIKSON'S THEORY OF PSYCHOSOCIAL DEVELOPMENT

Erikson (1963) expanded on Freud's psychosexual theory to develop his psychosocial theory, which is defined as the interpersonal and interpersonal responses of a person to external events (Schuster & Ashburn, 1992). Erikson concluded that societal, cultural, and historic factors as well as biophysical processes and

TABLE 4-1   Freud's Psychosexual Stages of Development

Stage	Approximate Age	Psychosexual Developments
Oral	0–1½ years	Pleasure derived from the mouth such as sucking, eating, chewing, biting, and vocalizing serve to reduce the infant's tension. The *id* controls this stage.
Anal	1½–3 years	Pleasure involves the elimination of feces. As the *ego* develops, the child decides to expel or retain the bowel movement.
Phallic	3–6 years	Pleasure is derived from the genital region. This can involve exploring and manipulating the genitals of self and others. A child can express curiosity about how a baby is "made" and born. The *superego* emerges from interactions with parents. Parents insist that the child controls biologic impulses. *Oedipal* (for males) and *Electra* (for females) complexes appear.
Latency	6–11 years	Abeyance of sexual urges occurs as the child develops more intellectual and social skills. It is a time of school activities, hobbies, sports, and in developing friendships with members of the same sex. The *superego* continues to develop. Defense mechanisms appear.
Genital	Adolescence	Puberty allows sexual impulses to reappear. Once conflicts with parents are resolved and if no major *fixations* have occurred, the individual will develop heterosexual attachments outside the family. Romantic love can lead to successful marriage and parenting.

Information from Freud, S. (1935). *A general introduction to psychoanalysis* (J. Riviere, Trans.). New York: Liveright and Freud, S. (1949). *An outline of psychoanalysis* (J. Strachey, Trans.). New York: W. W. Norton & Company, Inc.

cognitive function influence personality development (Erikson, 1968). He declared that the *ego* not only mediated between the *id's* abrupt impulses and the *superego's* moral demands, but also it can positively affect the person's development as more skills and experience are gained. Unlike Freud, Erikson believed that personality development continues to evolve throughout the lifespan. Whereas Freud attempted to explain reasons for pathology, Erikson searched for foundations of healthy personality development. He identified eight stages of the lifespan through which a person may sequentially develop (see Table 4-2). Each stage (or achievement level) proposed has a central developmental task composed of opposing viewpoints, which are dilemmas called *crises* (e.g., *basic trust vs. basic mistrust*). If the person resolves the challenge in favor of the more positive of the two viewpoints (e.g., emphasis on *basic trust*) then that person achieves resolution of the developmental task. The person must negotiate a healthy balance between the two concepts in order to move to the next stage and eventually become a well-adjusted adult in society. For example, a person needs some *basic mistrust* in some situations (i.e., stay a safe distance from blazing flames, cautiously approach an unfamiliar animal). Positive resolution for a crisis in one stage is necessary for positive resolution in the next stage. Erikson proposed strengths emerge with the positive resolution of each *crisis*. If a task is only partially resolved, then the person experiences difficulty in subsequent developmental tasks. These issues must be remediated to realize one's psychosocial potential. Erikson did not define chronologic boundaries but assigned developmental levels throughout the lifespan, which a person develops at his own rate based on potential and experiences (see Table 4-2).

PIAGET'S THEORY OF COGNITIVE DEVELOPMENT

Dr. Piaget (1970) explained the growth and development of intellectual structures. He focused on *how* a person learns and recognized that interrelationships of physical maturity, social interaction, environmental stimulation, and experiences were necessary for cognitive development. To explain his theory, he applied the concepts of *schema* (plural: *schemata*), *assimilation*, *accommodation*, and *equilibration* (equilibrium). A *schema* is a unit of thought that may consist of a thought, emotional memory, movement of a part of the body, or a sensory experience (such as making use of sight, hearing, taste, smell, or touch). *Schemata* can be categorized using either *assimilation* or *accommodation*. *Assimilation* is an adaptive process whereby a stimulus or information

TABLE 4-2 Erik Erikson's Stages of Psychosocial Development

Developmental Level	Central Task	Focal Relationships/Issues	Negative Resolution	Positive Resolution (Basic Virtues)
Infant	Basic trust vs. basic mistrust	Mother, primary caregivers, feeding, *"feeling and being comforted,"* sleeping, teething, *"taking in,"* trusting self, others, and environment	Suspicious, fearful	Drive and hope
Toddler	Autonomy vs. shame and doubt	Parents, primary caregivers, toilet training, bodily functions, experimenting with *"holding on and letting go,"* having control without loss of self-esteem	Doubts abilities, feels ashamed for not trying	Self-confidence and willpower
Preschooler	Initiative vs. guilt	Family, play, exploring and discovering, learning how much assertiveness influences others and the environment, developing a sense of moral responsibility	May fear disapproval of own powers	Direction and purpose
Schoolager	Industry vs. inferiority	School, teachers, friends, experiencing physical independence from parents, neighborhood, wishing to accomplish, learning to create and produce, accepting when to cease a project, learning to complete a project, learning to cooperate, developing an attitude toward work	May feel sense of failure	Method and competence
Adolescent	Identity vs. role confusion	Peers and groups, experiencing emotional independence from parents, seeking to be the same as others yet unique, planning to actualize abilities and goals, fusing several identities into one	Confused, nonfocused	Devotion and fidelity

Continued on following page

TABLE 4-2 Erik Erikson's Stages of Psychosocial Development (Continued)

Developmental Level	Central Task	Focal Relationships/Issues	Negative Resolution	Positive Resolution (Basic Virtues)
Young Adult	Intimacy vs. isolation	Friends, lovers, spouses, community, work connections (networking), committing to work relationships, committing to social relationships, committing to intimate relationships	Loneliness, poor relationships	Affiliation and love
Middle Adult	Generativity vs. stagnation	Younger generation—often children (whether one's own or those of others), family, community, mentoring others, helping to care for others, discovering new abilities/talents, continuing to create, "giving back"	Shallow involvement with the world in general, selfish, little psychosocial growth	Production and care
Older Adult	Ego integrity vs. despair"	All mankind, reviewing one's life, acceptance of self-uniqueness, acceptance of worth of others, acceptance of death as an entity	Regretful, discontent, pessimism	Renunciation and wisdom

"Based on his experiences/research and as he continued to live longer, Erikson contemplated extending this phase of generativity and suggested that a ninth stage might be added to his theory. He posited that those who positively resolved generativity could move to a higher level that addressed a "premonition of immortality" (i.e, a new sense of self that transcends universe and time).

Information from Erikson, E.H. (1963). Childhood and society (2nd ed.). New York: W. W. Norton & Company, Inc; Erikson, E.H. (1968). Identity: Youth and crisis. New York: W. W. Norton & Company, Inc; Erikson, E.H., Erikson, J.M., & Kivnick, H.Q. (1986). Vital involvement in old age. New York: W. W. Norton & Company, Inc; Erikson, E.H. (1991). Erikson's stages of personality development. Childhood and society. New York: W. W. Norton & Company, Inc. and Schuster, and Ashburn, S.S. (1992). The process of human development: A holistic life-span approach (3rd ed.). Philadelphia: J. B. Lippincott Company.

is incorporated into an already existing *schema*. Another way of saying this is the person changes reality into what he already knows. For example a toddler, who knows his pet cat to be a "Kitty," sees a dog for the first time and thinks the new animal is called "Kitty." *Accommodation* is the creation of a new *schema* or the modification of an old one to differentiate more accurately a stimulus or a behavior from an existing *schema*. One changes the self to fit reality. The same toddler may meet other cats and modify "Kitty" to "cat" and eventually, with experience and guidance, meet more dogs and create the idea of "dog." *Equilibration* is the balance between assimilation and *accommodation*. When disequilibrium occurs, it provides motivation for the individual to *assimilate* or *accommodate* further. A person who only assimilated stimuli would not be able to detect differences in things; a person who only accommodated stimuli would not be able to detect similarities. Piaget emphasized that *schemata, assimilation, accommodation,* and *equilibration* are all essential for cognitive growth and development. Piaget (1970) postulated that a person may progress through four major stages of intellectual development beginning at birth. Ages are not attached to these stages since each person progresses at his own rate. At each new stage, previous stages of thinking are incorporated and integrated. If a person attained formal operational thinking (see Table 4-3), he declared that qualitative changes in thinking cease and quantitative changes in the content and function of thinking may continue.

KOHLBERG'S THEORY OF MORAL DEVELOPMENT

Lawrence Kohlberg, a psychologist, developed a theory of moral development. He proposed morality is a dynamic process that extends over one's lifetime, involving the affective and cognitive domains in determining what is "right" and "wrong." Dr. Kohlberg examined the *reasoning* a person used to make a decision, as opposed to the *action* that resulted after that decision was made. Moral development is influenced by cognitive structures but not the same as cognitive development. Kohlberg viewed *justice* (or fairness) as the goal of moral judgment.

Kohlberg (Colby, Kohlberg, Gibbs, & Lieberman, 1983) proposed three levels of moral development that encompass six stages (see Table 4-4, p. 67). He believed that few people progress past the second level. Asserting that moral development extends beyond adolescence, he saw moral decisions and reasoning becoming increasingly differentiated, integrated, and universalized (i.e., independent of culture) at each successive stage. A person must

Continued on page 66

TABLE 4-3 Jean Piaget's Stages of Cognitive Development

Stage	Approximate Age	Significant Characteristics
Sensorimotor	0–2 years	Thoughts are demonstrated by physical manipulation of objects/stimuli.
Substage 1: Making use of ready-made reflexes (pure assimilation)	0–1 month	Pure reflex adaptation (e.g., if lips are touched, baby sucks; if object placed in palm, baby grasps).
Substage 2: Primary circular reactions (assimilation, accommodation, and equilibrium are now used as individual grows and develops)	1–4 months	Actions centered on infant's body and endlessly repeated reflex activities become modified and coordinated with each other with experience. Infant repeats behaviors for sensual pleasure (e.g., kicks repetitively, plays with own hands and fingers, sucking for a long time). Early coordination of selected reflexes (e.g., sucking and swallowing) and schema (e.g., hearing and looking at same object).
Substage 3: Secondary circular reactionary	4–8 months	Center of interest is not on own body's action but the environmental consequences of those actions. Behavior becomes intentional. Baby repeats behaviors that produce novel (i.e., pleasing, interesting) effects on environment (e.g., crying to get caregivers attention). Increased voluntary coordination of motor skills enabling exploration (e.g., mouthing objects by combining grasping and sucking). Appearance of cognitive object constancy awareness that an object or person is the same regardless of the angle from which it is viewed (e.g., baby will anticipate eating when he sees bottle of formula even if it is upside down and across the room).

TABLE 4-3   **Jean Piaget's Stages of Cognitive Development** (Continued)

Stage	Approximate Age	Significant Characteristics
Substage 4: Coordination of secondary circular reactions in new situations	8–12 months	Infant consciously uses an action that is a means to an end and solves simple problems (e.g., will reach for a toy and then will use that toy to retrieve another toy originally out of reach). *Object permanence* appears at approximately 8 months. This is the awareness that an object continues to exist even though one is not in direct contact with that object (e.g., when infant sees someone hide a favorite toy under a blanket, he will attempt to retrieve it from under the blanket). Imitate simple behaviors of others.
Substage 5: Tertiary circular reactions	12–18 months	Child now "experiments" (much trial and error) in order to discover new properties of objects and events. Varies approaches to an old situation or applies old approaches to a new problem. Must physically solve a problem to understand cause–effect relationship. Imitates simple novel behaviors.
Substage 6: Invention of new means through mental combinations	18–24 months	Invention of new means can occur without actual physical experimentation. Occasional new means through physical experimentation—still much trial and error problem solving. Child begins to *mentally represent* object/events before physically acting (e.g., can solve "detour" problems to go one small distance to another). Engages in early symbolic play. Both immediate and deferred imitation of actions and words noted.
Preoperational • Divided into two substages:	2–7 years	Increasing ability to make a mental representation for something not immediately present using language as a major tool. Eventually, the child is able to give his reasons for beliefs and rationales for action; however, they remain biased and immature. Magical thought (wishing something will make it so) predominates.

Continued on following page

TABLE 4-3 Jean Piaget's Stages of Cognitive Development (Continued)

Stage	Approximate Age	Significant Characteristics
• Preconceptional (2–4 years) and Intuitive (4–7 years).		The following characteristics (although they go through modification as the child develops from 2–7 years of age) serve as some obstacles to "adult logic."
• During the preconceptual substage, the child inconsistently assigns any word to several similar stimuli (e.g., child calls all four-legged mammals by his pet cat's name.)		• Fundamental egocentrism—never thinks that anything is other than the way he perceives it (e.g., "If I'm going to bed now, every child is going to bed now").
• During the intuitive stage, the child begins to realize the ability of a word to truly represent a specific object, event, or action.		• Centration—tends to focus on one aspect of an object or experience (e.g., when asked to compare two rows of like objects with one row containing six pennies and the other, a longer row containing three pennies, would answer that the longer row is "more").
		• Limited transformation—is not able to comprehend the steps of how an object is changed from one state to another (e.g., could not explain the sequence of events that occurs when an ice cube melts and turns into a puddle of water).
		• Action rather than abstraction—perceives an event as if actually participating in the event again (e.g., when asked about riding in her toy car, may imitate turning the steering wheel when she thinks about it).
		• Irreversibility—unable to follow a line of reasoning back to its beginning (e.g., if child is taken on a walk, especially one with a turn, he is unable to retrace his steps and return to the original point).

TABLE 4-3   Jean Piaget's Stages of Cognitive Development (Continued)

Stage	Approximate Age	Significant Characteristics
		• *Transductive reasoning*—thinks specific to specific; if two things are alike in one aspect, child thinks they are alike in all aspects (e.g., child thinks beetle seen on a picnic in the park is the same beetle seen in his backyard).
		• *Animism*—believes that inert objects are alive with feelings and can think and function with intent (e.g., child thinks that if vacuum cleaner "eats" the dirt, then it can "eat" him).
Concrete Operational	7–11 years	Begins to think and reason logically about objects in the environment. Can mentally perform actions that previously had to be carried out in actuality. Reasoning is limited to concrete objects and events ("what is") but not yet abstract objects and events ("what might be"). *Inductive* reasoning (specific to general) has begun. Can consider viewpoints of others. Understands and uses time on a clock. Understands days of week, months of year. Best understands years within life experience. Can de-center, understands transformations. Can reverse thoughts. Progressively able to *conserve* (understand that properties of substances will remain the same despite changes made in shape or physical arrangement) numbers, mass, weight, and volume in that order. Begins to understand relationship between distance and speed. Learns to add, subtract, multiply, and divide. Can organize, then classify objects. Progressively capable of money management.

Continued on following page

TABLE 4-3   **Jean Piaget's Stages of Cognitive Development** (Continued)

Stage	Approximate Age	Significant Characteristics
Formal Operational	11–15+ years	Develops ability to problem solve about both the real as well as the possible. Can logically and flexibly think about the past, present, and future. Possesses ability to think about symbols that represent other symbols (e.g., $x = 1$, $y = 2$). Can think abstractly when presented with information in verbal (as opposed to written) form.
		Able to envision and systematically test many possible combinations in reaching a conclusion. Is able to generate multiple potential solutions while considering the possible positive/negative effects of each solution. Can perform *deductive* reasoning (general to specific). Can hypothesize ("If…then" thinking).
		Can think about thinking (metacognition).

Information from Piaget, J. (1952). *The origins of intelligence in children* (M. Cook, Trans.). New York: International Universities Press; Piaget, J. (1969). *The language and thought of the child* (M. Gabain, Trans.). New York: Meridian Books; Piaget, J., & Inhelder, B. (1969). *The psychology of the child* (H. Weaver, Trans.). New York: Basic Books, Inc.; Piaget, J. (1981). *The psychology of intelligence* (M. Piercy and D. E. Berlyne, Trans.). Totowa, NJ: Littlefield & Adams; Piaget, J. (1982). *Play, dreams and imitation in children* (C. Gattengo and F. M. Hodgson, Trans.). New York: Norton and Schuster, C.S., & Ashburn, S.S. (1992). *The process of human development: A holistic life-span approach* (3rd ed.). Philadelphia: J. B. Lippincott Company.

enter his moral stage hierarchy in an ordered and irreversible sequence with no relationship to biologic age. He concluded that a person may never attain a higher stage of moral development and thus not ascend this proposed hierarchy of stages. He believed part of this was determined by how much a person is challenged with decisions of a higher order. Kohlberg did not theorize that infants and young toddlers were capable of moral reasoning. He viewed them as being naïve and egocentric.

TABLE 4-4 Lawrence Kohlberg's Stages of Moral Development

Level	Stage	Average Age	Characteristic Moral Reasoning That May Influence Behavior
Preconventional (premoral)	1. Orientation to punishment and obedience	Preschool through early school age	Finding it difficult to consider two points of view in a moral dilemma, individual ignores, or is unaware of meaning, value or intentions of others and instead focuses on fear of authority. Will avoid punishment by obeying what told to do by caregiver/supervisor. The physical consequences of individual actions determine "right" or "wrong." Punishment means action was "wrong."
	2. Orientation to instrumental relativism (individual purpose)	Late preschool through late school age	Slowly becoming aware that people can have different perspectives in a moral dilemma. Individual views "right" action as what satisfies personal needs, and believes others act out of self-interest. No true feelings of loyalty, justice, or gratitude. Individual conforms to rules out of self interest or in relation to what others can do in return. Desires reward for "right" action.
Conventional (maintain external expectations of others)	3. Orientation to interpersonal concordance (unity and mutuality)	School age through adulthood	Attempting to adhere to perceived norms; desires to maintain approval; and affection of friends, relatives, and significant others. Wants to avoid disapproval and be considered a "good person" who is trustworthy, loyal, respectful, and helpful. Capable of viewing a two person relationship as an impartial observer (beginning to judge the intentions of others—may or may not be correct in doing so).

Continued on following page

TABLE 4-4 Lawrence Kohlberg's Stages of Moral Development (Continued)

Level	Stage	Average Age	Characteristic Moral Reasoning That May Influence Behavior
	4. Orientation to maintenance of social order ("law and order")	Adolescence through adulthood	Attempting to make decisions and behave by strictly conforming to fixed rules and the written law—whether these be of a certain group, family, community, or the nation. "Right" consists of "doing one's duty."
Postconventional (maintain internal principles of self—Piaget's concept of formal operations must be employed at this level)	5. Orientation to social contract legalism	Middlescence through older adulthood (Only 10–20% of the dominant American culture attain this stage.)	Regarding rules and laws as changeable with due process. "Right" is respecting individual rights while emphasizing the needs of the majority. Outside of legal realm, will honor an obligation to another individual or group, even if the action is not necessarily viewed as the correct thing to do by friends, relatives, or numerous others.
	6. Orientation to universal ethical principle	Middlescence through older adulthood (Few people either attain or maintain this stage.)	Making decisions and behaving based on internalized rules, on conscience instead of social law and on self-chosen ethical principles that are consistent, comprehensive, and universal. Believes in absolute justice, human equality, reciprocity, and respect for the dignity of every individual person. Is willing to act alone and be punished (or actually die) for belief. Such behavior may be seen in times of crisis.

TABLE 4-4   **Lawrence Kohlberg's Stages of Moral Development** (Continued)

*Shortly before his death, Kohlberg added a seventh stage of moral reasoning titled *Orientation to Self-Transcendence and Faith.* Kohlberg proposed that this stage moved beyond the concept of justice and the goal was to achieve a sense of unity with the cosmos, nature, or God. The person attaining this stage views everyone and everything as being connected; thus, any action of a person affects everyone and everything with any consequences of that person's action ultimately returning to him. According to Garsee and Schuster (1992), the person in stage six may be willing to *die* for his principles whereas the person in stage seven is willing to *live* for his beliefs.

Information from Colby, A., Kohlberg, L., Gibbs, J., & Lieberman, M. (1983). A longitudinal study of moral behavior. *Monographs of the Society of Research in Child Development*, 48(1–2), 1–124; Garsee, J.W., & Schuster, C.S. (1992). Moral development. In C.S. Schuster & S.S. Ashburn (Eds.), *The process of human development: A holistic life-span approach.* Philadelphia: J.B. Lippincott Company; Kohlberg, L. (1984). *Essays on moral development: Vol. 2.* San Francisco: Harper & Row; Kohlberg, L. (1981). *The philosophy of moral development.* San Francisco: Harper & Row; Kohlberg, L., & Ryncarz, R. (1990). Beyond justice reasoning: Moral development and consideration of a seventh stage. In C. Alexander & E. Langer (Eds.), *Higher stages of human development* (pp. 191–207). New York: Oxford University Press; Levene, C., Kohlberg, L., & Hewer, A. (1985). The current formulation of Kohlberg's theory and a response to critics. *Human Development*, 28(2), 94–100 and Schuster, C.S., & Ashburn, S.S. (1992). *The process of human development: A holistic life-span approach* (3rd ed.). Philadelphia, PA: J.B. Lippincott Company.

Nursing Assessment

COLLECTING SUBJECTIVE DATA

Ask the patient about the following: Age, birthplace, number of years in current country, residence, cultural group, primary language, highest level of education, employment history, if retired or unemployed means of making a living or maintenance of everyday needs (food, shelter, etc.), current health concerns or changes, body weight, major stressors, coping patterns, support systems, difficulty making decisions, current life changes, description of self, strengths, weaknesses, best way to learn, history of psychiatric or psychological problems, treatment and outcome, use of medications (prescribed or OTC), counseling, weight changes, eating patterns, elimination patterns, exercise patterns, sleep patterns, chronic illnesses, treatment and outcome, perception who one calls "family," recall of growing up as a child, siblings and relationships, significant genetic predisposition or characteristic trait or disorder that you believe you have inherited, lifestyle and health practices.

OBJECTIVE ASSESSMENT OF DEVELOPMENTAL LEVEL: PSYCHOSOCIAL STATUS

The following assessment table offers guidance for the objective assessment of the client's psychosocial, cognitive, and moral development.

ASSESSMENT OF FREUD'S STAGES OF PSYCHOSEXUAL DEVELOPMENT

ASSESSMENT PROCEDURE	NORMAL FINDINGS	ABNORMAL FINDINGS
Determine the client's psychosocial level by asking the following suggested questions. Does the young adult • still live with parent(s) at home? • accept roles and responsibilities at place of residence? • have experience of growing up in a single parent home? • have unresolved issues with parent(s)? • have a satisfying sexual relationship with a significant other? • have gainful employment?	Many young adults today still live with parent(s) to continue higher education, become established in a career, or decrease financial hardship (Parker, 2012). Others return home to recover from divorce, obtain support with their children, or regain financial stability. It is important that the young adult assume different roles than those performed during the earlier years of development. Freud emphasized the significance of first maternal then later paternal influences on the person's ability to fulfill a socially acceptable gender role. Generation Y (born between 1982 and 2001) is much more accepting of same-gender relationships. Freud declared that it was normal for young people to marry . Single parent families were not common during the time of Freud. Many independent people today choose to remain single. Freud believed that healthy young adults should expend their genital energies in a hetero-sexual relationship and then marriage followed by parenthood. He believed reproduction within a heterosexual marriage was a	If a young adult demonstrates extreme dependence on a parent (e.g., assumes no responsibility for household which they share), Freud would state the *id*, *ego*, and *super ego* would not be fully developed and that the body organ that dominated that person's mode of interaction would influence the person's behavior. This young adult may make poor relationship choices, experience gender role confusion and more than mild anxiety, and suffer from low self-esteem. Defense mechanisms including projection (attributing one's unacceptable feelings, thoughts, impulses, wishes, or to another person). If the young adult does not possess a sense of healthy sexuality, social and emotional isolation may occur.

ASSESSMENT PROCEDURE	NORMAL FINDINGS	ABNORMAL FINDINGS
	socially acceptable reason to engage in sexual intercourse. His values do not correlate with the well-adjusted person who is content with an "alternate life style" including homosexuality. In the twenty-first century a healthy sexual relationship includes practicing "safe sex." The young adult is more likely to possess a sense of positive self-preservation if he or she can meet some financial expenses. Today, healthy young adults experience mild anxiety while attempting to balance employment, education, and relationships. Although Freud affirmed that women should remain in the home, many women now have multiple roles.	This person has difficulty establishing healthy relationships with others. The young adult concerned about finances without a career may experience depression, anxiety, poor eating habits, insomnia, or vivid dreams.
Does the middle-aged adult • demonstrate nervous mannerisms? • frequently derived pleasure from selected activities? • cope effectively with stress? • have a satisfying sexual relationship?	Copes with stress in a socially acceptable manner. All people experience stress throughout the life cycle. Mild anxiety (remaining attentive and alert to relevant stimuli) is normal throughout adulthood providing motivation. Adaptive defense (coping) mechanisms may be used. Positive coping makes use of previously successful actions to decrease stress. Healthy middle-aged adults may vent frustration to significant others and effectively communicates in relationships, seeking assistance as needed. Meets socially accepted norms and maintains a balance	Nervous mannerisms could indicate an unhealthy psychosexual state in many stages of the life cycle. For example, Freud might interpret fixation at the oral stage if a person is engaged in at least one of the following behaviors: Overreacting, excessive talking, smoking, thumb sucking, and nail biting. Likewise he would attribute other socially unacceptable behaviors

Continued on following page

ASSESSMENT OF FREUD'S STAGES OF PSYCHOSEXUAL DEVELOPMENT (Continued)

ASSESSMENT PROCEDURE	NORMAL FINDINGS	ABNORMAL FINDINGS
• believe physical changes of aging have affected any relation-ships?	of responsibilities and leisure activities. Experiences "mid-life crisis" differently, effectively prioritizing issues as they arise create to adapt a mid-life transition. Freud would say a person who is successful in this period uses repression (involuntary exclusion of anxiety producing feelings, thoughts, and impulses from awareness) and/or sublimation (substitution of a socially acceptable behavior for an unacceptable sexual or aggressive drive or impulse). Common middle age stressors include assisting adolescents to be more independent, caring for aging parents, grieving the lost of parent/grandparent and maintaining career/social status. A healthy middle-aged person according to Freud has attained and maintained the genital stage and purported that a satisfying sexual relationship was fundamental to a successful marriage. Freud might label the decision to not engage in an extramarital affair as suppression (exclusion of something from consciousness). Freud emphasized the importance of "romance." The sexual response cycle slows with age, focusing more on quality of a sexual relationship than the quantity of sexual intercourse.	for negative habits as being fixated at one of his other stages (anal, phallic, latency, or genital). Freud discussed fetishes as a way the libido attaches to objects other than a socially acceptable love object. Freud would label the person who engages in an extramarital affair(s) as narcissistic. He would say the same of the person with a body-image disturbance related to grieving the loss of a youthful physical appearance. Some unhealthy middle-aged adults refrain from social relationships/outings because they no longer look the same as they did when younger.

ASSESSMENT PROCEDURE	NORMAL FINDINGS	ABNORMAL FINDINGS
Does the older adult • engage in sexual activity? • positively cope with loss? • believe any changes in cognition have occurred? • believe any significant changes have occurred in interests/relationships?	Many older adults are capable of enjoying sexual intimacy. Many older adults make effective use of communication and companionship to have a healthy sense of sexuality (Fig. 4-1). Freud might interpret alternative ways of satisfying sexual needs as compensation (overachievement in one area to offset deficiencies real or imagined, or to overcome failure or frustration in another area). It is not uncommon to occasionally forget (e.g., lose keys, misplace a pen or glasses, not recall a person's name). The older adult makes effective use of previous experiences, self, and others to grieve loss. Experiencing more than one loss does not make a subsequent loss less painful.	The unhealthy older adult may avoid relationships and society. Chronic depression is not normal in older adulthood. Freud often interpreted the misplacing of objects as intentional. Current research on effects of stress and symptoms of dementia has not supported this belief ("Is it forgetfulness or dementia?" 2009; "Forgetfulness: Knowing when to ask for help" 2009; "Memory loss and forgetfulness…" 2012).

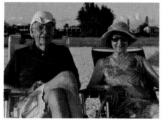

FIGURE 4-1 Stereotypical images of the older adult as narrow-minded, forgetful, sexless, and dependent are untrue for most of the older adult population. This older couple exhibits the vitality, joy, and spontaneity of a young couple.

Continued on following page

ASSESSMENT OF ERIKSON'S PSYCHOSOCIAL DEVELOPMENT

ASSESSMENT PROCEDURE	NORMAL FINDINGS	ABNORMAL FINDINGS
Determine the client's psychosocial developmental level by answering the following questions. Does the young adult— • accept self—physically, cognitively, and emotionally? • have independence from the parental home? • express love responsibly, emotionally, and sexually? • have close or intimate relationships with a partner? • have a social group of friends? • have a physiology of living and life? • have a profession or a life's work that provides a means of contribution?	**Intimacy** The young adult should have achieved self-efficacy during adolescence and is now ready to open up and become intimate with others (Fig. 4-2). Although this stage focuses on the desire for a special and permanent love relationship, it also includes the ability to have close, caring relationships with friends of both genders and a variety of ages. Spiritual love also develops during this stage. Having established an identity apart from the childhood family, the young adult is now able to form adult friendships with his parents and siblings. However, the young adult will always be a son or daughter.	**Isolation** If the young adult cannot express emotion and trust enough to open up to others, social and emotional isolation may occur. Loneliness may cause the young adult to turn to addictive behaviors such as alcoholism, drug abuse, or sexual promiscuity. Some people try to cope with this developmental stage by becoming very spiritual or social, playing an acceptable role, but never fully sharing who they are or becoming emotionally involved with others. When adults successfully navigate this stage, they have stable and satisfying relationships with important others.

ASSESSMENT PROCEDURE	NORMAL FINDINGS	ABNORMAL FINDINGS

• solve problems of life that accompany independence from the parental home?

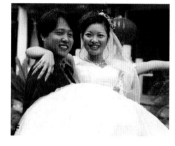

FIGURE 4-2 This young couple has reached Erikson's stage of intimacy. They have developed a loving relationship apart from their original families and fused their identity with one another.

Does the middle-aged adult
• have healthful life patterns?
• derive satisfaction from contributing to growth and development of others?
• have an abiding intimacy and long-term relationship with a partner?

Generativity
During this stage, the middle-aged adult is able to share self with others and establish nurturing relationships. The adult will be able to extend self and possessions to others.

Although traditionalists tend to think of generativity in terms of raising one's children and guiding their lives, generativity can be realized in several ways even without having children. Generativity implies mentoring and giving to future generations

Stagnation
Without this important step, the gift is not given and the stage does not come to successful completion. Stagnation occurs when the middle-aged person has not accomplished one or more of the previous developmental tasks, and is unable to give to future generations.

Continued on following page

ASSESSMENT OF ERIKSON'S PSYCHOSOCIAL DEVELOPMENT (Continued)

ASSESSMENT PROCEDURE	NORMAL FINDINGS	ABNORMAL FINDINGS
• maintain a stable home? • find pleasure in an established work or profession? • take pride in self and family accomplishments and contributions? • contributes to the community to support its growth and development?	(Fig. 4-3). This can be accomplished by producing ideas, products, inventions, paintings, writings, books, films, or any other creative endeavors that are then given to the world for the unrestricted use of its people. Generativity also includes teaching others, children or adults, mentoring young workers, or providing experience and wisdom to assist a new business to survive and grow. Also implied in this stage is the ability to guide, then let go of one's creations. Successful movement through this stage results in a fuller and more satisfying life and prepares the mature adult for the next stage.	Severe losses may result in withdrawal and stagnation. Then a person may have total dependency on work, a favorite child, or even a pet, and be incapable of giving to others. Goals (i.e., projects, schooling) may never be finished because the person cannot let go. Without a creative outlet, a paralyzing stagnation sets in.

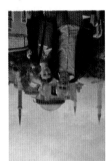

FIGURE 4-3 This father, in his early middle adult years, enjoys traveling with his teenage daughter and sharing with her his knowledge of history and culture.

ASSESSMENT PROCEDURE	NORMAL FINDINGS	ABNORMAL FINDINGS
Does the older adult • adjust to the changing physical self? • recognize changes present as a result of aging, in relationships and activities? • maintain relationships with children, grandchildren, and other relatives? • continue interests outside of self and home? • complete transition from retirement at work to satisfying alternative activities? • establishes relationships with others who are his or her own age? • adjust to deaths of relatives, spouse, and friends?	**Integrity** According to Erikson (1950), a person in this stage looks back and either finds that life was good or despairs because goals were not accomplished. This stage can extend over a long time and include excursions into previous stages to complete unfinished business. Successful movement through this stage does not mean that one day a person wakes up and says, "My life has been good"; rather, it encompasses a series of reminiscences in which the person may be able to see past events in a new and more positive light. This can be a very rich and rewarding time in a person's life, especially if there are others with whom to share memories and who can assist with reframing life experiences (Fig. 4-4). For some people, resolution and acceptance do not come until the final weeks of life, but this still allows for a peaceful death.	**Despair** If the older person cannot feel grateful for his or her life, cannot accept those less desirable aspects as merely part of living, or cannot integrate all of the experiences of life, then the person will spend his or her last days in bitterness and regret and will ultimately die in despair.

Continued on following page

ASSESSMENT OF ERIKSON'S PSYCHOSOCIAL DEVELOPMENT (Continued)

ASSESSMENT PROCEDURE	NORMAL FINDINGS	ABNORMAL FINDINGS
• maintain a maximum level of physical functioning through diet, exercise, and personal care? • find meaning in past life and face inevitable mortality of self and significant others? • integrate philosophical or religious values into self-understanding to promote comfort? • review accomplishments and recognize meaningful contributions he or she has made to community and relatives?	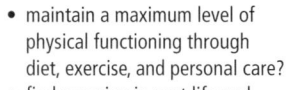 FIGURE 4-4 Older adulthood can be a rich and rewarding time to review life events.	

ASSESSMENT OF PIAGET'S COGNITIVE DEVELOPMENT

Determine the clients' cognitive level by asking the following questions: Does the young adult

• assume responsibility for independent decision making?

The young adult who has attained formal operational thought continues to use sensorimotor thought and learning. Being alert to both internal and external stimuli assists information processing. Cognitive regression occurs in all individuals throughout the life cycle under conditions of stress. However,

The young adult who has not attained formal operations will operate at the stage in which cognitive arrest occurred. This person will have difficulty with abstract thinking when information is presented in written

ASSESSMENT PROCEDURE	NORMAL FINDINGS	ABNORMAL FINDINGS
• realistically self-evaluate strengths and weaknesses? • identify and explore multiple options and potential outcomes? • seek assistance as necessary? • place decision into long-range context? • make realistic plans for the future? • seek career mentors?	it should be regained in a timely manner. Formal operations incorporate deductive reasoning. The young adult can evaluate the validity of reasoning. This person who performs self-evaluation must be able to make objective judgment. All people learn at their own pace and with their own style. The young adult is interested in learning that which is considered relevant and worthy of use. These people are capable of making realistic plans for the future.	form. This young adult will find it difficult to understand and process the information in some high school and definitely college level textbooks.
Does the middle-aged adult • differentiate discrepancies among goals, wishes, and realities? • identify factors that give life meaning and continuity? • effectively share knowledge and experience with others? • separate emotional (affective) issues from the cognitive domain for decision making?	The middle-aged adult using formal operational thought is capable of readjusting/modifying goals as necessary. Improving active and developing latent interests and talents increases creativity. The healthy middle-aged person provides mentorship to others due to increased problem solving abilities and experiences (Fig. 4-5, p. 80). Seeking new information maintains currency and promotes continued self-development and responsibility. This is especially true regarding rapid progress in technology and emphasis on computerization. The older members of generation X (born between 1965 and 1981) wish to learn to	The middle-aged adult who has not attained/maintained formal operational thought experiences in maintaining current at work and meeting expectations in all aspects of life in general. This person has not made adequate realistic plans for the future. The middle-aged client who has not attained formal operational thought may be able to teach other "hands-on" skills that don't require in-depth explanation and rationale.

Continued on following page

ASSESSMENT OF PIAGET'S COGNITIVE DEVELOPMENT (Continued)

ASSESSMENT PROCEDURE	NORMAL FINDINGS	ABNORMAL FINDINGS
• seek new ways to improve/add to knowledge? • adapt quickly to change and new knowledge? 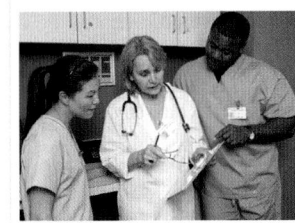	advance in their careers and other responsibilities. The "baby boomers" (born between 1946 and 1964) learn to adapt to fast change. Many of these adults have been called the *"sandwich generation"* (Schuster & Ashburn, 1992, p.786; Touhy & Jett, 2012, p. 4) because they try to meet the needs of their teenagers/adult children (who have often returned to live at home and bring grandchildren) as well as caring for aging parents/grandparents. They are attempting to guide young people who are seeking independence while manage the older persons who are experiencing loss of independence.	

FIGURE 4-5 The middle-aged adult is able to mentor young adults in the workplace because he or she has increased problem solving abilities and life experience.

ASSESSMENT PROCEDURE	NORMAL FINDINGS	ABNORMAL FINDINGS
Does the older adult • maintain maximal independence with activities of daily living? • problem solve ways to find satisfaction with life? • determine realistic plans for future, including own mortality?	The older adult who uses formal operational thinking, shares expertise with others remembering events from earlier years. He or she teaches others about the history and continuities of life. Many older adults prefer gradual transitions rather than abrupt changes. One who has seen much change, can demonstrate flexibility and is able to make realistic decisions regarding activities, self-care, living arrangements, transportation, medical regimen, and finances. "Traditionalists" (born before 1946) value achievement and are often fiscally conservative due to experiences with rationing during wars and the great depression. Capable of gradually transferring social/civic responsibilities to others. Solidifies the concepts of life and death. Piaget believed new learning can continue to occur.	The older adult who does not possess formal operational thinking eventually profits from assistance from others, especially in obtaining activities of daily living, correctly taking medication, and maintaining one's highest level of wellness.

ASSESSMENT OF KOHLBERG'S MORAL DEVELOPMENT

Determine the client's moral level by asking the following suggested questions.	According to Kohlberg's theory, which was based on male behavior, the young adult who has at least reached Piaget's stage of concrete operations may have attained the conventional	The young adult who continues to make decisions and behave for sole-satisfaction has not attained the conventional level.

Continued on following page

ASSESSMENT OF KOHLBERG'S MORAL DEVELOPMENT (Continued)

ASSESSMENT PROCEDURE	NORMAL FINDINGS	ABNORMAL FINDINGS
Does the young adult • state priorities to be considered when making a moral decision? • perceive being approved by family? • perceive being approved by peers? • perceive being approved by supervisor/teachers/authority figures? • perceive being approved by significant other? • consider self to be a "good person"? Why or why not? • able to judge the intentions of others?	level of moral reasoning. As the young adult attempts to take on new roles (adult student, exclusive sexual relationship, vocation, marriage, parent), attempts are made to maintain expectations and rules of the family, group, partnership, or society. This young adult obeys the law because it is respect for authority. Guilt can be a motivator to do the "right" thing. Decisions and behaviors are based on concerns about gaining approval from others. Some young adults who are capable of Piaget's formal operations will vacillate between the conventional and postconventional levels. For example, a young adult may intentionally break the law and join a protest group to stop medical research and experimentation on animals, believing that the principle of being humane to animals justifies the revolt. That same person may, however, exhibit more conventional reasoning when making decisions about "doing one's duty" at work, fulfilling the role of accountable student, and responsibly parenting a child.	Continued behavior that negatively affects the comfort zone of others or infringes on the rights of others is not normal (Fig. 4-6). Those persons experiencing extreme stress overload may demonstrate moral regression. 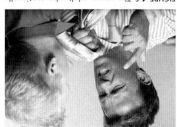 **FIGURE 4-6** The young adult who continually exhibits behavior that negatively affects the comfort zone of others or infringes on the rights of others is not normal.

ASSESSMENT PROCEDURE	NORMAL FINDINGS	ABNORMAL FINDINGS
Does the middle-aged adult • state priorities to be considered when making a moral decision? • focus more on law and order or individual rights when making a decision? • express willingness to stop unhealthy behavior and change lifestyle patterns to foster a higher level of wellness?	Kohlberg found that although many adults are capable of Piaget's stage of formal operations few demonstrated the postconventional level of behavior and, if healthy, were more than likely at the conventional level. Kohlberg believed that if a person was capable of formal operations and experienced additional positive personal moral choices, then that person could reach a higher level of moral development. Many older middle-aged adults questioned authority and challenged the status quo during their young adult years. There are many healthy middle-aged people who feel that they have learned from mistakes made earlier during young adulthood.	The person who has consistently used maladaptive coping will not reach the postconventional level. Such a person could regress as far as the premoral (or even amoral) level. This person fears authority and hopes to "not get caught."
Does the older adult • state priorities to be considered when making a moral decision? • view rules and laws as change-able using legal means? ·	Kohlberg believed very few people attain and maintain the highest stage of the postconventional level. During the fifth stage, the person believes in respect for individuals while still emphasizing that the needs of the majority are more important. During the sixth stage, the person believes in absolute justice for every individual and is willing to make a decision or perform an action risking external punishment. It may be that the older	It is difficult to assess anyone as normal or abnormal unless that person is harming self or others. Kohlberg hypothesized that older adults who were still at the preconventional level obey rules to avoid the disapproval of others. Kohlberg believed that older adults at the conventional level adhere to society's

Continued on following page

ASSESSMENT OF KOHLBERG'S MORAL DEVELOPMENT (Continued)

ASSESSMENT PROCEDURE	NORMAL FINDINGS	ABNORMAL FINDINGS
• make decisions consistently on internalized rules and in terms of conscience? • believe in equality for every person?	adult perceives more authority, time and courage to "speak one's mind." Today's senior citizen may have developed belief patterns during a time very different than the twenty-first century. A few older adults, as they ponder their mortality, may enter Kohlberg's seventh stage. Such a person would analyze the "whole picture" and conclude that all organisms are interconnected.	rules and laws because they believe this is what others expect of them.

 PEDIATRIC VARIATIONS

For a review of the stages associated with each developmental theory, see Tables 4-1, 4-2, 4-3, and 4-4 (pp. 57–69).

Psychosexual Development (Freud)

• Question children of all ages about sexual abuse. This may be elicited by asking, "Has anyone ever touched you where or when you did not want to be touched?"

• Oral stage (birth to 18 months): Ask the parents or caregiver the following questions: Does your infant have any problems with nursing or sucking from a bottle? Has your infant started chewing foods? Does he or she bite? Does your infant express himself by crying and a variety of vocalizations?

• Anal stage (8 months to 4 years): Ask the parents or caregiver the following questions: Does your toddler have any problems with toilet training? Does your toddler masturbate?

• Phallic stage (3 to 7 years): Ask the parents or caregiver the following questions: Does your preschooler masturbate? Does your preschooler know what sex he or she is? Has your preschooler asked questions about sex, childbirth, and the like?

- Latency period (5 to 12 years): Ask the parents or caregiver the following questions: Does your school-age child interact with same-sex peers? What has your school-age child been told about puberty and sex?
- Genital stage (12 to 20 years): Ask the adolescent the following questions: A full, confidential sexual/sexuality history should be obtained from adolescents and include: What is your sexual preference? How do you feel about becoming a man/woman? Are you sexually active? Do you use contraception? What forms?

Psychosocial Development (Erikson)

- Trust versus mistrust (birth to 1 year): Ask the parents or caregiver the following questions: How do you usually respond to your infant when they cry? Who usually cares for your infant when you are not around? Does your infant have a special blanket or toy that they often seek out for comfort or sleeping time?
- Autonomy versus shame and doubt (1 to 3 years): Ask the parents or caregiver the following questions: Does your toddler try to do things for himself or herself (e.g., feed, dress)? Does your toddler have temper tantrums? How are they handled? Does your toddler frequently use the word "no"? At what age was your toddler completely toilet trained? Does your toddler actively explore the environment?
- Initiative versus guilt (3 to 6 years): Ask the parents or caregiver the following questions: Does your preschooler have an active imagination? Does your preschooler imitate adult activities? Does your preschooler engage in fantasy play? Does your preschooler frequently ask questions? Does your preschooler enjoy new activities?
- Industry versus inferiority (7 to 11 years): Ask the parents or caregiver the following questions: What are your school-age child's interests/hobbies? Does your school-age child interact well with teachers, peers? Does your school-age child enjoy accomplishments? Does your school-age child shame self for failures? What is your school-age child's favorite activity?
- Identity versus role diffusion (11 to 18 years): Ask the parents or caregiver the following questions: Does your adolescent have a peer group? Does your adolescent have a best friend? Does your adolescent exhibit rebellious behavior at home? How does your adolescent see self as fitting in with peers? What does your adolescent want to do with her life?

Cognitive and Language Development (Piaget)

- Sensorimotor stage (birth to 18 months): Ask the parents or caregiver the following questions: Does your child have different types of crying? Explain. Does your infant coo, babble, make consonant sounds, combine syllables such as mama or dada? What does your infant do when you say "no-no"? What words does your infant use?

- Sensorimotor phase (12 to 24 months): Ask the parents or caregiver the following questions: Can your toddler name some body parts? Can your toddler state first and last name? Does your toddler imitate adults? Does your toddler put two words together to form sentence? (e.g., "me go")?

- Preoperational thought (2 to 7 years): Ask the parents or caregiver the following questions: Does your preschooler tell fantasy stories or have an imaginary friend? Does your preschooler have an invisible friend? Can your preschooler make simple classifications? (e.g., dogs, cats)? Is your preschooler "chatty"? Does your preschooler frequently ask "why?" Can your preschooler name at least four colors?

- Concrete operations (7 to 11 years): Ask the parents or caregiver: Can your school-age child see another's point of view? Does your child collect things? (e.g., baseball cards, dolls)? Does your child try to solve problems? How well does your child do in school? How well does your child read?

- Formal operations (11 to 15 years): Ask the parents or caregiver the following questions: Do you consider your adolescent to be a problem solver? How well does your adolescent do in school? Also ask the adolescent and compare the responses.

Moral Development (Kohlberg)

- Infants: Although Kohlberg's theory of moral development begins with toddlerhood, infants cannot be overlooked. Child moral development begins with the value and belief system of the parents and the infant's own development of trust.

- First substage of the preconventional stage (1 to 2 years): What forms of discipline do you use with your child? How do you praise your child?

- Preconventional stage of moral development (3 to 10 years): What forms of discipline do you use with your child when they do something not acceptable? How do you reward your child? How does he respond to discipline and rewards?

- Conventional level of the role conformity stage (10 to 13 years): How does your child try to please others? Who do they try to please the most?
- Postconventional stage of morality (greater than 13 years): Ask the parents or caregiver the following questions: Does your child understand the difference between right and wrong? Do you discuss family values with your child? Do you have family rules? How are they implemented? How are disciplinary measures handled? Has your child ever had problems with lying, cheating, or stealing? Has your child ever required disciplinary action at school? Has your child ever violated the law?

 GERIATRIC VARIATIONS

Psychosexual Development (Freud)

Does the older adult engage in sexual activity? Positively cope with loss? Believe any changes in cognition have occurred? Believe any significant changes have occurred in interests/relationships?

Psychosocial Development (Erikson)

Ego integrity versus despair: Does the older adult accept self as unique, accept others, and accept death an entity?

Cognitive Development (Piaget)

Does the older adult: Maintain maximal independence with activities of daily living? Problem solve ways to find satisfaction with life? Determine realistic plans for future, including own mortality?

Moral Development (Kohlberg)

Does the older adult state priorities to be considered when making a moral decision? View rules and laws as changeable using legal means? Make decisions consistently on internalized rules and in terms of conscience? Believe in equality for every individual?

 CULTURAL VARIATIONS

It is important to recognize and respect cultural diversity. Ask the client: With what cultural group(s) do you most identify? What is your primary language? When do you speak it? Are you fluent in other languages? Language is initially promulgated via culture. Freud (1930) and Erikson (1950) acknowledged differences of behavior caused by cultural conditions. Piaget (1981) postulated that cultural factors contribute significantly to differences in cognitive development. Kohlberg (Kohlberg & Gilligan, 1971) noted that cultures teach different beliefs, but that the stage sequence is universal and not affected by cultural difference.

POSSIBLE COLLABORATIVE PROBLEMS—RISK OF

- Anxiety
- Depression
- Suicide
- Neurosis
- Psychosis

Teaching Tips for Selected Nursing Diagnoses

Nursing Diagnosis: *Readiness for Enhanced Parenting related to giving birth to first child*

Teach new parents ways (bonding, interacting, playing, reading) to promote healthy physical, psychosocial, and cognitive development. Explain the variation in developmental milestones with individual children to alleviate anxiety.

 Nursing Diagnosis: *Caregiver Role Strain related to caring for dependent older parent*

Teach available resources to assist with the financial, physical, and psychosocial care of the older parent. Discuss the importance of engaging in healthy activities of daily living to stay healthy to meet one's own developmental goals.

 Nursing Diagnosis: *Social Isolation related to loss of driver's license, poor vision, and hearing.*

Assist and teach client ways to access community resources (i.e., Meals on Wheels, senior centers, transportation for the disabled, local church organizations). Refer to organizations (i.e., American Foundation for the Blind, Hearing Loss Association of America) to acquire assistance with obtaining tools (i.e., magnifying glasses, large print reading materials and checks, hearing devices) to enhance activities of daily living.

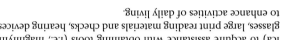 **Nursing Diagnosis:** *Compromised Family Coping related to family developmental crisis adjusting to infant/child development*

Discuss social development of the child. Assess the parent's knowledge and understanding of the developmental milestones for the child and educate them regarding normal parameters for the developmental stage of their child and the tasks that need to be achieved for the child to move to the next level. Infant's "stranger anxiety" is normal. Teach parents ways to assist infant to warm up to strangers. Encourage verbalization, reassurance, and cuddling. Help parent assess child's readiness to begin school and to discuss any school problems with child. Teach parent the importance of spending quality time with child and ways to promote effective communication with child. Encourage the parent to identify parenting strategies that will enhance parenting skills and communication between the parent and child. Identify strengths, weaknesses, and new coping skills that will improve communication and family dynamics between parent and child throughout the developmental changes of the lifespan.

CHAPTER 5

Assessing Mental Status and Substance Abuse

Conceptual Foundations

Mental status refers to a client's level of cognitive and emotional functioning and stability. Mental status is reflected in one's speech, appearance, and thought patterns. The ability to think clearly and respond appropriately to daily stressors of life is necessary to function effectively in the activities of daily

living. One cannot be totally healthy without "mental health." Mental health is an essential part of one's total health and is more than just the absence of mental disabilities or disorders. It is reflected in one's appearance, behavior, speech, thought patterns, and decision making, and in one's ability to function in an effective manner in relationships in a variety of settings (home, work, social, recreational). The structure and function of the neurologic system can affect one's mental and psychosocial status. Cerebral abnormalities disturb the client's intellectual ability, communication ability, or emotional behaviors. Refer to Chapter 21, Assessing Neurologic System, for review of the structure and function of the cerebral cortex. In addition, several factors may influence the client's mental health or put him or her at risk for impaired mental health. These factors include economic and social factors, unhealthy lifestyle choices, exposure to violence, personality factors, spiritual factors, cultural factors, and/or changes or impairments in the structure and function of the neurologic system.

Nursing Assessment

COLLECTING SUBJECTIVE DATA

Past mental health diagnoses? Counseling services? Head injury, meningitis, encephalitis, stroke? Headaches? Served active duty in armed forces? Difficulty breathing, dizziness, nausea and vomiting, heart palpitations? Eating and bowel habits, family history of mental health disease, Alzheimer? Coping patterns? Pattern activities of daily living (energy level, sleep patterns, eating habits)? Use of over-the-counter and prescribed drugs? Use of alcohol? Use the CAGE Assessment Questionnaire (available at http://www.mercycarehealthplans.com/ace-files/Provider%20Reference%20Guide/6_screening_tools.pdf) to detect alcohol dependence in trauma center populations. It is recommended that the CAGE be used with alcohol testing to identify at risk patients (Soderstrom, et al., 1997). The AUDIT questionnaire (available at http://whqlibdoc.who.int/hq/2001/who_msd_msb_01.6a.pdf) may also be used to assess alcohol-related disorders by asking the client questions and then calculating a score. Use of recreational drugs such as marijuana, tranquilizers, barbiturates, or cocaine? Relationship patterns with others? Marital status? Educational level? Socioeconomic level? Exposure to environmental toxins? Cultural practices? Religious practices? Support systems? Feelings about the future?

COLLECTING OBJECTIVE DATA

Equipment Needed

- Pencil and paper
- Glasgow Coma Scale (p. 101)
- Saint Louis University Mental Status (SLUMS) Examination Tool (p. 102)

ASSESSMENT PROCEDURE	NORMAL FINDINGS	ABNORMAL FINDINGS
Observe level of consciousness. • Note response to calling the client's name. • If the client does not respond, call the name louder. If necessary, shake the client gently. • If the client still does not respond, apply a painful stimulus.	• Alert and awake with eyes open and looking at examiner; client responds appropriately.	• Lethargy: Opens eyes, answers questions, and falls back asleep. • Obtunded: Opens eyes to loud voice, responds slowly with confusion, seems unaware of environment. • Stupor: Awakens to vigorous shake or painful stimuli, but returns to unresponsive sleep.

• Quick Inventory of Depressive Symptomatology (Self-Report) (p. 103)
• SAD PERSONS Suicide Risk Assessment Tool (p. 107)
• CAGE Assessment Questionnaire (available at http:// www.mercycarehealthplans.com/ace-files/Provider%20 Reference%20Guide/6_screening_tools.pdf)
• AUDIT Questionnaire (available at http://whqlibdoc.who .int/hq/2001/who_msd_msb_01.6a.pdf)

Physical Assessment

Perform an assessment of mental status by observing the client and asking questions. Much of this information may have already been assessed during the initial interview and general survey. There are several parts of the examination, which include assessment of the client's level of consciousness, posture, gait, body movements, dress, grooming, hygiene, facial expressions, behavior and affect, speech, mood, feelings, expressions, thought processes, perceptions, and cognitive abilities.

ASSESSMENT PROCEDURE	NORMAL FINDINGS	ABNORMAL FINDINGS
		• Coma: Remains unresponsive to all stimuli; eyes stay closed. Client with lesions of the corticospinal tract draws hands up to chest (*decorticate* or abnormal flexor posture) when stimulated.
		• Client with lesions of the diencephalon, mid-brain, or pons extends arms and legs, arches neck, and rotates hands and arms internally (*decorticate* or abnormal extensor posture) when stimulated.
• Use the Glasgow Coma Scale (GCS) for clients who are at high risk for rapid deterioration of the nervous system (Box 5-1, p. 101).	• GCS score of 14 indicates an optimal level of consciousness.	• GCS score of less than 14 indicates some impairment of consciousness. A score of 3, the lowest possible score, indicates deep coma.
• Administer the Saint Louis University Mental Status (SLUMS) Examination (Box 5-2, p. 102) and The Confusion Assessment Method (CAM) for a complete in-depth mental status examination.	• For a high school educated client, a score of 27–30 on the SLUMS Examination is normal, and for less than high school educated a score of 20–30 is normal.	• A SLUMS score of 20–27 for a high school educated client, or 14–19 for a less than high school educated client, indicates that mental cognition is impaired and the client should be referred for further testing.

Continued on following page

ASSESSMENT PROCEDURE	NORMAL FINDINGS	ABNORMAL FINDINGS
		• A score of 1–19 for a high school educated client, or of 1–14 for a less than high school educated client, indicates dementia and the client should be referred for further testing.
Observe **appearance and movement.**		
• Posture	• Relaxed, with shoulders back and both feet stable	• Tense, rigid, slumped, asymmetrical posture. Slumped posture is seen with depression or organic brain disease.
• Gait	• Smooth, coordinated movements; client alters position occasionally.	• Uncoordinated—staggering, shuffling, stumbling.
• Motor movements	• Same as above	• Jerky, uncoordinated; tremors, tics, fast or slow movements. Bizarre movements are seen with schizophrenia; tense, fidgety, and restless behavior in anxious patients.
• Dress	• Clothes fit and are appropriate for occasion and weather.	• Clothes extra large or small and inappropriate for occasion. Inappropriate dress is seen with depression, dementia, Alzheimer disease, and schizophrenia.

ASSESSMENT PROCEDURE	NORMAL FINDINGS	ABNORMAL FINDINGS
• Hygiene	• Skin clean, nails clean and trimmed	• Dirty, unshaven; dirty nails; foul odors. Poor hygiene is seen with depression, dementia, Alzheimer disease, and schizophrenia; meticulous, finicky grooming in obsessive–compulsive disorder.
• Facial expression	• Good eye contact, smiles/frowns appropriately	• Poor eye contact is seen in apathy or depression; mask-like expression in Parkinson disease; extreme anger or happiness in anxious clients.
• Speech	• Clear with moderate pace	• High pitched; monotonal; hoarse; very soft or weak. Slow, repetitive speech is present in depression or Parkinson disease; loud and rapid in manic phases; irregular, uncoordinated speech in multiple sclerosis; dysphonia in impairment of CN X; dysarthria in Parkinson or cerebellar disease; aphasia in lesions of dominant hemisphere.

Continued on following page

ASSESSMENT PROCEDURE	NORMAL FINDINGS	ABNORMAL FINDINGS
Observe **mood** by asking, "How are you feeling?" or "What are your plans for the future?"		
• Feelings (vary from joy to anger)	• Responds appropriately to the topic discussed; expresses feelings appropriate to the situation.	• Expresses feelings inappropriate to the situation (e.g., extreme anger or euphoria)
• Expressions	• Expresses good feelings about self, others, and life; verbalizes positive coping mechanisms (talking, support systems, counseling, exercise, etc.)	• Expresses dissatisfaction with self, others, and life in general; verbalizes negative coping mechanisms (use of alcohol, drugs, etc.); prolonged negative feelings seen with depression; elation and high energy seen with manic phases; excessive worry seen in obsessive–compulsive disorders; eccentric moods not relevant to situation are seen in schizophrenia.
Use Box 5-3: Quick Inventory of Depressive Symptomatology (Self-Report) on page 103 to determine if the client is at risk for depression and needs to be referred to a primary care health provider for further evaluation.	Inventory scores of 0–5 = No risk of depression	Inventory scores of 6–10 = Mild 11–15 = Moderate 16–20 = Severe 21–27 = Very Severe

ASSESSMENT PROCEDURE	NORMAL FINDINGS	ABNORMAL FINDINGS
Observe **thought process and perceptions** by stating, "Tell me your understanding of your current health situation."		
• Clarity and content	• Expresses full and free-flowing thoughts during interview.	• Expressed thoughts are jumbled, confusing, and not reality oriented. Repetition and expression of illogical thoughts are seen with schizophrenia; rapid flight of ideas with manic phases; irrational fears with phobias; delusions seen with psychotic disorders, delirium, and dementia; illusions seen with acute grief, stress reactions, schizophrenia, and delirium; hallucinations with organic brain disease or psychotic illness.
• Perceptions	• Follows directions accurately; perceptions realistic and consistent with yours and others	• Is unable to follow through with directives; perceptions unrealistic and inconsistent with yours and others.
• Judgment	• Answers to questions are based on sound rationale.	• Impaired judgment may be seen in organic brain syndrome, emotional disturbances, mental retardation, or schizophrenia.

Continued on following page

ASSESSMENT PROCEDURE	NORMAL FINDINGS	ABNORMAL FINDINGS
• Identify possibly destructive or suicidal tendencies in client's thought processes and perceptions by asking, "How do you feel about the future?" or "Have you ever had thoughts of hurting yourself or doing away with yourself?" or "How do others feel about you?" • Use Box 5-4, the SAD PERSONS Suicide Risk Assessment Guide on page 107, to determine the risk factors the client may have that may put him or her at risk for suicide.	Verbalizes positive, healthy thoughts about the future and self. No risk factors present on the SAD PERSONS factors.	Clients who are suicidal may share past attempts of suicide, give plan for suicide, verbalize worthlessness about self, joke about death frequently. Clients who are depressed or feel hopeless are at higher risk for suicide. Clients who have depression early in life have a twofold-increased risk for dementia (Byers & Yaffe, 2011). Evaluate any risk factors on the SAD PERSONS. Suicide is the 10th leading cause of death in the United States for all ages and is four times more prevalent in men. Firearms accounted for 17,352 deaths, suffocation 8,161 deaths, and poisoning 6,358 deaths (Hammer, Moynihan, & Pagliaro, 2013).
Observe cognitive abilities. • Orientation—Ask client name, hour, date, season, where he or she lives now.	Aware of self, others, place, time; has address	Unable to express where he or she is, time, and who others are; does not follow instructions. Reduced level of orientation is seen with organic brain disorders.

ASSESSMENT PROCEDURE	NORMAL FINDINGS	ABNORMAL FINDINGS
• Length of concentration	• Listens to you and responds with full thoughts	• Fidgets; does not listen attentively to you; expresses incomplete thoughts. Distraction and inability to focus are noted with anxiety, fatigue, attention deficit disorders, and altered states due to drug or alcohol intoxication.
• Memory—Ask client, "What did you eat today?" (recent) and "When is your birthday?" (past)	• Correctly answers questions about current day's activities; recalls significant past events.	• Unable to recall any recent events with delirium, dementia, depression, and anxiety; unable to recall past events with cerebral cortex disorders.
• Abstract reasoning—Ask client to explain a proverb, for example, "A stitch in time saves nine."	• Explains proverb accurately	• Unable to give abstract meaning of proverb with schizophrenia, mental retardation, delirium, or dementia.
• Ability to make sound judgments—Ask client question such as "Why did you come to the hospital?" or "What do you do when you have pain?"	• Answers to questions based on sound rationale	• Answers to questions are not based on sound rationale in organic brain syndrome, emotional disturbances, mental retardation, or schizophrenia.

Continued on following page

ASSESSMENT PROCEDURE	NORMAL FINDINGS	ABNORMAL FINDINGS
• Ability to identify similarities—Ask client questions such as "How are birds and bees alike?"	• Identifies similarity	• Unable to identify similarity with schizophrenia, mental retardation, delirium, or dementia.
• Sensory perception and coordination—Ask client to write name and draw the face of a clock or copy simple figures such as:	• Writes name, draws clock and/or simple figures.	• Does not write name or draw clock/figures accurately with mental retardation, dementia, or parietal lobe dysfunction.

BOX 5-1 GLASGOW COMA SCALE

The Glasgow Coma Scale is useful for rating one's response to stimuli. The client who scores 10 or lower needs emergency attention. The client with a score of 7 or lower is generally considered to be in a coma.

	Score	
Eye Opening Response	Spontaneous opening	4
	To verbal command	3
	To pain	2
	No response	1
Most Appropriate Verbal Response	Oriented	5
	Confused	4
	Inappropriate words	3
	Incoherent	2
	No response	1
Most Integral Motor Response (Arm)	Obeys verbal commands	6
	Localizes pain	5
	Withdraws from pain	4
	Flexion (decorticate rigidity)	3
	Extension (decerebrate rigidity)	2
	No response	1
Total Score		3–15

From Teasdale, G., & Jennett, B. (1974). Assessment of coma and impaired consciousness: A practical scale. The Lancet, 2(7872), 81–84. Used with permission.

BOX 5-2   MENTAL STATUS EXAMINATIONS TOOLS

Saint Louis University
Mental Status (SLUMS) Examination

Name _____ Age _____ Level of education _____

Is patient alert? _____

_/1	**1. What day of the week is it?**
_/1	**2. What is the year?**
_/1	**3. What state are we in?**
	4. Please remember these five objects. I will ask you what they are later.
	Apple Pen Tie House Car
_/3	**5. You have $100 and you go to the store and buy a dozen apples for $3 and a tricycle for $20.**
	How much did you spend?
_/3	How much do you have left?
	6. Please name as many animals as you can in 1 minute.
_/3	❶ 0–5 animals ❷ 5–10 animals ❸ 10–15 animals ❹ 15+ animals
_/1	**7. What were the 5 objects I asked you to remember? 1 point for each one correct.**
	8. I am going to give you a series of numbers and I would like you to give them to me backwards
_/2	For example, if I say 42, you would say 24.
	❶ 87 ❷ 649 ❸ 8537
	9. This is a clock face. Please put in the hour markers and the time at 10 minutes
	to 11 o'clock.
_/2	Hour markers okay
_/2	Time correct

10. Please place an X in the triangle.

Which of the above figures is largest?

11. I am going to tell you a story. Please listen carefully because afterwards I'm going to ask you some questions about it.

Jill was a very successful stockbroker. She made a lot of money on the stock market. She then met Jack, a devastatingly handsome man. She married him and had three children. They lived in Chicago. She then stopped work and stayed at home to bring up her children. When they were teenagers, she went back to work. She and Jack lived happily ever after.

_/8	**What was the female's name?** **What work did she do?**
	When did she go back to work? **What state did she live in?**

Scoring

	High School Education		Less than High School Education
Normal	27–30	....	26–30
MNCD*	21–26	....	20–25
Dementia	19–20	....	14–19
	....		

*Mild Neurocognitive Disorder

For further information on using the tool, visit http://www.elderguru.com/
downloads/SLUMS_instructions.pdf.

BOX 5-3 QUICK INVENTORY OF DEPRESSIVE SYMPTOMATOLOGY (SELF-REPORT)

PLEASE CHECKMARK THE ONE RESPONSE TO EACH ITEM THAT IS MOST APPROPRIATE TO HOW YOU HAVE BEEN FEELING OVER THE PAST 7 DAYS.

1. **Falling asleep:**
   - ☐ 0 I never took longer than 30 minutes to fall asleep.
   - ☐ 1 I took at least 30 minutes to fall asleep, less than half the time (3 days or less out of the past 7 days).
   - ☐ 2 I took at least 30 minutes to fall asleep, more than half the time (4 days or more out of the past 7 days).
   - ☐ 3 I took more than 60 minutes to fall asleep, more than half the time (4 days or more out of the past 7 days).

2. **Sleep during the night:**
   - ☐ 0 I didn't wake up at night.
   - ☐ 1 I had a restless, light sleep, briefly waking up a few times each night.
   - ☐ 2 I woke up at least once a night, but I got back to sleep easily.
   - ☐ 3 I woke up more than once a night and stayed awake for 20 minutes or more, more than half the time (4 days or more out of the past 7 days).

3. **Waking up too early:**
   - ☐ 0 Most of the time, I woke up no more than 30 minutes before my scheduled time.
   - ☐ 1 More than half the time (4 days or more out of the past 7 days), I woke up more than 30 minutes before my scheduled time.
   - ☐ 2 I almost always woke up at least one hour or so before my scheduled time, but I got back to sleep eventually.
   - ☐ 3 I woke up at least one hour before my scheduled time, and couldn't get back to sleep.

4. **Sleeping too much:**
   - ☐ 0 I slept no longer than 7–8 hours/night, without napping during the day.
   - ☐ 1 I slept no longer than 10 hours in a 24-hour period including naps.
   - ☐ 2 I slept no longer than 12 hours in a 24-hour period including naps.
   - ☐ 3 I slept longer than 12 hours in a 24-hour period including naps.

5. **Feeling sad:**
   - ☐ 0 I didn't feel sad.
   - ☐ 1 I felt sad less than half the time (3 days or less out of the past 7 days).
   - ☐ 2 I felt sad more than half the time (4 days or more out of the past 7 days).
   - ☐ 3 I felt sad nearly all of the time.

Continued on following page

BOX 5-3 QUICK INVENTORY OF DEPRESSIVE SYMPTOMATOLOGY (SELF-REPORT) (Continued)

PLEASE CHECKMARK THE ONE RESPONSE TO EACH ITEM THAT IS MOST APPROPRIATE TO HOW YOU HAVE BEEN FEELING OVER THE PAST 7 DAYS.

Please complete either 6 or 7 (not both)

6. Decreased appetite:

☐ 0 There was no change in my usual appetite.

☐ 1 I ate somewhat less often or smaller amounts of food than usual.

☐ 2 I ate much less than usual and only by forcing myself to eat.

☐ 3 I rarely ate within a 24-hour period, and only by really forcing myself to eat or when others persuaded me to eat.

7. Increased appetite:

☐ 0 There was no change in my usual appetite.

☐ 1 I felt a need to eat more frequently than usual.

☐ 2 I regularly ate more often and/or greater amounts of food than usual.

☐ 3 I felt driven to overeat both at mealtime and between meals.

Please complete either 8 or 9 (not both)

8. Decreased weight (within the last 14 days):

☐ 0 My weight has not changed.

☐ 1 I feel as if I've had a slight weight loss.

☐ 2 I've lost 2 pounds (about 1 kilo) or more.

☐ 3 I've lost 5 pounds (about 2 kilos) or more.

9. Increased weight (within the last 14 days):

☐ 0 My weight has not changed.

☐ 1 I feel as if I've had a slight weight gain.

☐ 2 I've gained 2 pounds (about 1 kilo) or more.

☐ 3 I've gained 5 pounds (about 2 kilos) or more.

10. Concentration/decision-making:

☐ 0 There was no change in my usual ability to concentrate or make decisions.

☐ 1 I occasionally felt indecisive or found that my attention wandered.

☐ 2 Most of the time, I found it hard to focus or to make decisions.

☐ 3 I couldn't concentrate well enough to read or I couldn't make even minor decisions.

11. Perception of myself:
- ☐ 0 I saw myself as equally worthwhile and deserving as other people.
- ☐ 1 I put the blame on myself more than usual.
- ☐ 2 For the most part, I believed that I caused problems for others.
- ☐ 3 I thought almost constantly about major and minor defects in myself.

12. Thoughts of my own death or suicide:
- ☐ 0 I didn't think of suicide or death.
- ☐ 1 I felt that life was empty or wondered if it was worth living.
- ☐ 2 I thought of suicide or death several times for several minutes over the past 7 days.
- ☐ 3 I thought of suicide or death several times a day in some detail, or I made specific plans for suicide or actually tried to take my life.

13. General interest:
- ☐ 0 There was no change from usual in how interested I was in other people or activities.
- ☐ 1 I noticed that I was less interested in other people or activities.
- ☐ 2 I found I had interest in only one or two of the activities I used to do.
- ☐ 3 I had virtually no interest in the activities I used to do.

14. Energy level:
- ☐ 0 There was no change in my usual level of energy.
- ☐ 1 I got tired more easily than usual.
- ☐ 2 I had to make a big effort to start or finish my usual daily activities (for example: shopping, homework, cooking or going to work).
- ☐ 3 I really couldn't carry out most of my usual daily activities because I just didn't have the energy.

15. Feeling more sluggish than usual:
- ☐ 0 I thought, spoke, and moved at my usual pace.
- ☐ 1 I found that my thinking was more sluggish than usual or my voice sounded dull or flat.
- ☐ 2 It took me several seconds to respond to most questions and I was sure my thinking was more sluggish than usual.
- ☐ 3 I was often unable to respond to questions without forcing myself.

Continued on following page

BOX 5-3 QUICK INVENTORY OF DEPRESSIVE SYMPTOMATOLOGY (SELF-REPORT) (Continued)

PLEASE CHECKMARK THE ONE RESPONSE TO EACH ITEM THAT IS MOST APPROPRIATE TO HOW YOU HAVE BEEN FEELING OVER THE PAST 7 DAYS.

16. Feeling restless (agitated, not relaxed, fidgety):

☐ 0 I didn't feel restless.

☐ 1 I was often fidgety, wringing my hands, or needed to change my sitting position.

☐ 2 I had sudden urges to move about and was quite restless.

☐ 3 At times, I was unable to stay seated and needed to pace around.

QUICK INVENTORY OF DEPRESSIVE SYMPTOMATOLOGY (SCORE SHEET)

NOTE: THIS SECTION IS TO BE COMPLETED BY THE STUDY PERSONNEL ONLY.

_____ Enter the highest score on any 1 of the 4 sleep items (1–4)

_____ Item 5

_____ Enter the highest score on any 1 of the appetite/weight items (6–9)

_____ Item 10

_____ Item 11

_____ Item 12

_____ Item 13

_____ Item 14

_____ Enter the highest score on either of the 2 psychomotor items (15 and 16)

_____ Total Score (Range: 0–27)

Interpretation of scores

0–5 = No risk of depression

6–10 = Mild

11–15 = Moderate

16–20 = Severe

21–27 = Very Severe

Rush et al, Biol Psychiatry (2003) 54: 573–83.

BOX 5-4 SAD PERSONS SUICIDE RISK ASSESSMENT TOOL

This box can be used to assess the likelihood of a suicide attempt. Consider risk factors within the context of the clinical presentation. Campbell (2004) recommends that scoring not be used, but the examiner should look at the risk factors and respond accordingly.

RISK FACTORS

- Sex
- Age
- Depression
- Previous attempt
- Ethanol abuse
- Rational thinking loss
- Social supports lacking
- Organized plan
- No spouse
- Sickness

(Adapted from Patterson, W. M., Dohn, H. H., Bird J., Patterson, G. A. (1983). Evaluation of suicidal patients: the SAD PERSONS scale. Psychosomatics, 24(4), 343–345, 348–349.)

 PEDIATRIC VARIATIONS

Focus questions would include the following.

- How have feelings/activities changed over the past week?
- Difficulty with concentrating with school tasks.
- Decrease or increase in eating habits.
- Difficulty with sleeping.
- Social isolation.
- Decreased self-esteem.
- Extreme mood changes (happiness/sadness/acting out/ temper tantrums).
- Feelings of fear, confusion.
- Change in relationships with peers, family.
- Use of drugs/alcohol.

 GERIATRIC VARIATIONS

- May seem confused in a new or acute care setting owing to slowed thought processes and slowed responses to questions; however, is oriented to person, time, and place.
- Decreased ability to recall directions.
- Slight decline in short-term memory.
- Slowed reaction time.

- Likes to reminisce and tends to wander from topic at hand.
- May have hesitation with short-term memory.
- Clients greater than 80 years should be able to recall two to four words after a 5-minute time period.
- Use the GDS-5/15 Geriatric Depression Scale to screen older adults for depression.

CULTURAL VARIATIONS

The stroke rate in most industrialized countries has been decreasing, but it remains high among African Americans and across the U.S. stroke belt (most southeastern states, Missouri, and Nevada (CDC, 2012d). Hispanics fall between African Americans and Caucasian Americans, and it is possible that education, rates of diabetes, hypertension, smoking, and poor health insurance coverage affect these rates (CDC, 2013e).

POSSIBLE COLLABORATIVE PROBLEMS—RISK FOR COMPLICATION

- Depression
- Suicide attempt
- Alcohol abuse
- Drug abuse

Teaching Tips for Selected Nursing Diagnoses

Nursing Diagnosis: Disturbed Thought Processes related to neurologic changes (aging, head injury, stroke, etc.)

Inform client or caregiver of the purpose and benefits of community agencies that offer support. Refer client as necessary. Assist family in coping, and explain how to communicate accurately using short sentences.

Nursing Diagnosis: Ineffective Individual Coping related to inadequate opportunity to prepare for stressor

Teach client the use of appropriate stress-reducing measures (e.g., relaxation techniques, biofeedback, exercise, hobbies). Inform client of beneficial effects of decreasing coffee, sugar, and salt in diet and maintaining adequate B and C vitamins in diet and normal functioning of the endocrine and nervous systems. Refer client to community agencies and support groups as necessary.

Nursing Diagnosis: *Impaired Memory*

Teach client memory-enhancing techniques.

Nursing Diagnosis: *Readiness for enhanced critical thinking*

Teach client critical-thinking skills. Assist client to obtain resources to enhance critical thought processes.

 Nursing Diagnosis: *Compromised Family Coping related to family developmental crisis adjusting to infant/child development*

Discuss social development of the child. Infant's "stranger anxiety" is normal. Teach parents' ways to assist infant to warm up to strangers. Encourage verbalization, reassurance, and cuddling. Help parent assess child's readiness to begin school and to verbalize any school problems with child.

 Nursing Diagnosis: *Ineffective coping related to inadequate social support or disturbance in pattern of appraisal of threat*

Teach positive coping strategies to the child, such as relaxation and guided imagery. Identify family and friends that are supportive of the child and include them identifying strategies to help improve self-esteem.

 Nursing Diagnosis: *Hopelessness related to long-term stress.*

Identify feelings of hopelessness, sadness, and pain. Encourage the child to discuss these feelings and develop strategies to use when these feelings are present.

Use play therapy for younger children to help identify these feelings and teach them resources and techniques to use when needed. Include parents/friends, especially for younger children, that will redirect the child's actions/thoughts when these feelings are exhibited.

CHAPTER 6

Assessing General Status and Vital Signs

Structure and Function Overview

The general survey is the first part of the physical examination that begins the moment the nurse meets the client to obtain an overall impression about the client's general health status. The general survey includes observation of the client's physical development, body build, gender, apparent age as compared to reported age, skin condition and color, dress and hygiene, posture and gait, level of consciousness, behaviors, body movements, affect, facial expressions, speech patterns and clarity, and vital signs.

The client's vital signs are the body's indicators of health. Traditionally, vital signs have included the client's temperature, pulse, respirations, and blood pressure. Today, "pain" is considered to be the "fifth vital sign." For the body to function on a cellular level, a core body temperature between 35.5 °C and 37.7 °C (96 °F and 99.9 °F orally) must be maintained. Arterial or peripheral pulses are shock waves produced when the heart contracts and forcefully pumps blood out of the ventricles into the aorta. The body has many arterial pulse sites. One of them—the radial pulse—gives a good overall picture of the client's health status. The respiratory rate and character are additional clues to the client's overall health status. Blood pressure reflects the pressure exerted on the walls of the arteries. This pressure varies with the cardiac cycle, reaching a high point with systole and a low point with diastole. Therefore, blood pressure is a measurement of the pressure of the blood in the arteries when the ventricles are contracted (systolic blood pressure) and when the ventricles are relaxed (diastolic blood pressure). Blood pressure is expressed as the ratio of the systolic pressure over the diastolic pressure. *Cardiac output, distensibility of the arteries, blood volume, blood velocity, and blood viscosity (thickness)* all affect a client's blood pressure. The difference between systolic and diastolic pressure is termed the *pulse pressure*. Determine the pulse pressure after measuring the blood pressure because it reflects the stroke volume—the volume of blood ejected with each heartbeat.

Finally, pain screening is essential for an overall impression of the client. See Chapter 7 for an in-depth Pain Assessment.

Nursing Assessment

COLLECTING SUBJECTIVE DATA

Name, address, current age, birthdate, reason for seeking health care? Major concern about current health? Current age, height, and weight? Recent weight change? High fevers? Change in pulse or heart rate? Usual blood pressure? Blood pressure last checked? Problem with hypertension or hypotension? Difficulty breathing? At rest? With mild or strenuous exercise? Any pain? How does it feel (dull, sharp, aching, throbbing)? How does area of pain look (shiny, bumpy, red, swollen, bruised)? Onset: when did it begin? Location: where is it? Does it radiate? Duration: how long does it last? Does it recur? Severity: how bad is it? Associated factors: what makes it better? What makes it worse? What other symptoms occur with it? See Chapter 7 for further assessment of pain. Over-the-counter and prescribed medications? Allergies? Family history of heart disease, diabetes, thyroid disease, lung disease, high blood pressure, cancer, or others? Educational background, employment? Disabilities, satisfaction with current life; frequency for seeking health care; use of tobacco products including cigarettes, chewing tobacco, snuff, or dip? Drink alcohol (amount, frequency, and type)? Use of illicit drugs (type and frequency)? Usual diet? Exercise (type and frequency)?

COLLECTING OBJECTIVE DATA

Equipment Needed

- Thermometer: tympanic thermometer, temporal artery thermometer, electronic oral and/or axillary thermometer, or rectal thermometer
- Protective, disposable covers for the type of thermometer used
- Aneroid or mercury sphygmomanometer or electronic blood pressure measuring equipment
- Stethoscope
- Watch with a second hand
- If available, use a mobile monitoring system, such as "DINAMAP," which can be taken room to room to perform multiple vital signs simultaneously. These devices often have a thermometer, electronic sphygmomanometer, oxygenation saturation detector, and pulse monitor (Fig. 6-1)

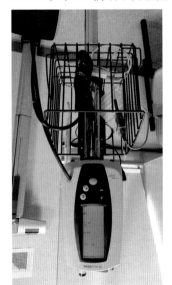

FIGURE 6-1 Mobile monitoring system.

Physical Assessment

When you meet the client, observe the client from head-to-toe to note any gross abnormalities in appearance or behavior. Assess vital signs (temperature, pulse, respirations, and blood pressure) to detect any severe deviations and to acquire baseline data. Then weigh the client and measure height with shoes and heavy clothing removed.

GENERAL PHYSICAL SURVEY		
PROCEDURE	**NORMAL FINDINGS**	**ABNORMAL FINDINGS**
Observe the following: • Physical development for age	• Appears to be stated chronologic age	• Appears older than age with hard manual labor, chronic illness, or alcoholism/smoking.
• Dress	• Dressed for occasion	• Dress bizarre and inappropriate for occasion seen in mentally ill, grieving, depressed, or poor clients.
• Posture and gait	• Erect posture. Gait is rhythmic, smooth, steady, and coordinated with arms swinging at side.	• Curvatures of the spine (lordosis, scoliosis, or kyphosis) may indicate a musculoskeletal disorder. Stiff, rigid movements are common in arthritis or Parkinson disease. Slumped shoulders may signify depression. Clients with chronic pulmonary obstructive disease tend to lean forward and brace themselves with their arms.

Continued on following page

GENERAL PHYSICAL SURVEY (Continued)

PROCEDURE	NORMAL FINDINGS	ABNORMAL FINDINGS
• Body build	• A wide variety of body types fall within a normal range: from small amounts of fat and muscle to larger amounts of fat and muscle to larger amounts of fat and developed muscle. Body proportions are normal. Arm span (distance between finger tips with arms extended) is approximately equal. The distance from the head crown to the symphysis pubis is approximately equal to the distance from the symphysis pubis to the sole of the client's foot.	• Lack of subcutaneous fat with prominent bones seen in the malnourished, abdominal ascites seen in starvation, abundant fatty tissue seen in obesity. Extreme weight loss is seen in anorexia nervosa. Decreased height and delayed puberty, with chubbiness, are seen in hypopituitary dwarfism. Skeletal malformations with a decrease in height are seen in achondroplastic dwarfism. In gigantism, there is increased height and weight with delayed sexual development. Overgrowth of bones in the face, head, hands, and feet with normal height is seen in hyperpituitarism (acromegaly). Arm span is greater than height, and pubis to sole measurement exceeds pubis to crown measurement in Marfan syndrome. Excessive body fat that is evenly distributed is referred to as exogenous obesity. Central body

PROCEDURE	NORMAL FINDINGS	ABNORMAL FINDINGS
		weight gain with excessive cervical obesity (Buffalo's hump), also referred to as endogenous obesity, is seen in Cushing syndrome.
• Gender and sexual development	• Appropriate for age and gender	• Delayed or advanced puberty for stated age; male client with female characteristics, and female client with male characteristics.
• Skin color and condition	• Varies from light to dark skinned. Color is even without obvious lesions: light to dark beige-pink in light-skinned client; light tan to dark brown or olive in dark-skinned clients. Underlying red tones from good circulation give a liveliness or healthy glow to all shades of skin color.	• Extreme pallor, flushed, yellow skin in light-skinned client; loss of red tones and ashen gray cyanosis in dark-skinned client.
Monitor temperature with electronic thermometers. They may be used for tympanic, oral, rectal, axillary, or continuous temperatures depending on the model and type of probe used.	Body temperature is usually lowest in early AM and highest in late PM: 35.5–37.7 °C (96–99.9 °F).	Temperatures below 36.7 °C (98 °F) represent hypothermia and can be a result of prolonged exposure to cold, hypoglycemia, hypothyroidism, starvation, neurologic dysfunction, or shock.

Continued on following page

GENERAL PHYSICAL SURVEY (Continued)

PROCEDURE	NORMAL FINDINGS	ABNORMAL FINDINGS
Tympanic. Tympanic membrane thermometers are gentle and noninvasive. Place the probe very gently at the opening of the ear canal for 2–3 seconds until the temperature appears in the digital display (Fig. 6-2).	Several factors may cause normal variations in the core body temperature. Body temperature is lowest early in the morning (4 to 6 AM) and highest late in the evening (8 PM to midnight). Strenuous exercise, stress, and ovulation may elevate temperature to 38.3 °C (101 °F). Hot fluids, smoking, and gum chewing may elevate temperature, while cold fluids may lower it. Normal tympanic temperature range is 36.7–38.3 °C (98–100.9 °F). The tympanic membrane temperature is normally about 0.8 °C (1.4 °F) higher than the normal oral temperature.	Temperatures above 38.3 °C (100.9 °F) represent hyperthermia and can indicate bacterial, viral, or fungal infections, an inflammatory process, malignancies, trauma, or various blood, endocrine, and immune disorders. Tympanic temperature is under 36.7 °C (98 °F) or over 38.3 °C (100.9 °F).

PROCEDURE	NORMAL FINDINGS	ABNORMAL FINDINGS

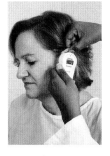

FIGURE 6-2 Taking a tympanic temperature.

PROCEDURE	NORMAL FINDINGS	ABNORMAL FINDINGS
Oral. Use an electronic thermometer with a disposable protective probe cover. Place the thermometer under the client's tongue to the right or left of the frenulum deep In the posterlor sublingual pocket. Ask the client to close their lips around probe. Hold the probe until you hear a beep. Remove the probe and dispose of its cover by pressing the release button.	Oral temperature is between 35.9 °C and 37.5 °C (96.6 °F and 99.5 °F).	Oral temperature is below 35.9 °C (96.6 °F) or over 37.5 °C (99.5 °F).

Continued on following page

GENERAL PHYSICAL SURVEY (Continued)

PROCEDURE	NORMAL FINDINGS	ABNORMAL FINDINGS
Electronic thermometers give a digital reading in about 2 minutes.		
Rectal. Lubricate clean thermometer with water-soluble lubricant and insert 2.5–5.08 cm (1–2 in) into rectum for 3 minutes. *Note: Use this method only when other routes are not practical (e.g., client cannot cooperate, is comatose, cannot close mouth, or tympanic thermometer is unavailable). Never force ther- mometer into rectum and never use a rectal thermometer for clients with severe coagula- tion disorders, recent rectal, anal, vaginal or prostate surgeries, diarrhea, hemorrhoids, colitis, or fecal impaction.*	The rectal temperature is between 0.4 °C and 0.5 °C (0.7 °F) and 1 °F) higher than the normal oral temperature. Normal rectal temperature range is 36.3–37.9 °C (97.4–100.3 °F).	Rectal temperature below 36.3 °C (97.4 °F) or above 37.9 °C (100.3 °F).
Axillary. Insert thermometer under axilla with arm down and across chest for 5–10 minutes.	Normal axillary temperature range is 35.4–37 °C (95.6–98.5 °F). The axillary temperature is 0.5 °C (1 °F) lower than the oral temperature.	Axillary temperature is below 35.4 °C (95.6 °F) or above 37 °C (98.5 °F).

PROCEDURE	NORMAL FINDINGS	ABNORMAL FINDINGS
Temporal arterial. *Note: Temporal arterial temperature is measured by the thermometer reading the infrared heat waves released by the temporal artery through the skin.* Remove the protective cap and place the thermometer over the client's forehead. While holding and pressing the scan button, gently stroke the thermometer across the client's forehead over the temporal artery to a point directly behind the ear. You will hear beeping and a red light will blink to indicate a measurement is taking place. Release the scan button and remove the thermometer from the forehead. Read the temperature on display. *Note: Temporal artery temperature measurement takes approximately 6 seconds.*	The temporal artery temperature is approximately 0.4 °C (0.8 °F) higher than oral (Titus, 2009). Normal temporal artery temperature range is 36.3–37.9 °C (97.4–100.3 °F).	Temporal artery temperature is below 36.3 °C (97.4 °F) or above 37.9 °C (100.3 °F).

Continued on following page

GENERAL PHYSICAL SURVEY (Continued)

PROCEDURE	NORMAL FINDINGS	ABNORMAL FINDINGS
Monitor for pulse.	60–100 beats/minute is normal for adults.	*Tachycardia* (>100 beats/minute) may occur with fever, certain medications, stress, and other abnormal states, such as cardiac dysrhythmias.
Palpate radial pulse for rhythm and rate. Use the pads of your two middle fingers and lightly palpate the radial artery on the lateral aspect of the client's wrist (Fig. 6-3). Count the number of beats you feel for 30 seconds if the pulse rhythm is regular. Multiply by two to get the rate. Count for a full minute if the rhythm is irregular. Then, verify by taking an apical pulse as well.	Tachycardia may be normal in clients who have just finished strenuous exercise. Bradycardia may be normal in well-conditioned athletes.	*Bradycardia* (<60 beats/minute) may be seen with sitting or standing for long periods causing blood to pool decreasing pulse rate, with heart block or dropped beats.
Note: Perform cardiac auscultation of the apical pulse if the client exhibits any abnormal findings.		

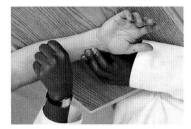

FIGURE 6-3 Timing the radial pulse rate.

PROCEDURE	NORMAL FINDINGS	ABNORMAL FINDINGS
Palpate arterial elasticity.	Artery feels straight, resilient, and springy.	Artery feels rigid.
Palpate apical pulse. Auscultate heart sounds for 1 minute with stethoscope for the following.		
• Rate	• 60–100 beats/minute	• More than 100 beats/minute equals tachycardia; less than 60 beats/minute equals bradycardia.
• Rhythm	• Regular	• Irregular; pulse deficit (difference between apical and radial pulse) may indicate atrial fibrillation, atrial flutter, premature ventricular contractions, and various degrees of heart block.
Monitor respirations 1 full minute for the rate, rhythm, and depth (see Table 6-1, p. 124). Observe the client's chest rise and fall with each breath. Count respirations for 30 seconds and multiply by two. If you place the client's arm across the chest while palpating the pulse, you can also count respirations. Do this by keeping your fingers on the client's pulse even after you have finished taking it.		

Continued on following page

GENERAL PHYSICAL SURVEY (Continued)

PROCEDURE	NORMAL FINDINGS	ABNORMAL FINDINGS
Measure blood pressure on dominant arm first. Take blood pressure in both arms when recording it for the first time. Take subsequent readings in arm with highest measurement. *Note:* Advise client to avoid nicotine and caffeine for 30 minutes prior to measurement. Ask client to empty bladder before evaluating and avoid talking to the client while taking the reading to prevent elevating blood pressure before/during readings (Mayo Clinic, 2012c). • Rate • Rhythm • Depth	• 12–20 breaths/minute • Rhythm is regular • Equal bilateral chest expansion of 2.5–5.08 cm (1–2 in) Systolic pressure is <120 mm Hg. Diastolic pressure is <80 mm Hg; varies with individuals. A pressure difference of 10 mm Hg between arms is normal. Varies throughout the day due to external influences, including time of day, caffeine or nicotine intake, exercise, emotions, pain, and temperature, and with body and arm positions. Usually slightly higher in a client who is standing due to compensation for the effects of gravity and slightly lower in a reclining client because of decreased resistance.	• Fewer than 12 breaths/minute or more than 20 breaths/minute. • Irregular (if irregular, count for 1 full minute). • Unequal, shallow, or extremely deep chest expansion, labored or gasping breaths. Higher or lower than normal systolic and diastolic readings. Tables 6-2 and 6-3 on page 125 provide blood pressure classifications and recommended follow-up criteria. More than a 10 mm Hg pressure difference between arms may indicate coarctation of the aorta or cardiac disease.

PROCEDURE	NORMAL FINDINGS	ABNORMAL FINDINGS
Assess the pulse pressure, which is the difference between the systolic and diastolic blood pressure levels. Record findings in mm Hg. For example, if the blood pressure was 120/80, then the pulse pressure would be 120 minus 80 or 40 mm Hg.	Pulse pressure is 30 to 50 mm Hg.	Pulse pressure lower than 30 mm Hg or higher than 50 mm Hg may indicate cardiovascular disease.
If the client takes antihypertensive medications or has a history of fainting or dizziness, **assess for possible orthostatic hypotension** by measuring the blood pressure and pulse with the client in a standing or sitting position after measuring the blood pressure with the client in a supine position.	A drop of less than 20 mm Hg from recorded sitting position.	A drop of 20 mm Hg or more from the recorded sitting blood pressure may indicate orthostatic (postural) hypotension. Pulse will increase to accommodate the drop in blood pressure. Orthostatic hypotension may be related to a decreased baroreceptor sensitivity, fluid volume deficit (e.g., dehydration), or certain medications (i.e., diuretics, antihypertensives). Symptoms of orthostatic hypotension include dizziness, lightheadedness, and falling. Further evaluation and referral to the client's primary care provider are necessary.

Continued on following page

GENERAL PHYSICAL SURVEY (Continued)

PROCEDURE	NORMAL FINDINGS	ABNORMAL FINDINGS
Observe comfort level.	Client assumes a relatively relaxed posture without excessive position shifting. Facial expression is alert and pleasant. No subjective report of pain.	Facial expression indicates discomfort (grimacing, frowning). Client may brace or hold a body part that is painful. Breathing pattern indicates distress (e.g., shortness of breath, shallow, rapid breathing).
Ask the client if he or she has any pain.		Explore any subjective report of pain. Refer to Chapter 7 for further assessment of pain.

TABLE 6-1   Types of Respirations

Description	Pattern	Description	Pattern
Normal	12–20 breaths/minute and regular		Hypoventilation	Decreased rate and decreased depth	
Apnea	Absence of respiration		Cheyne-Stokes	Periods of apnea and hyperventilation	
Bradypnea	Slow, shallow respiration		Kussmaul	Very deep with normal rhythm	
Tachypnea	More than 20 breaths/minute and regular				
Hyperventilation	Increased rate and increased depth				

TABLE 6-2   Categories for Blood Pressure Levels in Adults (Ages 18 and Older)

	Blood Pressure Level (mm Hg)	
Category	Systolic	Diastolic
Normal	<120	<80
Prehypertension	120–139	80–89
Stage 1 hypertension	140–159	90–99
Stage 2 hypertension	≥160	≥100

Adapted from: These categories are from the National High Blood Pressure Education Program; National Heart, Lung, and Blood Institute; National Institutes of Health. Available at www.nhlbi.nih.gov/hbp/detect/categ/htm.

 PEDIATRIC VARIATIONS

Equipment Needed

- Tape measure
- Growth charts for specific age comparisons (see Appendix 8)
- Thermometer
- Stethoscope

TABLE 6-3   Recommendations for Follow-Up Based on Initial Blood Pressure Measurements for Adults Without Acute End-Organ Damage

Initial Blood Pressure, mm Hg[a]	Follow-Up Recommended[b]
Normal	Recheck in 2 years
Prehypertension	Recheck in 1 year[c]
Stage 1 hypertension	Confirm within 2 months[c]
Stage 2 hypertension	Evaluate or refer to source of care within 1 month. For those with higher pressures (e.g., >180/110 mm Hg), evaluate and treat immediately or within 1 week depending on clinical situation and complications.

[a]If systolic and diastolic categories are different, follow recommendations for shorter time follow-up (e.g., 160/86 mm Hg should be evaluated or referred to source of care within 1 month).
[b]Modify the scheduling of follow-up according to reliable information about past BP measurements, other cardiovascular risk factors, or target organ disease.
[c]Provide advice about lifestyle modifications.
Adapted from: National High Blood Pressure Education Program; National Heart, Lung, and Blood Institute; National Institutes of Health. Available at: www.nhlbi.nih.gov/hbp/detect/categ/htm.

Subjective Data: Focus Questions

- Inquire about child's development milestones (see Appendix 5, p. 706)

- Inquire about immunizations (see Appendix 6, p. 714)
- Inquire about parent–child relationships (see Appendix 4, p. 700)

Objective Data: Assessment Techniques

PROCEDURE	NORMAL VARIATIONS
Observe **physical level of development** and compare with chronologic age.	See Appendix 5, p. 706.
Note: When taking vital signs in infants, measure the respiratory and pulse rates first as taking a temperature (especially a rectal temperature) may cause the infant to cry, which will and alter the pulse and respiratory rates.	
Monitor temperature.	Temperature fluctuates markedly in infants and young children.
In infants **<6 months old,** use axillary, tympanic, or rectal measurements.	
In infants and children **>6 months old,** use temporal, tympanic, axillary, rectal, or oral measurements.	
Temporal Arterial. May be used in healthy infants **<90 days old.** Contraindicated in infants **<90 days old** who have illness, fever, etc. May be used in infants and children **>90 days old** with or without fever, illness, etc. *Note: The measurement technique is the same as for the adult client.*	<38 °C (100.4 °F)

PROCEDURE	NORMAL VARIATIONS
Rectal. The rectal temperature should be used in infants and older children when other routes are not acceptable. Examples of these circumstances include a child who is critically ill, an uncooperative child, a child that is unconscious or at risk for seizures. Rectal measurement is contraindicated for premature infants, children with a medical history of GI bleed, or other GI abnormalities (cancer, etc.). (Society of Pediatric Nurses, 2008.)	<38 °C (100.4 °F) Rectal temperatures measure higher in infants and children versus other routes. Rectal temperature may also measure higher in the late afternoon/evening and/or after playing/ vigorous activity.
Procedure. Position child prone, supine, or side lying (may use parent's lap). Insert lubricated thermometer no more than 2.5 cm (1 in) into rectum. For children <6 months of age, insert thermometer only 0.63–1.2 cm (1/4–1/2 in). Never force thermometer into rectum against resistance.	
Tympanic. Recommended for newborns, infants, toddlers through adolescence. Contraindicated in critically ill children younger than 7 years old. Procedure: Instruct child/parent on securing child's head to prevent movement while performing temperature. Pull pinna down and back and proceed with the same measurement technique as is used for the adult client.	<38 °C (100.4 °F)
Axillary. When taking axillary temperature, place tip of thermometer into axilla and hold arm down close to the body.	<37.2 °C (99 °F)
Note: Measurement technique is the same as for the adult client.	

Continued on following page

PROCEDURE	NORMAL VARIATIONS
Oral. Starting at approximately 4 years old, use of oral thermometers may be used in children; however this will depend on the cooperation of the child. Instruct child to place probe under tongue and avoid biting on the probe. When using an electronic probe, cover it with a disposable probe cover to prevent breaking the probe cover to prevent or causing injury. *Note: Measurement technique is the same as for the adult client.* **Monitor pulse.** Take apical (not radial) pulse in children younger than 2 years (Fig. 6-4). Count pulse for 1 full minute.	<37.8 °C (100 °F) Awake and resting pulse rates vary with the age of the child: 1 week–3 months, 100–160; 3 months–2 years, 80–150; 2–10 years, 70–110; 10 years–adult, 55–90. Athletic adolescents tend to have lower pulse rates.

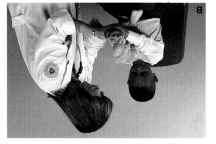
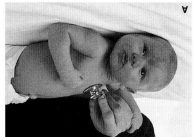

FIGURE 6-4 **A:** Auscultating apical pulse rate in child less than 2 years. **B:** Measuring radial pulse in child greater than 2 years. (Photo by B. Proud.)

PROCEDURE	NORMAL VARIATIONS
Monitor respirations by observing abdominal movement in infants and younger children	Respiratory rates: birth–6 months, 30–50; 6 months–2 years, 20–30; 3–10 years, 20–28; 10–18 years, 12–20.
Monitor blood pressure. Blood pressure is not routinely performed on children younger than 3 years old. Recommend annual screening beginning at 3 years of age and as indicated for high risk children. Width of cuff should cover two thirds of upper arm or be 20% greater than diameter of the extremity. Length of bladder should encircle without overlapping. Take blood pressure while child is calm and quiet. For infants and children younger than 3 years of age, use an electronic DINAMAP that is designed to interpret blood pressure according to size and weight of young children.	Blood pressure rates: *Systolic:* 1–7 years, age in years + 90; 8–18 years, (2 × age in years) + 90; *Diastolic:* 1–5 years, 56; 6–18 years, age in years + 52.
• Measure height, weight and head circumference and plot on growth chart.	
• Height	• See Appendix 8, page 730, for normal height ranges.
Children less than 24 months: Measure length from vertex of head to heel in recumbent position.	
Children greater than 24 months: Measure standing height in bare feet.	
• Weight: For infants and young children up to 3 years old, use infant or platform balance scale. Weigh child with only clean diaper on. At approximately 3 years, or, once child is able to stand, the upright scale may be used.	• See Appendix 8. At 1 year of age, the child's weight is usually three times the birth weight.

Continued on following page

PROCEDURE

- Head circumference (HC)

  Children less than 24 months: Measure slightly above eyebrows, pinna of ears over occipital prominence of skull (see Fig. 6-5).

NORMAL VARIATIONS

- Plot head circumference on standard growth chart (Appendix 8, p. 730). Head circumference measurement should fall between the 5th and 95th percentiles, and should be comparable with the child's height and weight percentiles. Those greater than 95% may indicate macrocephaly. Those under the 5th percentile may indicate microcephaly. Increased head circumference in children older than 3 years may indicate separation of cranial sutures due to increased intracranial pressure.

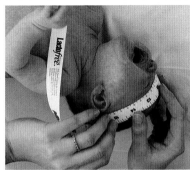

FIGURE 6-5 Measuring the circumference of an infant's head. (Photo by B. Proud.)

GERIATRIC VARIATIONS

- Dress may be heavier because of a decrease in body metabolism and a loss of subcutaneous fat.
- Osteoporotic thinning and collapse of the vertebrae secondary to bone loss may result in kyphosis.
- In older men, gait may be wider based with arms held outward.
- Older women tend to have a narrow base and may waddle to compensate for a decreased sense of balance.
- Mobility may be decreased, and gait may be rigid.
- Steps in gait may shorten with decreased speed and arm swing.
- Temperature may range from 35 to 36.3 °C (95 to 97.5 °F). Therefore, the older client may not have an obviously elevated temperature with an infection or be considered hypothermic below 35.5 °C (96 °F). Normal body temperature values for all routes in older adults are consistently lower than values reported in younger populations (Lu, Leasure, & Dai, 2010).
- Arteries are more rigid, hard, and bent.
- More rigid, arteriosclerotic arteries account for higher systolic blood pressure.
- Systolic pressure over 140 mm Hg but diastolic pressure under 90 mm Hg is called isolated systolic hypertension.
- Systolic murmurs may be present.
- Widening of the pulse pressure is seen with aging due to less-elastic peripheral arteries.

CULTURAL VARIATIONS

- Caucasian men tend to be 1.2 cm (0.5 in) taller than African American men.
- African American women consistently weigh more than Caucasian women (Lee, 2008).
- Blood pressure percentiles of prepubertal children in nonindustrialized countries may fall well below Western percentiles.
- Asians and Native Americans have fewer sweat glands and so, less obvious body odor than Caucasians and Black Africans.

POSSIBLE COLLABORATIVE PROBLEMS—RISK OF

- Hyperthermia
- Hypothermia
- Hypertension
- Hypotension
- Infection
- Dysrhythmia
- Dyspnea

Teaching Tips for Selected Nursing Diagnoses and Collaborative Problems

Nursing Diagnosis: *Readiness for Enhanced Self-Health Management: Expresses desire to learn more about health promotion.* *Teach client self-assessment procedures (e.g., breast self-exam, testicular self-exam) and the importance of regular medical checkups. Refer to community wellness resources and support groups as they relate to client.*

Collaborative Problem: *Potential complication–hypertension*

Explain the relationships between body weight, diet, exercise, stress, and blood pressure. Explain the possible effects of a low-fat, low-cholesterol diet along with vigorous exercise in reducing the atherosclerotic process. Explain the methods of preparing food low in sodium and fat, and high in potassium. Teach clients who drink alcohol to limit their intake. (See Tables 6-2 and 6-3 p. 125 for follow-up and referral.)

Nursing Diagnosis: *Impaired Walking related to deconditioning (inability) to climb stairs) after illness*

Teach client to increase muscle conditioning slowly. Refer to physician for physical therapy if necessary.

Nursing Diagnosis: *Risk for imbalanced Body Temperature related to febrile illness*

Instruct parents on proper method to assess temperature and detect fever. Teach proper method of giving tepid sponge baths and using antipyretics to reduce fever. Teach parents to avoid aspirin or aspirin products in children. Explain the use of quiet play and increasing fluids during this time. Teach parents to monitor for dehydration by assessing oral mucous membranes as needed.

Instruct parent to notify physician in case of high fever.

Nursing Diagnosis: *Ineffective Protection related to loss of passive immunity of placenta (age 6 to 12 months)*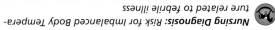

Instruct parents to clothe infant well to decrease exposure to others with illnesses. Encourage use of good hand-washing techniques for parents and children. Encourage parents to comply with the CDC recommendations on children's immunizations throughout childhood.

Nursing Diagnosis: *Risk for Delayed Development related to inadequate nutrition*

Instruct parents on adequate nutrient intake for developmental age of child. Refer to dietician if necessary. Educate parents on the recommended dietary intake of the child for the appropriate age and changes to expect as the child gets older. Identify and discuss cultural beliefs related to dietary intake of the child and strategies to meet child's dietary needs. Teach parents normal eating behaviors of children, such as toddlers grazing with finger foods, etc. Identify community resources, as appropriate (early intervention, WIC, etc.) to assist the family in providing additional financial resources to support the family in purchasing healthy meals.

 Collaborative Problem: *Potential Complication—Postural Hypotension*

Identify postural hypotension in elderly (difference of 20 mm Hg systolic BP and 10 mm Hg diastolic BP from a lying to a standing position). Instruct client to reduce risk of falls by moving from a lying to a sitting position slowly, then standing for 2 to 3 minutes before proceeding.

 Nursing Diagnosis: *Risk for Imbalanced Body Temperature—Hypothermia related to decreased cardiac output and decreased subcutaneous tissue secondary to aging processes*

Encourage good heating in homes and added clothing in cold weather. Teach family to observe for signs of hypothermia, including facial edema, pallor, clouding of vision, decreased blood pressure, and decreased heart rate. Refer to community agencies that may provide shelter, clothing, and food when needed.

 Nursing Diagnosis: *Risk for Imbalanced Body Temperature related to age greater than 90 years and inappropriate clothing for environmental temperature*

Discuss with client decreasing ability to sense environmental temperature extremes with aging and effects of decreased efficiency of circulation to maintain body temperature. Teach client to seek assistance in determining adequate/appropriate clothing to match environment.

CHAPTER 7

Assessing Pain: The 5th Vital Sign

Conceptual Foundations

The International Association for the Study of Pain (IASP) has defined pain as "an unpleasant sensory and emotional experience which we primarily associate with tissue damage or describe in terms of such damage" (IASP, 2011). The most important definition of pain as it is experienced is that by McCaffery and Pasero (1999): "Pain is whatever the person says it is." It is important to remember this definition when assessing and treating pain. Recent literature has emphasized the importance and undertreatment of pain and has recommended that pain be the fifth vital

sign. Some states have passed laws necessitating the adoption of an assessment tool and documenting pain assessment in client records along with temperature, pulse, heart rate, and blood pressure (see Chapter 6). In addition, TJC has established standards for pain assessment and management (see http://www.jointcommission.org/standards_information/standards.aspx).

PATHOPHYSIOLOGY OF PAIN

The pathophysiologic phenomena of pain are associated with the central and the peripheral nervous systems. The source of pain stimulates the peripheral nerve endings (nociceptors) which transmit the sensations to the central nervous system. They are sensory receptors that detect signals from damaged tissue and to chemicals released from the damaged tissue. Nociceptors are sensitive to intense mechanical stimulation, temperature, or noxious stimuli (chemical, thermal, or mechanical). Nociceptors are distributed in the body, in the skin, subcutaneous tissue, skeletal muscle, joints, peritoneal surfaces, pleural membranes, dura mater, and blood vessel walls. Note that they are not located in the parenchyma of visceral organs. Physiologic processes involved in pain perception (or nociception) include transduction, transmission, perception, and modulation (see Fig. 7-1). These processes serve as means for the stimuli to be sent to various parts of the spinal cord and to the brain, where they are perceived and can be responded to. The modulation process, which changes or inhibits transmission, is poorly understood but affects the level of pain perceived (see Chapter 9 in the textbook for details of the physiology and processes of pain).

PHYSIOLOGIC RESPONSES TO PAIN

Pain elicits a stress response in the human body, triggering the sympathetic nervous system, resulting in physiologic responses such as the following.

- Anxiety, fear, hopelessness, sleeplessness, thoughts of suicide

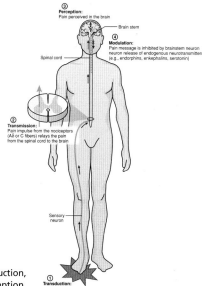

FIGURE 7-1 Transduction, transmission, perception, and modulation of pain.

- Focus on pain, reports of pain, cries and moans, frowns and facial grimaces
- Decrease in cognitive function, mental confusion, altered temperament, high somatization, dilated pupils
- Increased heart rate, peripheral, systemic, and coronary vascular resistance
- Increased respiratory rate and sputum retention resulting in infection and atelectasis
- Decreased gastric and intestinal motility
- Decreased urinary output, resulting in urinary retention, fluid overload, depression of all immune responses
- Increased antidiuretic hormone, epinephrine, norepinephrine, aldosterone, and glucagon; decreased insulin and testosterone
- Hyperglycemia, glucose intolerance, insulin resistance, protein catabolism
- Muscle spasm resulting in impaired muscle function and immobility, perspiration

CLASSIFICATION OF PAIN

Pain has many different classifications. Common categories of pain include acute, chronic nonmalignant, and cancer pain.

- **Acute pain:** usually associated with an injury with a recent onset and duration of less than 6 months and usually lasts less than a month
- **Chronic nonmalignant pain:** usually associated with a specific cause or injury and is described as a constant pain that persists for more than 6 months
- **Cancer pain:** often due to the compression of peripheral nerves or meninges or from the damage to these structures following surgery, chemotherapy, radiation, or tumor growth and infiltration

Pain is also described as transient pain, tissue injury pain (surgical pain, trauma-related pain, burn pain, or iatrogenic pain as a result of an intervention), and chronic neuropathic pain.

Pain is also viewed in terms of its location and intensity. Pain location classifications include the following.

- **Cutaneous pain** (skin or subcutaneous tissue)
- **Visceral pain** (abdominal cavity, thorax, cranium)
- **Deep somatic pain** (ligaments, tendons, bones, blood vessels, nerves)

Another aspect of pain locations is whether or not it is perceived at the site of the pain stimuli.

- **Radiating** (perceived both at the source and extending to other tissues)
- **Referred** (perceived in body areas away from the pain source; see Fig. 7-2).

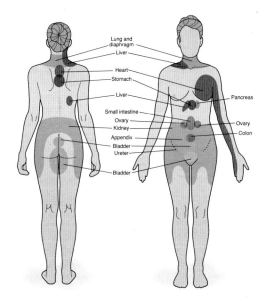

FIGURE 7-2 Areas of referred pain. **Top:** Anterior view. **Bottom:** Posterior view.

- **Phantom pain** (perceived in nerves left by a missing, amputated, or paralyzed body part).

Other descriptions of pain include the following.

- **Neuropathic pain** causes an abnormal processing of pain messages and results from past damage to peripheral or central nerves due to sustained neurochemical levels.
- **Intractable pain** is defined by its high resistance to pain relief.

THE SEVEN DIMENSIONS OF PAIN

Silkman (2008) describes the multidimensional complexity of pain in seven dimensions: physical, sensory, behavioral, sociocultural, cognitive, affective, and spiritual.

- **Physical dimension:** physical causes, body's reaction to the stimulus, and the patient's perception of the pain and the body's reaction to the stimulus.
- **Sensory dimension:** the quality of the pain and how severe the pain is perceived to be, including perception of the pain's location, intensity, and quality.
- **Behavioral dimension:** the verbal and the nonverbal behaviors that the patient demonstrates in response to the pain.
- **Sociocultural dimension:** the influences of the patient's social context and cultural background on the patient's pain experience.

- **Cognitive dimension:** "beliefs, attitudes, intentions, and motivations related to the pain and its management" (p. 14).
- **Affective dimension:** feelings, sentiments, and emotions related to the pain experience.
- **Spiritual dimension:** the meaning and purpose that the person "attributes to the pain, self, others, and the divine" (p. 15).

Nursing Assessment

COLLECTING SUBJECTIVE DATA

There are few objective findings on which the assessment of pain can rely. Pain is a subjective phenomenon and thus the main assessment lies in the client's reporting. The client's description of pain is quoted. The exact words used to describe the experience of pain are used to help in the diagnosis and management. The pain and its onset, duration, causes, and alleviating and aggravating factors are assessed. Then the quality, intensity, and effects of pain on the physical, psychosocial, and spiritual aspects are questioned. Past experience with pain in addition to past and current therapies are explored.

Preparing the Client

In preparation for the interview, clients are seated in a quiet, comfortable, and calm environment with minimal interruption. Explain to the client that the interview will entail questions to clarify the picture of the pain experienced in order to develop the plan of care.

Pain Assessment Tools

There are many assessment tools, some of which are specific to special types of pain. The main issues in choosing the tool are its reliability and its validity. Moreover, the tool must be clear and, therefore, easily understood by the client, and requires little effort from the client and the nurse.

Select one or more pain assessment tools appropriate for the client. There are many pain assessment scales such as the following:

- Visual Analog Scale (VAS)
- Numeric Rating Scale (NRS) (Fig. 7-3)
- Numeric Pain Intensity Scale (NPIS)
- Verbal Descriptor Scale
- Simple Descriptive Pain Intensity Scale
- Graphic Rating Scale
- Verbal Rating Scale
- Faces Pain Scales, Faces Pain Scales—Revised (FPS, FPS-R).

You can look at all of these and other scales at http://www.partnersagainstpain.com/hcp/pain-assessment/tools.aspx. Most of these scales have been shown to be reliable measures of client pain. The three most popular scales are the NRS, the Verbal

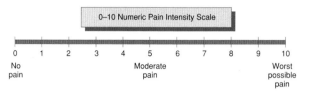

FIGURE 7-3 Numeric Rating Scale (NRS). From: Acute Pain Management: Operative or Medical Procedures and Trauma, Clinical Practice Guideline No. 1. AHCPR Publication No. 92-0032; February 1992; with permission.

Descriptor Scale, and the FPS, although VASs are often mentioned as very simple. The NRS has been shown to be the best for older adults with no cognitive impairment and the FPS-R for cognitively impaired adults (Flaherty, 2008).

A universal pain assessment tool integrating several assessment tools and verbal translation to several languages has been developed (UCLA, n.d.). Included within this tool is the Faces Pain Scale (see Box 7-1).

Two pain assessment tools that serve well for the patient's initial assessment are the Initial Pain Assessment Tool (see Box 7-2) (McCaffery & Pasero, 1999) and the Brief Pain Inventory (Short Form) (Cleeland, 1992).

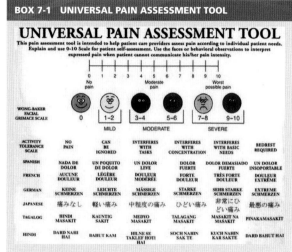

BOX 7-1 UNIVERSAL PAIN ASSESSMENT TOOL

(From: Department of Anesthesiology, David Geffen School of Medicine at UCLA. Available at http://www.anes.uda.edu/pain/index.htm)

BOX 7-2 McCAFFERY INITIAL PAIN ASSESSMENT TOOL

McCaffery Initial Pain Assessment Tool

Patient's Name _____ Age _____ Date _____

Diagnosis _____ Physician _____ Room _____

Nurse _____

1. LOCATION: Patient or nurse marks drawing.

2. INTENSITY: Patient rates the pain. Scale used _____

   Present: _____

   Worst pain gets: _____

   Best pain gets: _____

   Acceptable level of pain: _____

3. QUALITY: (Use patient's own words, e.g., prick, ache, burn, throb, pull sharp) _____

4. ONSET, DURATION, VARIATIONS, RHYTHMS: _____

5. MANNER OF EXPRESSING PAIN? _____

6. WHAT RELIEVES THE PAIN? _____

7. WHAT CAUSES OR INCREASES THE PAIN? _____

8. EFFECTS OF PAIN: (Note decreased function, decreased quality of life.)

   Accompanying symptoms (e.g., nausea) _____

   Sleep _____

   Appetite _____

   Physical activity _____

   Relationship with others (e.g., irritability) _____

   Emotions (e.g., anger, suicidal, crying) _____

   Concentration _____

   Other _____

9. OTHER COMMENTS: _____

10. PLAN: _____

May be duplicated for use in clinical practice. From McCaffery M, Pasero C: Pain: Clinical manual, p. 60. Copyright ©1999, Mosby, Inc.

PRESENT HEALTH CONCERNS

QUESTION	RATIONALE
Are you experiencing pain now or have you in the past 24 hours?	This helps to establish the presence or absence of perceived pain.
Where is the pain located?	The location of pain helps to identify the underlying cause.
Does it radiate or spread?	Radiating or spreading pain helps to identify the source. For example, chest pain radiating to the left arm is most probably of cardiac origin, while pain that is pricking and spreading in the chest muscle area is probably musculoskeletal in origin.
Are there any other concurrent symptoms accompanying the pain?	Accompanying symptoms also help to identify the possible source. For example, right lower quadrant pain associated with nausea, vomiting, and the inability to stand up straight is possibly associated with appendicitis.
When did the pain start?	The onset of pain is an essential indicator for the severity of the situation and suggests a source.
What were you doing when the pain first started?	This helps to identify the precipitating factors and what might have exacerbated the pain.

Continued on following page

PRESENT HEALTH CONCERNS (Continued)

QUESTION	RATIONALE
Is the pain continuous or intermittent?	The pain pattern helps to identify the nature of the pain and may assist in identifying the source.
If intermittent pain, how often do the episodes occur and for how long do they last?	Understanding the course of the pain provides a pattern that may help to determine the source.
Describe the pain in your own words.	Clients are quoted so that terms used to describe their pain may indicate the type and source. The most common terms used are throbbing, shooting, sharp, stabbing, gnawing, hot/burning, aching, heavy, tender, splitting, tiring/exhausting, sickening, fearful, and punishing.
What factors relieve your pain?	Relieving factors help to determine the source and the plan of care.
What factors increase your pain?	Identifying factors that increase pain helps to determine the source and helps in planning to avoid aggravating factors.
Are you on any therapy to manage your pain?	This question establishes any current treatment modalities and their effect on the pain. This helps in planning the future plan of care.
Is there anything you would like to add?	An open-ended question allows the client to mention anything that has been missed or the issues that were not fully addressed by the above questions.

PERSONAL HEALTH HISTORY	
QUESTION	**RATIONALE**
Have you had any previous experience with pain?	Past experiences of pain may shed light on the previous history of the client in addition to possible positive or negative expectations of pain therapies.

FAMILY HISTORY	
QUESTION	**RATIONALE**
Does anyone in your family experience pain?	This helps to assess the possible family-related perceptions or any past experiences with persons in pain.
How does pain affect your family?	This helps to assess how much the pain is interfering with the client's family relations.

LIFESTYLE AND HEALTH PRACTICES	
QUESTION	**RATIONALE**
What are your concerns about pain?	Identifying the client's fears and worries helps in prioritizing the plan of care and providing adequate psychological support.

Continued on following page

LIFESTYLE AND HEALTH PRACTICES (Continued)

QUESTION	RATIONALE
How does your pain interfere with the following? • General activity • Mood/emotions • Concentration • Physical ability • Work • Relations with other people • Sleep • Appetite • Enjoyment of life	These are the main lifestyle factors that pain interferes with. The more the pain interferes with the client's ability to function in his or her daily activities, the more it will reflect on the client's psychological status and thus the quality of life.

COLLECTING OBJECTIVE DATA

Physical Assessment

Objective data for pain are collected by observing the client's movement and responses to touch or descriptions of the pain experience. Many of the pain assessment tools incorporate a section to evaluate the objective responses to pain. Key points to remember during a physical examination for pain include the following:

• Choose an assessment tool that is reliable and valid to the client's culture.
• Explain to the client the purpose of rating the intensity of pain.

- Ensure the client's privacy and confidentiality.
- Respect the client's behavior toward pain and the terms used to express it.
- Understand that different cultures express pain differently and maintain different pain thresholds and expectations.

Note: Refer to Chapter 3, Performing Physical Assessment Skills, appropriate to affected body area. Body system assessments will include techniques for assessing pain (e.g., palpating the abdomen for tenderness or palpating the joints for tenderness or pain).

GENERAL OBSERVATION

ASSESSMENT PROCEDURE	NORMAL FINDINGS	ABNORMAL FINDINGS
Observe posture.	Posture is upright when the client appears to be comfortable, attentive, and without excessive changes in position and posture.	Client appears to be slumped with the shoulders not straight (indicates being disturbed/uncomfortable). Client is inattentive and agitated. Client might be guarding affected area and have breathing patterns reflecting distress.
Observe facial expression.	Client smiles with appropriate facial expressions and maintains adequate eye contact.	Client's facial expressions indicate distress and discomfort, including frowning, moans, cries, and grimacing. Eye contact is not maintained, indicating discomfort.
Inspect joints and muscles.	Joints appear normal (no edema); muscles appear relaxed.	Edema of a joint may indicate injury or arthritis. Pain may result in muscle tension.
Observe skin for scars, lesions, rashes, changes, or discoloration.	No inconsistency, wounds, or bruising are noted.	Bruising, wounds, or edema may be the result of injuries or infections, which may cause pain.

VITAL SIGNS

PROCEDURE	NORMAL FINDINGS	ABNORMAL FINDINGS
Measure heart rate.	Heart rate ranges from 60–100 beats per minute.	Increased heart rate may indicate discomfort or pain.
Measure respiratory rate.	Respiratory rate ranges from 12–20 beats per minute.	Respiratory rate may be increased and breathing may be irregular and shallow.
Measure blood pressure.	Blood pressure ranges from 100–130 mm Hg (systolic) and 60–80 mm Hg (diastolic).	Increased blood pressure often occurs in severe pain.

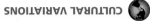 PEDIATRIC VARIATIONS

It is hard to evaluate pain in neonates and infants. Behaviors that indicate pain are used to assess their pain. One tool for such assessment is the N-PASS: Neonatal Pain, Agitation, and Sedation Scale (Hummel & Puchalski, 2000). Another popular tool for assessing pediatric pain is the FLACC Scale (Face, Legs, Activity, Cry, and Consolability); see Box 7-3.

A pain assessment tool that serves well for the patient's initial assessment is the Initial Pain Assessment for Pediatric Use Only (Otto, Duncan, & Baker, 1996).

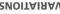 GERIATRIC VARIATIONS

Older people often suffer from pain related to chronic disorders, which is often undertreated. Untreated pain can lead to anxiety, depression, isolation, functional decline, and confusion. Aggressive or combative behaviors in the demented elderly may be the result of untreated pain.

 CULTURAL VARIATIONS

Cultures vary in the meaning of pain, how it is expressed, and how it is treated.

BOX 7-3 FLACC SCALE FOR PEDIATRIC PAIN ASSESSMENT

Item	Score 0	Score 1	Score 2
FACE	No particular expression or smile	Occasional grimace or frown, withdrawn, disinterested *appears sad or worried*	Frequent to constant frown, clenched jaw, quivering chin *distress-looking face: expression of fright or panic*
LEGS	Normal position or relaxed	Uneasy, restless, tense *occasional tremors*	Kicking, or legs drawn up *marked increase in spasticity, constant tremors, or jerking*
ACTIVITY	Lying quietly, normal position moves easily	Squirming, shifting back and forth, tense *mildly agitated (e.g., head back and forth, aggression); shallow, splinting respirations, intermittent sighs*	Arched, rigid, or jerking *severe agitation, head banging, shivering (not rigors); breath-holding, gasping or sharp intake of breath; severe splinting*
CRY	No cry (awake or asleep)	Moans or whimpers, occasional complaint *occasional verbal outburst or grunt*	Crying steadily, screams or sobs, frequent complaints, *repeated outbursts, constant grunting*
CONSOLABILITY	Content, relaxed	Reassured by occasional touching, hugging, or being talked to, distractable	Difficult to console or comfort *pushing away caregiver, resisting care or comfort measures*

Continued on following page

BOX 7-3   FLACC SCALE FOR PEDIATRIC PAIN ASSESSMENT (Continued)

Each of the five categories (F) Face; (L) Legs; (A) Activity; (C) Cry; (C) Consolability is scored from 0–2, which results in a total score between 0 and 10.

The revised FLACC can be used for children with cognitive disability. The additional descriptors (in italics) are included with the original FLACC. Review with parents the descriptors within each category. Ask them if there are additional behaviors that are better indicators of pain in their child. Add these behaviors to the tool in the appropriate category.

Procedure:

Patients who are awake: Observe for at least 1–2 minutes. Observe legs and body uncovered. Reposition patient or observe activity, assess body for tenseness and tone. Initiate consoling interventions if needed.

Patients who are asleep: Observe for at least 2 minutes or longer. Observe body and legs uncovered. If possible, reposition the patient. Touch the body and assess for tenseness and tone.

- *Meaning:* Asians may associate pain with atoning for sins. Many Westerners believe pain is a sign of physical illness. Some Westerners of traditional religions believe pain can enhance spiritual well-being.

- *Expression:* Some cultures, such as Asian, Irish, and others, assume a stoic approach and avoid expressing pain. Latin cultures and others express pain openly and loudly with moaning, crying, etc.

- *Treatment:* Many cultures promote folk, alternative, or complimentary therapies as pain treatment, or use them in addition to pain medications.

POSSIBLE COLLABORATIVE PROBLEMS—RISK OF

Angina
Decreased cardiac output
Paralytic ileus/small bowel
   obstruction
Sickling crisis
Peripheral nerve compression
Corneal ulceration

Endocarditis
Peripheral vascular
   insufficiency
Osteoarthritis
Joint dislocation
Pathologic fractures
Renal calculi

Teaching Tips for Selected Nursing Diagnoses

Nursing Diagnosis: *Readiness for Enhanced Spiritual Well-Being related to coping with prolonged physical pain*

- Encourage the client to request interactions with spiritual leaders and to request forgiveness from family, friends, and others.
- Encourage the client to express reverence and awe and to participate in religious activities.
- Encourage the client to spend time outdoors and to display creative energy (i.e., writing, drawing, poetry, etc.).

Nursing Diagnosis: *Readiness for Enhanced Comfort*

- Teach the client to identify comfortable positions.
- Teach the client to identify uncomfortable postures and to attempt to minimize their occurrences.

CHAPTER 8

Assessing for Violence

Conceptual Foundations

Family violence can be defined as "a situation in which one family member causes physical or emotional harm to another family member. At the center of this violence is the abuser's need to gain power and control over the victim" (Violence wheel, 2009). Family violence includes intimate partner violence (IPV), child abuse, and elder mistreatment. Family violence affects people of all ages, sexes, religions, ethnicities, and socioeconomic levels.

IPV includes a range of behaviors including physical abuse, emotional abuse, economic abuse, psychological abuse, and sexual assault. The Child Abuse Prevention and Treatment Act (CAPTA) defines child abuse as "any recent act or failure to act, resulting in imminent risk of serious harm, death, serious physical or emotional harm, sexual abuse, or exploitation of a child (a person less than the age of 18 years, unless the child protection law of the State in which the child resides specifies a younger age for cases not involving sexual abuse) by a parent or caretaker (including any employee of a residential facility or any staff person providing out-of-home care) who is responsible for the child's welfare" (Child Abuse Prevention & Treatment Act [2003], Public Law 104–235, §111; 42 U.S.C. 510 g). Elder mistreatment includes physical abuse, neglect, exploitation, abandonment, or prejudicial attitudes that decrease the quality of life and are demeaning to those greater than the age of 65 years.

TYPES OF FAMILY VIOLENCE

- **Physical abuse:** Pushing, shoving, slapping, kicking, choking, punching, burning; methods of restraint including holding, tying; attacks with household items (lamps, radios, ashtrays, irons, etc., or knives, guns)
- **Psychological abuse:** Constant use of insults or criticism, blaming the victim for things that are not the victim's faults, threats to hurt children or pets, isolation from supporters (family, friends, or coworkers), deprivation, humiliation, and intimidation
- **Economic abuse:** Preventing the victim from getting or keeping a job, controlling money and limiting access to funds, and controlling knowledge of family finances
- **Sexual abuse:** Forcing the victim to perform sexual acts against his or her will, pursuing sexual activity after the victim has said no, using violence during sex, and using weapons vaginally, orally, or anally

Nursing Assessment

Assessment for family violence mostly consists of the collection of adequate subjective data followed by a physical assessment. Before screening, discuss any legal, mandatory reporting requirements or other limits to confidentiality. Convey a concerned and nonjudgmental attitude. Show appropriate empathy.

To assess for the presence of family violence effectively, first examine your feelings, beliefs, and biases regarding violence. No one under any circumstances should be physically, sexually, or emotionally abused. It is imperative that you become active in interrupting or ending cycles of violence. Be aware of "red flags" that may indicate the presence of family violence.

Universal screening for family violence and IPV has been recommended by a number of agencies, but actual compliance with the recommendations is very low (Colarossi, Breitbart, & Betancourt, 2010). Nelson, Bougatsos, and Blazina (2012) review screening for IVP and find there are many instruments that accurately identify women at risk and there is minimal risk of adverse effects. The Family Violence Prevention Fund (2009) recommends that all female clients, aged 14 and older, be screened for abuse when seen in emergency departments, urgent care centers, or primary health care clinics. Battered

COLLECTING SUBJECTIVE DATA

women account for 22% to 35% of all women seeking care in emergency departments.

Screen for a history of current and past abuse at initial and annual health care visits regardless of the presence or absence of abuse indicators. Screen at each health care visit if there is a history of abuse. Screen all pregnant women at least once per trimester and once postpartum (Committee on Health Care for Underserved Women of ACOG, 2012). Screen mothers during well-child visits to the pediatrician. Also screen for abuse if the client is in a new relationship or if there are signs or symptoms indicating the presence of abuse.

Recommendations by the AMA and ANA (AMA, 2008) and Stop Relationship Abuse Organization (n.d.) for all providers are the following.

1. Routinely screen for IPV.
2. Acknowledge the victim's experience and assess the abuse for acute and chronic health effects.
3. Document the abuse through detailed charting, body maps, and photos.
4. Assess the risk for future injury or lethality. Perform a risk assessment and ascertain client's level of safety before the client leaves.
5. Review options and refer as necessary. Safety planning should be done with every patient with positive history of IPV before leaving the clinical setting.

See the Pediatric and Geriatric Variations (pp. 160–162) for information on child abuse and elder abuse.

ASSESSMENT PROCEDURE	NORMAL FINDINGS	ABNORMAL FINDINGS (INDICATORS OF VIOLENCE OR POTENTIAL VIOLENCE)
Review past health history and physical examination records.	No indicators of abuse are present.	Documentation of past assaults. Unexplained injuries, symptoms of pain, nausea and vomiting, or choking. Repeated visits to emergency department. Signs and symptoms of anxiety. Use of sedatives or tranquilizers.

ASSESSMENT PROCEDURE	NORMAL FINDINGS	ABNORMAL FINDINGS (INDICATORS OF VIOLENCE OR POTENTIAL VIOLENCE)
		Injuries during pregnancy. History of drug or alcohol abuse, depression, and/or suicide attempts.
If partner/parent/caregiver is present at the visit, observe client's interactions with partner.	Client is not afraid of partner. Client answers questions independently. Partner appears supportive.	Partner criticizes client about appearance, feelings, and/or actions and is not sensitive to client's needs. Partner refuses to leave client's presence and speaks for client. Client is anxious and afraid of partner; is submissive to negative comments from partner.
Perform the rest of the examination without the partner, parent, or caregiver present.		
Ask all clients: • Has anyone in your home ever hurt you? • Do you feel unsafe in your home? • Are you afraid of anyone in your home? • Has anyone made you do anything you didn't want to do? • Has anyone ever touched you without your permission? • Has anyone ever threatened you?	Client answers no to all questions.	"Yes" to any of the questions indicates abuse.

Continued on following page

ASSESSMENT PROCEDURE	NORMAL FINDINGS	ABNORMAL FINDINGS (INDICATORS OF VIOLENCE OR POTENTIAL VIOLENCE)
For IPV, begin the screening by telling the woman that it is important to screen all women routinely for IPV because it affects so many women and men in our society. Ask the client to fill out or help the client fill out the Abuse Assessment Screen in Box 8-1. **CLINICAL TIP** Sometimes, no matter how carefully you prepare the client and ask the questions, she may not disclose abuse.	Client answers "no" to all three questions (see Box 8-1). If the client replies "no" to screening questions and is not being abused, it is important for the client to know that you are available if she ever experiences abuse in the future. Make statements that build trust such as: "I am happy to hear that you are not being abused. If that should ever change, this is a safe place to talk."	"Yes" to any of the questions strongly indicates initial disclosure of abuse. You should do the following: • Acknowledge the abuse and her courage. • Use supportive statements such as "I'm sorry this is happening to you. This is not your fault. You are not responsible for his behavior. You are not alone. You don't deserve to be treated this way. Help is available to you." • Acknowledge her autonomy and right to self-determination. • Reiterate confidentiality of disclosure.

COLLECTING OBJECTIVE DATA

Equipment Needed

- All equipment for a complete head-to-toe physical examination
- Safe and secure private screening area (Do not screen in an area that poses any safety concerns for the client or yourself.)

Physical Assessment

During examination of a client who you suspect or know has been abused, it is essential to provide privacy for the client and keep your hands warm to promote the client's comfort during the examination. Also, remain nonjudgmental regarding the client's habits, lifestyle, and any revelations about abuse. At the same time, educate and inform about risks and possibilities for assistance.

BOX 8-1 ABUSE ASSESSMENT SCREEN

1. WITHIN THE LAST YEAR, have you been hit, slapped, kicked, or   YES   NO
otherwise physically hurt by someone?
If YES, by whom? _____
Total number of times _____

2. SINCE YOU'VE BEEN PREGNANT, have you been hit, slapped,   YES   NO
kicked, or otherwise physically hurt by someone?
If YES, by whom? _____
Total number of times _____

MARK THE AREA OF INJURY ON THE BODY MAP. SCORE EACH INCIDENT ACCORDING TO THE FOLLOWING SCALE.
    SCORE
    1 = Threats of abuse including use of a weapon _____
    2 = Slapping, pushing: no injuries and/or lasting pain _____
    3 = Punching, kicking, bruises, cuts, and/or continuing pain _____
    4 = Beating up, severe contusions, burns, broken bones _____
    5 = Head injury, internal injury, permanent injury _____
    6 = Use of weapon; wound from weapon _____
    If any of the descriptions for the higher number apply, use the higher number.

3. WITHIN THE LAST YEAR, has anyone forced you to have sexual activities?   YES   NO
If YES, who? _____
Total number of times _____

Developed by the Nursing Research Consortium on Violence and Abuse. Readers are encouraged to reproduce and use this assessment tool.

ASSESSMENT PROCEDURE	NORMAL FINDINGS	ABNORMAL FINDINGS
Perform a general survey. Observe general appearance and body build.	Client appears stated age and well-developed.	Abused children may appear younger than stated age due to developmental delays or malnourishment. Older clients may appear thin and frail due to malnourishment.
Note dress and hygiene.	Client is well-groomed and dressed appropriately for season and occasion.	Poor hygiene and soiled clothing may indicate neglect. Long sleeves and pants in warm weather may be an attempt to cover bruising or other injuries. Victims of sexual abuse may dress provocatively.
Assess the following:		
• Mental status	• Client is coherent and relaxed. A child shows proper developmental level for age.	• Client is anxious, depressed, suicidal, or withdrawn, or has difficulty concentrating. Client has poor eye contact or soft, passive speech. Client is unable to recall recent or past events. Child does not meet developmental expectations.
• Vital signs	• Vital signs are within normal limits.	• Hypertension may be seen in victims of abuse.
• Skin	• Skin is clean, dry, and free of lesions or bruises. Skin fragility increases with age; bruising may occur with pressure and may mimic bruising associated with abuse. Be careful to distinguish between normal and abnormal findings.	• Client has scars, bruises, burns, welts, or swelling on face, breasts, arms, chest, abdomen, or genitalia.

ASSESSMENT PROCEDURE	NORMAL FINDINGS	ABNORMAL FINDINGS
• Head and neck	• Head and neck are free of injuries.	• Client has hair missing in clumps, subdural hematomas, or rope marks or finger/hand strangulation marks on neck.
• Eyes	• Eyes are free of injury.	• Client has bruising or swelling around eyes, unilateral ptosis of upper eyelids (due to repeated blows causing nerve damage to eyelids), or a subconjunctival hemorrhage.
• Ears	• Ears are clean and free of injuries.	• Client has external or internal ear injuries.
• Abdomen	• Abdomen is free of bruises and other injuries and is nontender.	• Client has bruising in various stages of healing. Assessment reveals intra-abdominal injuries. A pregnant client has received blows to abdomen.
• Genitalia and rectal area	• Client is free of injury.	• Client has irritation, tenderness, bruising, bleeding, or swelling of genitals or rectal area. Discharge, redness, or lacerations may indicate abuse in young children. Hemorrhoids are unusual in children and may be caused by sexual abuse. Extreme apprehension during examination may indicate physical or sexual abuse.
• Musculoskeletal system	• Client shows full range of motion and has no evidence of injuries.	• Dislocation of shoulder; old or new fractures of face, arms, or ribs; and poor range of motion of joints are indicators of abuse.

Continued on following page

ASSESSMENT PROCEDURE	NORMAL FINDINGS	ABNORMAL FINDINGS
• Neurologic system	• Client demonstrates normal neurologic function.	• Abnormal findings include tremors, hyperactive reflexes, and decreased sensations to areas of old injuries secondary to neurologic damage.
Further Assessment for Positive IPV Findings		
If screening for IPV is positive, ask the client to fill out a danger assessment questionnaire (Box 8-2). If screening for IPV is positive and the client's answers on the danger assessment questionnaire indicate a high probability for serious violence, ask the client if she has a safety plan and where she would like to go when she leaves your agency (Box 8-3, p. 161). Be sure to schedule a follow-up appointment and/or refer the client as appropriate.	Client has a safety plan to prevent further abuse and injury.	If the client says she prefers to return home, ask her if it is safe for her to do so and have her respond to the questions in Box 8-3, p. 161. Provide the client with contact information for shelters and groups. Encourage her to call with any concerns.

BOX 8-2 SELF-ASSESSMENT: DANGER ASSESSMENT

Several risk factors have been associated with increased risk of homicides (murders) of women and men in violent relationships. We cannot predict what will happen in your case, but we would like you to be aware of the danger of homicide in situations of abuse and for you to see how many of the risk factors apply to your situation.

Using the calendar, please mark the approximate dates during the past year when you were abused by your partner or ex-partner. Write on that date how bad the incident was according to the following scale:

1. Slapping, pushing; no injuries and/or lasting pain
2. Punching, kicking; bruises, cuts, and/or continuing pain
3. "Beating up"; severe contusions, burns, broken bones
4. Threat to use weapon; head injury, internal injury, permanent injury
5. Use of weapon; wounds from weapon

(If any of the descriptions for the higher number apply, use the higher number.)

Mark Yes or No for each of the following. ("He" refers to your husband, partner, ex-husband, ex-partner, or whoever is currently physically hurting you.)

1. Has the physical violence increased in severity or frequency over the past year?
2. Does he own a gun?
3. Have you left him after living together during the past year?
3a. (If you have *never* lived with him, check here_____)
4. Is he unemployed?
5. Has he ever used a weapon against you or threatened you with a lethal weapon? (If yes, was the weapon a gun?)
6. Does he threaten to kill you?
7. Has he avoided being arrested for domestic violence?
8. Do you have a child that is not his?
9. Has he ever forced you to have sex when you did not wish to do so?
10. Does he ever try to choke you?
11. Does he use illegal drugs? By drugs, I mean "uppers" or amphetamines, speed, angel dust, cocaine, "crack," street drugs, or mixtures.
12. Is he an alcoholic or problem drinker?
13. Does he control most or all of your daily activities? For instance, does he tell you who you can be friends with, when you can see your family, how much money you can use, or when you can take the car? (If he tries, but you do not let him, check here: _____)

Continued on following page

BOX 8-2 SELF-ASSESSMENT: DANGER ASSESSMENT (Continued)

14. Is he violently and constantly jealous of you? (For instance, does he say "If I can't have you, no one can"?)
15. Have you ever been beaten by him while you were pregnant? (If you have never been pregnant by him, check here: _____)
16. Have you ever threatened or tried to commit suicide?
17. Has he ever threatened or tried to commit suicide?
18. Does he threaten to harm your children?
19. Do you believe he is capable of killing you?

20. Does he follow or spy on you, leave threatening notes or messages on your answering machine, destroy your property, or call you when you don't want him to?
Total "Yes" Answers

Thank you. Please talk to your nurse, advocate, or counselor about what the Danger Assessment means in terms of your situation.

Campbell, J.C., PhD, RN. Copyright, 2003. Humphreys, J., & Campbell, J. C. (2004). Family violence and nursing practice. Philadelphia: Lippincott Williams & Wilkins.

🐎 PEDIATRIC VARIATIONS

In 2010, 5.9 million children were referred to child protective services and 695,000 were determined to be victims of child abuse (physical, sexual, psychological abuse, or neglect), and of these, 1,560 children die ("Child Abuse and Neglect Stats," 2012). The following are important to keep in mind when assessing for abuse in children.

- For any client greater than the age of 3 years, ask any screening questions in a secure, private setting with no one else present in the room.

- Receive any information the child may disclose to you in an interested, calm, and accepting manner. Avoid showing surprise or distaste.
- Do not coerce the child to answer questions by offering rewards.
- Establish the child's level of understanding by asking simple questions (name, how to spell name, age, birth date, how many eyes do you have, etc.). Then formulate questions the child can comprehend.

BOX 8-3 ASSESSING A SAFETY PLAN

Ask the client, do you:
- Have a packed bag ready? Keep it hidden but make it easy to grab quickly?
- Tell your neighbors about your abuse and ask them to call the police when they hear a disturbance?
- Have a code word to use with your kids, family, and friends so they will know to call the police and get you help?
- Know where you are going to go, if you ever have to leave?
- Remove weapons from the home?
- Have the following gathered:
- Cash?
- Social security cards/numbers for you and your children?
- Birth certificates for you and your children?
- Driver's license?
- Rent and utility receipts?
- Bank account numbers?
- Insurance policies and numbers?
- Marriage license?
- Jewelry?
- Important phone numbers?
- Copy of protection order?
  Ask children, do you:
- Know a safe place to go?
- Know who is safe to tell you are unsafe?
- Know how and when to call 911? Know how to make a collect call?
  Inform children that it is their job to keep themselves safe; they should not interject themselves into adult conflict.
  If the client is planning to leave:
- Remind the client this is a dangerous time that requires awareness and planning.
- Review where the client is planning to go, shelter options, and the need to be around others to curtail violence.
- Review the client's right to possessions and list of possessions to take.

- The majority of children disclose to questions specific to the person suspected of abuse or related to the type of abuse (Hegar, Emans, & Muram, 2000).
- Use multiple-choice or open-ended questions and avoid "yes" or no" questions.
- The less information you supply in your questions and the more information the child gives in answering the questions increases the credibility of the collected data.
- Realize that girls who witness domestic violence are far more likely to become victims of domestic violence, and boys who witness domestic violence are also far more likely to become abusers, of both their spouses/partners and their children ("Domestic Violence: The Facts," 2012).
- Question the child about safety including physical abuse, sexual abuse, emotional abuse, and neglect. Positive find-ings to indicate a potentially abusive environment include the following.
  - Child indicates someone has hurt him or her (physi-cally, sexually, or emotionally).
  - Child appears neglected. The majority of children who suffers from psychological abuse often use effective coping mechanisms and will not exhibit any patho-logic behaviors.

GERIATRIC VARIATIONS

- The rate of violence against older adults for 2010 was 9.5% or nearly 6 million elders, and 68% of the cases were by family members ("Elder Abuse Statistics," 2012).
- The medical consequences of elder abuse include (1) inabil-ity of the frail elderly to handle the trauma, (2) inability to get food or medication because of neglect, (3) inability to pay for food or medication because of financial abuse, and (4) inability to deal with illness/malnutrition/problems because of depression associated with abuse.
- Statistics of economic abuse are difficult to find due to under-reporting by abused elders.
- Start out by asking the older adult client to tell you about a typical day in his or her life. Be alert for indicators placing the older client at a high risk for abuse or neglect. Then ask the following ("Yes" to any of the questions indicates abuse).
  - Has anyone ever made you sign papers that you did not understand?
  - Are you alone often?
  - Has anyone refused to help you when you needed help?
  - Has anyone ever refused to give you or let you take your medications?

- Has anyone ever taken your medications from you? Explain.

 CULTURAL VARIATIONS

Conducting a cultural assessment using assessment guidelines is necessary before attempting to understand family violence. Recent studies have supported reports of a high rate of child abuse among black children with the racial differences due to poverty levels and a "Hispanic paradox" of culturally based protective factors leading to lower rates of child abuse for Hispanics (Drake, et al., 2011).

POSSIBLE COLLABORATIVE PROBLEMS—RISK OF

- Bone fractures
- Concussion
- Subdural hematoma
- Subconjunctival hemorrhage
- Intra-abdominal injury
- Depression
- Suicide
- Death

Teaching Tips for Selected Nursing Diagnoses

Nursing Diagnosis: Risk for Altered Family Processes related to the presence of family violence

Teach the family about the availability of safe community resources.

Avoid giving the family print resources that may be accessed by the partner, who may respond in a violent manner to this information. Direct the client to online Internet resources as available.

Nursing Diagnosis: Ineffective Protection related to history of spousal abuse episodes

Teach the client that he or she is a victim and that no one deserves to be treated with violence in any situation or circumstance.

Teach the client ways to become empowered through healthy lifestyle practices including exercise, diet, and adequate rest and sleep.

Provide the client to victim assistance program contact information.

 ***Nursing Diagnosis: Risk for Self-Esteem Disturbance** related to feeling guilty and responsible for being a victim*

Explain to children that they are not responsible for the abusive behavior of the offender. Assess social and interpersonal relationships and identify a person that the child can depend on or call for support. Notify social services to assess family situation. Assess need for counseling for self-esteem.

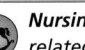 ***Nursing Diagnosis: Risk for Social Isolation** related to shame about family violence*

Identify high-risk relationships and encourage family and social support for the client. Teach the client problem-solving skills and strategies to avoid social isolation. Explain to the client that he/she is not responsible for the violence and encourage the client to discuss concerns he/she may have to work through conflicting feelings.

 ***Nursing Diagnosis: Risk for Powerlessness** related to control of relationships, control of children, and control of finances by an abusive significant other*

Teach the older client about the hazards of myths (e.g., teach that this is not the client's fault and that he or she has a right to feel safe).

Give the client simple choices to make him or her feel empowered.

Teach problem-solving and decision-making skills to empower the older client.

CHAPTER 9

Assessing Nutritional Status

Structure and Function Overview

Nutritional assessment helps identify the client's overall health status and need for health promotion. It also reveals risks for nutritional deficits, which leads to undernutrition or malnutrition or overnutrition and obesity. Hydration status is an important aspect of nutritional assessment that identifies the client at risk dehydration or overhydration.

Nutrition is a complex process by which nutrients are ingested, digested, absorbed, transported, used, and then excreted. Essential nutrients, including carbohydrates, proteins, fats, vitamins, minerals, and water, must be ingested in adequate amounts to maintain health.

Nutritional problems can result from unhealthy eating habits, inappropriate food choices, and reduced food availability. Diet-related chronic disorders and diseases including cardiovascular disease, hypertension, diabetes, various cancers, osteoporosis, and gastrointestinal disorders are heavily influenced by dietary factors. Certain diseases, disorders, or lifestyle behaviors can place clients at risk for undernutrition or malnutrition such as Crohn disease, cirrhosis, cancer, dementia, poor dental health, poor food choices, or inability to afford nutritious food.

Overnutrition is a huge problem in the United States. The United States Department of Agriculture (2011) and the Department of Health and Human Services (2011) reports that more than two thirds of adults and more than one third of children in the United States are overweight or obese. Obesity is a major risk factor for developing hypertension and diabetes, which lead to heart disease, stroke, congestive heart failure, and kidney disease.

Nursing Assessment

COLLECTING SUBJECTIVE DATA

Describe appetite and daily food intake. Special diet? Number of meals and snacks per day? Do you consider your diet to be healthy? Any food preferences or intolerances? Allergic to any foods? Explain. Who shops and prepares food in your household? Number of meals eaten out weekly? Use of special health foods, vitamins, or other supplements? Explain. Amount and type of daily fluid intake? Usual daily activities? Unintended weight loss or gain in past 6 months?

COLLECTING OBJECTIVE DATA

Equipment Needed

• Metric tape measure
• Balance beam scale
• Skinfold calipers

Physical Assessment

Assessment of the client's nutritional status consists of an overall inspection of muscle mass, distribution of fat, and skeleton. It is important to determine if abnormalities found during assessment of the skin, thyroid, mouth, lungs, abdomen, and nervous system are related to alterations in nutrition.

General Inspection

PROCEDURE	NORMAL FINDINGS	ABNORMAL FINDINGS
Observe muscle mass over temporal areas, dorsum of hands, and spine for the following: • Tone • Strength with voluntary movement • Body fat for distribution over waist, thighs, and triceps.	• Firm, developed • Strength equal bilaterally • Equal distribution; some fat under skin	• Flaccid, wasted, underdeveloped • Weak, sluggish, or unequal • Lack of fat under skin, increased bony prominences, emaciated, cachexic, abundant fatty tissue, abdominal ascites (due to fluid shift in protein).
• Posture • Energy level	• Erect, no malformations, smooth and coordinated gait • Energetic	• Poor posture, difficulty walking, bowlegged, knock-kneed • Fatigued, irritable
Observe skin for color, texture, and turgor.	Pink, smooth, turgor present (no tenting).	Pale, rough, dry, flaky, petechiae, lacks subcutaneous fat, loss of turgor (tenting) may indicate dehydration.
Observe nails for color and texture.	Nails firm; skin under nails pink.	Pale, brittle, opaque, spoon shaped, ridged.
Observe hair for texture.	Lustrous and shiny.	Brittle, dry.

Continued on following page

PROCEDURE	NORMAL FINDINGS	ABNORMAL FINDINGS
Observe lips for color and texture.	Pink, smooth, moist.	Swollen, puffy, lesions, fissures at corners of mouth.
Inspect tongue for color and texture.	Deep red with papillae.	Beefy red, smooth, atrophy, or hypertrophy; dry tongue seen with dehydration.
Inspect teeth for position and condition.	Straight with no cavities.	Missing, malpositioned, cavities.
Inspect gums for condition and color.	Smooth, firm, pink.	Inflamed, spongy, swollen, red, bleed easily.
Inspect eyes for moisture, lesions.	Clear, moist surfaces, transparent cornea.	Pale or red eye; membranes dry, increased vascularity, dull appearance of cornea; sunken eyeballs seen with dehydration.
Test reflexes.	Reflexes normal.	Loss of or decreased ankle and knee reflexes.
Measure pulse and blood pressure.	Normal heart rate and blood pressure for age.	Tachycardia, hypertension, irregular pulse; blood pressure that drops 20 mm Hg from lying to standing position may indicate fluid volume deficit.

Anthropometric Measurements

PROCEDURE	NORMAL FINDINGS	ABNORMAL FINDINGS
Measure height. Have client stand erect against wall without shoes. Record height in centimeters and inches.	Compare findings for normal adult height and weight.	Extreme shortness seen with achondroplastic dwarfism and Turner syndrome. Extreme heights are seen with Marfan syndrome, gigantism, and with excessive secretion of growth hormone.
Measure weight on a balance beam scale. Ask client to remove shoes and heavy outer clothing and to stand on the scale. **Record weight** (2.2 lb = 1 kg). If you are weighing a client at home, you may have to use a scale with an automatically adjusting true zero.	Healthy weights for men and women are listed in Table 9-1.	Weight does not fall within the range of desirable weights for women and men. Table 9-1 indicates weights in the overweight and obese categories.
Determine ideal body weight (IBW) and percentage of IBW. Use this formula to calculate IBW. *Female:* 45.3 kg (100 lb) for 152.4 cm (5 ft) + 2.26 kg (5 lb) for each inch over 152.4 cm (5 ft) ± 10% for small or large frame.	Body weight is within 10% of ideal range.	A current weight that is 80–90% of IBW indicates a lean client and possibly mild malnutrition. Weight that is 70–80% indicates moderate malnutrition; less than 70% may indicate

Continued on following page

PROCEDURE	NORMAL FINDINGS	ABNORMAL FINDINGS
Male: 48.08 kg (106 lb) for 152.4 cm (5 ft) + 2.72 kg (6 lb) for each inch over 152.4 cm (5 ft) ± 10% for small or large frame.		severe malnutrition possibly from systemic disease, eating disorders, cancer therapies, and other problems. Weight exceeding 10% of the IBW range is called overweight; weight exceeding 20% of IBW is called obesity.
Determine **Body Mass Index (BMI)** using one of these formulas. $$\frac{\text{Weight in kilograms}}{\text{Height in meters}^2} = \text{BMI}$$ or $$\frac{\text{Weight in pounds}}{\text{Height in inches}^2} \times 750 = \text{BMI}$$ or Quick Web BMI by accessing the National Institutes of Health's website: http://nhlbisupport.com/bmi/bmicalc.htm.	BMI between 18.5 and 24.9. Refer to Table 9-1 for the healthy weight.	BMI < 18.5 is associated with being underweight. BMI between 25 and 29.9 is considered overweight and may lead to health problems. BMI ≥ 30 is considered obese and indicates increased risk of developing health problems such as diabetes and cardiovascular disorders. Refer to Table 9-1.

PROCEDURE	NORMAL FINDINGS	ABNORMAL FINDINGS
Determine waist circumference. Have the client stand straight with feet together and arms at the sides. Place the measuring tape snugly around the waist at the umbilicus, yet not compressing the skin. Instruct the client to relax the abdomen and take a normal breath. When the client exhales, record the waist circumference. See Table 9-2 for an interpretation of waist circumference, BMI, and associated risks.	*Females:* Less than or equal to 88.9 cm (35 in) *Males:* Less than or equal to 101.6 cm (40 in) These findings are associated with reduced disease risk.	*Females:* Greater than 88.9 cm (35 in) *Males:* Greater than 102 cm (40 in) See Table 9-2. Adults with large amounts of visceral fat located mostly around the waist are more likely to develop health-related problems than adults with the fat located in the hips or thighs. Increased risk of type 2 diabetes, abnormal cholesterol and triglyceride levels, hypertension, and cardiovascular disease such as heart attack or stroke may occur.
Measure mid-arm circumference (MAC) (Fig. 9-1). The MAC measurement evaluates skeletal muscle mass and fat stores.	Compare the client's current MAC to prior measurements and compare to standard MAC measurements for the client's age and sex listed in Table 9-3. The standard reference is 29.3 cm for men and 28.5 cm for women.	Measurements less than 90% of the standard reference are in the category of moderately malnourished. Measurements less than 60% of the standard reference indicate severe malnourishment. See Table 9-3.

Continued on following page

PROCEDURE	NORMAL FINDINGS	ABNORMAL FINDINGS

Have the client dangle the nondominant arm freely next to the body. Locate the arm's midpoint (halfway between the top of the acromion process and the olecranon process). Mark the midpoint and measure the MAC, holding the tape measure firmly around, but not pinching, the arm.

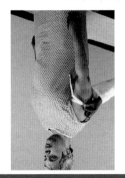

FIGURE 9-1 Measuring mid-arm circumference.

Measure triceps skinfold thickness (TSF) (Fig. 9-2).

Take the TSF measurement to evaluate the degree of fat stores. Instruct the client to stand and hang the nondominant arm freely. Grasp

Compare the client's current measurement to past measurements and to standard TSF measurements for the client's age and sex listed in Table 9-4. Standard reference is 12.5 mm for men and 16.5 mm for women.

Fat stores decrease in malnutrition and increase in obesity. See Table 9-6 for criteria indicating moderate to severe malnourishment. Measurements greater than 120% of the standard indicate obesity.

PROCEDURE	NORMAL FINDINGS	ABNORMAL FINDINGS

the skinfold and subcutaneous fat between the thumb and forefinger midway between the acromion process and the tip of the elbow. Pull the skin away from the muscle (ask client to flex arm—if you feel a contraction with this maneuver, you still have the muscle) and apply the calipers. Repeat three times and average the three measurements.

Note: A more accurate measurement can be obtained from the suprailiac region of the abdomen or the subscapular area.

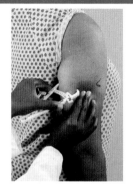

FIGURE 9-2 Measuring triceps skinfold thickness.

Continued on following page

PROCEDURE	NORMAL FINDINGS	ABNORMAL FINDINGS
Calculate mid-arm muscle circumference (MAMC). The MAMC calculation determines skeletal muscle reserves from MAC and TSF measurements by this formula. $$\text{MAMC (cm)} = \text{MAC (cm)} - (0.314 \times \text{TSF})$$	Compare the client's current MAMC to past measurements and to data for MAMCs for the client's age and sex listed in Table 9-5. Standard reference is 25.3 cm for men and 23.2 cm for women.	The MAMC decreases to the lower percentiles with malnutrition and in obesity if TSF is high. If the MAMC is in a lower percentile and the TSF is in a higher percentile, the client may benefit from muscle-building exercises that increase muscle mass and decrease fat. Malnutrition • Mild—MAMC of 90–99% • Moderate—MAMC 60–90% • Severe—MAMC < 60% as seen in protein–calorie malnutrition. See Table 9-5.

TABLE 9-1 **Adult Body Mass Index (BMI) Chart**

		Body Mass Index Table			
	Normal	Overweight	Obese	Extreme Obesity	

BMI	19	20	21	22	23	24	25	26	27	28	29	30	31	32	33	34	35	36	37	38	39	40	41	42	43	44	45	46	47	48	49	50	51	52	53	54
Height (inches)												Body Weight (pounds)																								
58	91	96	100	105	110	115	119	124	129	134	138	143	148	153	158	162	167	172	177	181	186	191	196	201	205	210	215	220	224	229	234	239	244	248	253	258
59	94	99	104	109	114	119	124	128	133	138	143	148	153	158	163	168	173	178	183	188	193	198	203	208	212	217	222	227	232	237	242	247	252	257	262	267
60	97	102	107	112	118	123	128	133	138	143	148	153	158	163	168	174	179	184	189	194	199	204	209	215	220	225	230	235	240	245	250	255	261	266	271	276
61	100	106	111	116	122	127	132	137	143	148	153	158	164	169	174	180	185	190	195	201	206	211	217	222	227	232	238	243	248	254	259	264	269	275	280	285
62	104	109	115	120	126	131	136	142	147	153	158	164	169	175	180	186	191	196	202	207	213	218	224	229	235	240	246	251	256	262	267	273	278	284	289	295
63	107	113	118	124	130	135	141	146	152	158	163	169	175	180	186	191	197	203	208	214	220	225	231	237	242	248	254	259	265	270	278	282	287	293	299	304
64	110	116	122	128	134	140	145	151	157	163	169	174	180	186	192	197	204	209	215	221	227	232	238	244	250	256	262	267	273	279	285	291	296	302	308	314
65	114	120	126	132	138	144	150	156	162	168	174	180	186	192	198	204	210	216	222	228	234	240	246	252	258	264	270	276	282	288	294	300	306	312	318	324
66	118	124	130	136	142	148	155	161	167	173	179	186	192	198	204	210	216	223	229	235	241	247	253	260	266	272	278	284	291	297	303	309	315	322	328	334
67	121	127	134	140	146	153	159	166	172	178	185	191	198	204	211	217	223	230	236	242	249	255	261	268	274	280	287	293	299	306	312	319	325	331	338	344
68	125	131	138	144	151	158	164	171	177	184	190	197	203	210	216	223	230	236	243	249	256	262	269	276	282	289	295	302	308	315	322	328	335	341	348	354
69	128	135	142	149	155	162	169	176	182	189	196	203	209	216	223	230	236	243	250	257	263	270	277	284	291	297	304	311	318	324	331	338	345	351	358	365
70	132	139	146	153	160	167	174	181	188	195	202	209	216	222	229	236	243	250	257	264	271	278	285	292	299	306	313	320	327	334	341	348	355	362	369	376
71	136	143	150	157	165	172	179	186	193	200	208	215	222	229	236	243	250	257	265	272	279	286	293	301	308	315	322	329	338	343	351	358	365	372	379	386
72	140	147	154	162	169	177	184	191	199	206	213	221	228	235	242	250	258	265	272	279	287	294	302	309	316	324	331	338	346	353	361	368	375	383	390	397
73	144	151	159	166	174	182	189	197	204	212	219	227	235	242	250	257	265	272	280	288	295	302	310	318	325	333	340	348	355	363	371	378	386	393	401	408
74	148	155	163	171	179	186	194	202	210	218	225	233	241	249	256	264	272	280	287	295	303	311	319	326	334	342	350	358	365	373	381	389	396	404	412	420
75	152	160	168	176	184	192	200	208	216	224	232	240	248	256	264	272	279	287	295	303	311	319	327	335	343	351	359	367	375	383	391	399	407	415	423	431
76	156	164	172	180	189	197	205	213	221	230	238	246	254	263	271	279	287	295	304	312	320	328	336	344	353	361	369	377	385	394	402	410	418	426	435	443

Source: Adapted from *Clinical Guidelines on the Identification, Evaluation, and Treatment of Overweight and Obesity in Adults: The Evidence Report* (1998). http://www.nhlbi.nih.gov/guidelines/obesity/bmi_tbl.pdf

TABLE 9-2   Disease Risk for Type 2 Diabetes, Hypertension, and Cardiovascular Diseases Relative to BMI and Waist Circumference

BMI	Waist Size Men: ≤ 101.6 cm (40 in) Women: ≤ 88.9 cm (35 in)	Waist Size Men: > 101.6 cm (40 in) Women: > 88.9 cm (35 in)
25–29.9	Increased	High
30–34.9	High	Very high
35–39.9	Very high	Very high
40 and above	Extremely high	Extremely high

Source: National Heart Lung and Blood Institute.

TABLE 9-3   Mid-Arm Circumference (MAC) Standard Reference

Adult MAC (cm)	Standard Reference	Moderately Malnourished— 60% of Standard Reference	Severely Malnourished
Men	29.3	26.3	17.6
Women	28.5	25.7	17.1

TABLE 9-4 Triceps Skinfold Thickness (TSF) Standard Reference

Adult TSF (mm)	Standard Reference	90% of Standard Reference—Moderately Malnourished	60% of Standard Reference—Severely Malnourished
Men	12.5	11.3	7.5
Women	16.5	14.9	9.9

TABLE 9-5 Mid-Arm Muscle Circumference (MAMC) Standard Reference

Adult MAMC (cm)	Standard Reference	90% of Standard Reference—Moderately Malnourished	60% of Standard Reference—Severely Malnourished
Men	25.3	22.8	15.2
Women	23.2	20.9	13.9

Dietary Assessment

Assess client's dietary requirements and intake by asking client to keep a 3-day diary of food and fluid intake. You may also use Box 9-1, p. 179 or Box 9-2, p. 180.

PROCEDURE	NORMAL FINDINGS	ABNORMAL FINDINGS
Estimate client's daily caloric requirements. See Table 9-6 for estimated daily caloric needs.	Meets caloric requirements.	Consumes more or less than caloric requirements for age, height, body build, and weight.
Compare intake with USDA-recommended food guidelines (Fig. 9-3).	See Table 9-6 for daily amount of food from each group.	Consumes more or less than recommended.

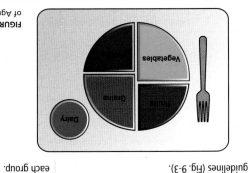

FIGURE 9-3 Choose MyPlate food Guide (Reprinted from *ChooseMyPlate.gov*, U.S. Department of Agriculture, Center for Nutrition Policy and Promotion).

BOX 9-1 SPEEDY CHECKLIST FOR NUTRITIONAL HEALTH

Some warning signs of poor nutritional health are noted in this checklist. Use it to find out if your client is at nutritional risk. Read the statements below. Circle the number in the yes column for those that apply to the client. For each yes answer, score the number in the box. Total the nutrition score.

	YES
Illness or condition that made the client change the kind and/or amount of food eaten	2
Eats fewer than two meals per day	3
Eats few fruits or vegetables, or milk products	2
Has three or more drinks of beer, liquor, or wine almost every day	2
Has tooth or mouth problems that make it hard to eat	2
Does not always have enough money to buy the food needed	4
Eats alone most of the time	1
Takes three or more different prescribed or over-the-counter drugs a day	1
Without wanting to, has lost or gained 4.5 kg (10 lb) in the last 6 months	2
Is not physically able to shop, cook, and/or feed self	2
TOTAL	

Total the nutritional score.

0–2	Good. Recheck the score in 6 months.
3–5	Moderate nutritional risk. See what can be done to improve eating habits and lifestyle. Recheck score in 3 months.
6 or more	High nutritional risk. Consult with physician, dietitian, or other qualified health or social service professional.

Note: Remember that warning signs suggest risk but do not represent diagnosis of any condition.

BOX 9-2 SELF-ASSESSMENT: SAMPLE FORM FOR A NUTRITION HISTORY

1. How many meals and snacks do you eat each day?

   Meals _____
   Snacks _____

2. How many times a week do you eat the following meals away from home?

   Breakfast _____
   Dinner _____
   Lunch _____

   What types of eating places do you frequently visit? (Check all that apply.)

   Fast-food _____
   Restaurant _____
   Diner/cafeteria _____
   Other _____

3. On average, how many pieces of fruit or glasses of juice do you eat or drink each day?

   Fresh fruit _____
   Juice (8-oz cup) _____

4. On average, how many servings of vegetables do you eat each day? _____

5. On average, how many times a week do you eat a high-fiber breakfast cereal? _____

6. How many times a week do you eat red meat (beef, lamb, veal) or pork? _____

7. How many times a week do you eat chicken or turkey? _____

8. How many times a week do you eat fish or shellfish? _____

9. How many hours of television do you watch every day? _____

   Do you usually snack while watching television? Yes _____ No _____

10. How many times a week do you eat deserts and sweets? _____

11. What types of beverages do you usually drink? How many servings of each do you drink a day?

    Water _____
    Juice _____
    Soda _____
    Diet soda _____
    Sports drinks _____
    Iced tea _____
    Iced tea with sugar _____

    Milk:
    Whole milk _____
    2% milk _____
    1% milk _____
    Skim milk _____

    Alcohol:
    Beer _____
    Wine _____
    Hard liquor _____

BOX 9-3   EDINBURGH FEEDING EVALUATION IN DEMENTIA QUESTIONNAIRE (EDFED-Q)[a]

Score answers to questions 1–10: never (0), sometimes (1), often (2)

1. Does the patient require close supervision while feeding?
2. Does the patient require physical help with feeding?
3. Is there spillage while feeding?
4. Does the patient tend to leave food on the plate at the end of the meal?
5. Does the patient ever refuse to eat?
6. Does the patient turn his head away while being fed?
7. Does the patient refuse to open his mouth?
8. Does the patient spit out his food?
9. Does the patient leave his mouth open allowing food to drop out?
10. Does the patient refuse to swallow?

Total Score:

(Total scores range from 0–20, with 20 being the most serious. Scores can be used to track change.)

11. Indicate appropriate level of assistance required by patient: supportive-educative; partly compensatory; wholly compensatory.

[a]Used with permission: Dr. Roger Watson.

TABLE 9-6 Estimated Calorie Needs per Day by Age, Gender, and Physical Activity Level

For each food group or subgroup,[a] recommended average daily intake amounts[b] at all calorie levels. Recommended intakes from vegetable and protein foods subgroups are per week. For more information and tools for application, go to MyPyramid.gov.

Calorie Level of Pattern[c]	1,000	1,200	1,400	1,600	1,800	2,000	2,200	2,400	2,600	2,800	3,000	3,200
Fruits	1 c	1 c	1½ c	1½ c	1½ c	2 c	2 c	2 c	2 c	2½ c	2½ c	2½ c
Vegetables[d]	1 c	1½ c	1½ c	2 c	2½ c	2½ c	3 c	3 c	3½ c	3½ c	4 c	4 c
Dark-green vegetables	½ c/wk	1 c/wk	1 c/wk	1½ c/wk	1½ c/wk	1½ c/wk	2 c/wk	2 c/wk	2½ c/wk	2½ c/wk	2½ c/wk	2½ c/wk
Red and orange vegetables	2½ c/wk	3 c/wk	3 c/wk	4 c/wk	5½ c/wk	5½ c/wk	6 c/wk	6 c/wk	7 c/wk	7 c/wk	7½ c/wk	7½ c/wk
Beans and peas (legumes)	½ c/wk	½ c/wk	½ c/wk	1 c/wk	1½ c/wk	1½ c/wk	2 c/wk	2 c/wk	2½ c/wk	2½ c/wk	3 c/wk	3 c/wk
Starchy vegetables	2 c/wk	3½ c/wk	3½ c/wk	4 c/wk	5 c/wk	5 c/wk	6 c/wk	6 c/wk	7 c/wk	7 c/wk	8 c/wk	8 c/wk
Other vegetables	1½ c/wk	2½ c/wk	2½ c/wk	3½ c/wk	4 c/wk	4 c/wk	5 c/wk	5 c/wk	5½ c/wk	5½ c/wk	7 c/wk	7 c/wk
Grains[e]	3 oz-eq	4 oz-eq	5 oz-eq	5 oz-eq	6 oz-eq	6 oz-eq	7 oz-eq	8 oz-eq	9 oz-eq	10 oz-eq	10 oz-eq	10 oz-eq
Whole grains	1½ oz-eq	2 oz-eq	2½ oz-eq	3 oz-eq	3 oz-eq	3 oz-eq	3½ oz-eq	4 oz-eq	4½ oz-eq	5 oz-eq	5 oz-eq	5 oz-eq
Enriched grains	1½ oz-eq	2 oz-eq	2½ oz-eq	2 oz-eq	3 oz-eq	3 oz-eq	3½ oz-eq	4 oz-eq	4½ oz-eq	5 oz-eq	5 oz-eq	5 oz-eq
Protein foods[d]	2 oz-eq	3 oz-eq	4 oz-eq	5 oz-eq	5 oz-eq	5½ oz-eq	6 oz-eq	6½ oz-eq	6½ oz-eq	7 oz-eq	7 oz-eq	7 oz-eq
Seafood	3 oz/wk	5 oz/wk	6 oz/wk	8 oz/wk	8 oz/wk	8 oz/wk	9 oz/wk	10 oz/wk	10 oz/wk	11 oz/wk	11 oz/wk	11 oz/wk
Meat, poultry, eggs	10 oz/wk	14 oz/wk	19 oz/wk	24 oz/wk	24 oz/wk	26 oz/wk	29 oz/wk	31 oz/wk	31 oz/wk	34 oz/wk	34 oz/wk	34 oz/wk
Nuts, seeds, soy products	1 oz/wk	2 oz/wk	3 oz/wk	4 oz/wk	4 oz/wk	4 oz/wk	4 oz/wk	5 oz/wk	5 oz/wk	5 oz/wk	5 oz/wk	5 oz/wk
Dairy[f]	2 c	2½ c	2½ c	3 c	3 c	3 c	3 c	3 c	3 c	3 c	3 c	3 c
Oils[g]	15 g	17 g	17 g	22 g	24 g	27 g	29 g	31 g	34 g	36 g	44 g	51 g
Maximum SoFAS[h] limit, calories (% of calories)	137 (14%)	121 (10%)	121 (9%)	121 (8%)	161 (9%)	258 (13%)	266 (12%)	330 (14%)	362 (14%)	395 (14%)	459 (15%)	596 (19%)

TABLE 9-6   **Estimated Calorie Needs per Day by Age, Gender, and Physical Activity Level** (Continued)

Notes:

[a]All foods are assumed to be in nutrient-dense forms, lean or low-fat and prepared without added fats, sugars, or salt. Solid fats and added sugars may be included up to the daily maximum limit identified in the table. Food items in each group and subgroup are:

Fruits

All fresh, frozen, canned, and dried fruits and fruit juices: for example, oranges and orange juice, apples and apple juice, bananas, grapes, melons, berries, raisins.

Vegetables

- Dark-green vegetables

  All fresh, frozen, and canned dark-green leafy vegetables and broccoli, cooked or raw: for example, broccoli; spinach; romaine; collard, turnip, and mustard greens.

- Red and orange vegetables

  All fresh, frozen, and canned red and orange vegetables, cooked or raw: for example, tomatoes, red peppers, carrots, sweet potatoes, winter squash, and pumpkin.

- Beans and peas (legumes)

  All cooked beans and peas: for example, kidney beans, lentils, chickpeas, and pinto beans. Does not include green beans or green peas. (See additional comment under protein foods group.)

- Starchy vegetables

  All fresh, frozen, and canned starchy vegetables: for example, white potatoes, corn, green peas.

- Other vegetables

  All fresh, frozen, and canned other vegetables, cooked or raw: for example, iceberg lettuce, green beans, and onions.

Grains

- Whole grains

  All whole-grain products and whole grains used as ingredients: for example, whole-wheat bread, whole-grain cereals and crackers, oatmeal, and brown rice.

- Enriched grains

  All enriched refined-grain products and enriched refined grains used as ingredients: for example, white breads, enriched grain cereals and crackers, enriched pasta, white rice.

Protein foods

All meat, poultry, seafood, eggs, nuts, seeds, and processed soy products. Meat and poultry should be lean or low-fat and nuts should be unsalted. Beans and peas are considered part of this group as well as the vegetable group, but should be counted in one group only.

Dairy

All milks, including lactose-free and lactose-reduced products and fortified soy beverages, yogurts, frozen yo-gurts, dairy desserts, and cheeses. Most choices should be fat-free or low-fat. Cream, sour cream, and cream cheese are not included due to their low calcium content.

[b]Food group amounts are shown in cup (c) or ounce-equivalents (oz-eq). Oils are shown in grams (g). Quantity equivalents for each food group are:

- Grains, 1 ounce-equivalent is: 1 one-ounce slice bread; 1 ounce uncooked pasta or rice; ½ cup cooked rice, pasta, or cereal; 1 tortilla (6″ diameter); 1 pancake (5″ diameter); 1 ounce ready-to-eat cereal (about 1 cup cereal flakes).
- Vegetables and fruits, 1 cup equivalent is: 1 cup raw or cooked vegetable or fruit; ½ cup dried vegetable or fruit; 1 cup vegetable or fruit juice; 2 cups leafy salad greens.
- Protein foods, 1 ounce-equivalent is: 1 ounce lean meat, poultry, seafood; 1 egg; 1 Tbsp peanut butter; ½ ounce nuts or seeds. Also, ¼ cup cooked beans or peas may also be counted as 1 ounce-equivalent.
- Dairy, 1 cup equivalent is: 1 cup milk, fortified soy beverage, or yogurt; 1½ ounces natural cheese (e.g., cheddar); 2 ounces of processed cheese (e.g., American).

Continued on following page

TABLE 9-6 Estimated Calorie Needs per Day by Age, Gender, and Physical Activity Level (Continued)

[a]See Appendix 6 [on the website] for estimated calorie needs per day by age, gender, and physical activity level. Food intake patterns at 1,000, 1,200, and 1,400 calories meet the nutritional needs of children ages 2 to 8 years. Patterns from 1,600 to 3,200 calories meet the nutritional needs of children ages 9 years and older and adults. If a child ages 4 to 8 years needs more calories and, therefore, is following a pattern at 1,600 calories or more, the recommended amount from the dairy group can be 2½ cups per day. Children ages 9 years and older and adults should not use the 1,000, 1,200, or 1,400 calorie patterns.

[b]Vegetable and protein foods subgroup amounts are shown in this table as weekly amounts, because it would be difficult for consumers to select foods from all subgroups daily.

[c]Whole-grain subgroup amounts shown in this table are minimums. More whole grains up to all of the grains recommended may be selected, with offsetting decreases in the amounts of enriched refined grains.

[d]The amount of dairy foods in the 1,200 and 1,400 calorie patterns have increased to reflect new RDAs for calcium that are higher than previous recommendations for children ages 4 to 8 years.

[e]Oils and soft margarines include vegetable, nut, and fish oils and soft vegetable oil table spreads that have no trans fats.

[f]SoFAs are calories from solid fats and added sugars. The limit for SoFAs is the remaining amount of calories in each food pattern after selecting the specified food group amounts in each food group in nutrient-dense forms (forms that are fat-free or low-fat and with no added sugars). The number of SoFAs is lower in the 1,200, 1,400, and 1,600 calorie patterns than in the 1,000 calorie pattern. The nutrient goals for the 1,200 to 1,600 calorie patterns are higher and require that more calories be used for nutrient-dense foods from the food groups.

Reprinted from *Dietary Guidelines for Americans* (2010), United States Department of Agriculture and Health and Human Services.

PEDIATRIC VARIATIONS

Physiologic Growth Patterns

- Growth is most rapid during the first year of life.
- Birth weight doubles at age 4 to 6 months and triples by 1 year.
- Length increases 50% the first year of life.
- Teeth erupt first year of life.
- Growth decreases from ages 1 to 6 years, but biting, chewing, and swallowing abilities increase.
- Muscle mass and bone density increase from ages 1 to 6 years.
- There is a latent uneven period of growth from ages 1 to 12 years.
- Permanent teeth erupt at ages 6 to 12 years.
- School-age children tolerate larger, less frequent meals.
- Nutritional needs increase during growth spurts (ages 10 to 15 years for girls and ages 12 to 19 years for boys).

Dietary Requirements

- Allow 1,000 calories plus 100 more per year of age (e.g., a 5-year-old needs 1,500 calories per day).

- Children need three milks, two meats, four fruits or vegetables, and four grains per day.
- Adolescents need four milks, two meats, four fruits or vegetables, and four grains per day.
- The American Academy of Pediatrics (2012) recommends exclusive breastfeeding for about 6 months, followed by breastfeeding as complementary foods are added into the infants' diet, with continuation of breastfeeding for 1 year or longer as mutually desired by mother and infant. Exclusive breastfeeding is sufficient for optimal growth and development for approximately the first 6 months. Solid foods should not be introduced before age 6 months. When they are introduced, solid foods should be iron enriched.

Physical Assessment

- Infants: Obtain weight, length, and head circumference. Identify type of feeding and iron source.
- Children and adolescents: Weigh child and obtain height. Identify adequacy of meals and snacks and sources of iron, calories, and protein.

 GERIATRIC VARIATIONS

- Older clients may have atrophy on dorsum of hands even with good nutrition.
- Assess for poor-fitting dentures and decreased ability to taste.
- Body weight may decrease with aging because of a loss of muscle or lean body tissue.
- Older adults tend to consume less food and eat more irregularly as they get older. This tends to increase with social isolation.
- Older adults have decreased peristalsis and nerve sensation, which may lead to constipation. Encourage fluids and dietary bulk to avoid laxative abuse.
- Caloric requirements decrease in response to a decreased basal metabolic rate, decreased activity, and change in body composition. A 10% decrease in calories is recommended for people aged 51 to 75 years and a 20% to 25% decrease in calories for people older than 75 years.
- A decrease in mobility and vision may impair the ability to purchase and prepare food. Sensory taste losses may lead to anorexia.
- Fifty percent of older adults are thought to be economically deprived. This factor may affect their nutrition if meat and milk are omitted from the diet to save money.

- Dietary recall may be difficult for older adults.
- Skinfold measurements are often inaccurate owing to changes in subcutaneous fat.

CULTURAL VARIATIONS

- Great variations may be seen in nutritional preferences, eating habits, and patterns of various groups.
- Foods, beverages, and medications are classified as hot/cold by many Asians and Hispanics (e.g., yin/yang by Chinese); it is very important to these clients to seek a balanced consumption based on these theories.
- Many people, especially of non-northern European descent, have some degree of lactose intolerance.*
- Classifications of "food" and "nonfood" items vary in cultures.
- Cultural or religious dietary rules or laws are of great importance to some groups (e.g., Orthodox Jews).
- Some groups may have diseases precipitated by certain foods or medications (e.g., glucose-6-phosphate dehydrogenase [G-6-PD] deficiency, lactose deficiency).

*Clients with lactose intolerance may be able to consume yogurt, buttermilk, fermented cheese, and acidophilus milk, or they may use products such as chewable tablets or liquid drops to act in place of the lactose enzyme.

Teaching Tips for Selected Nursing Diagnoses

Nursing Diagnosis: Readiness for enhanced nutritional–metabolic pattern

Encourage proper oral hygiene.
Teach nutritional guidelines.

- Eat a variety of foods.
- Balance the food you eat with physical activity—maintain or improve your weight. All adults should get at least 30 minutes of moderate physical activity most or all days of the week. Regular physical activity is important for a healthy body, enhancing psychological well-being, and preventing premature death (Healthy People, 2020 [2013]).
- Choose a diet with more dark green and orange vegetables, legumes, fruits, whole grains, and low-fat milk and milk products.
- Choose a diet with less total fats.
- Choose a diet with less added sugar and calories.
- Some cultural food preferences are contraindicated in specific disease states (e.g., Japanese client with hypertension who consumes high-sodium soy sauce).

- Choose a diet with less salt and sodium.
- If you drink alcoholic beverages, do so in moderation. According to Healthy People, 2020 (2013), alcohol as well as illegal drug use is linked to violence, injury, and HIV infection. Indicators set forth by Healthy People, 2020 (2013) include increasing the proportion of adolescents not using alcohol or any illicit drugs and reducing the proportion of adults using any illicit drug during the past 30 days.
- Teach client how to get the most for his/her food dollar, how to read food labels, and ways to maintain nutrients in foods.
- Buy frozen vegetables and ripe fresh produce when available.
- Encourage safe food storage and preparation to retain nutritional value and prevent food-borne illnesses.
- Prepare low-fat foods—suggest substituting applesauce or yogurt for butter when baking. Use bouillon or tomato juice instead of oil for sautéing. For added flavor, use herbs and spices to replace some or all the fat.
- Suggest using the online dietary and physical activity assessment tool *SuperTracker* to help plan, analyze, and track dietary choices and physical activity at www.choosemyplate.gov.
- Encourage use of Canada's Food Guide (2012) for Canadian residents. See Appendix 12.

Nursing Diagnosis: *Imbalanced Nutrition: more than body requirements*

Provide client with information on social support groups. Teach client self-assessment and rewarding techniques when proper nutrition is followed. Teach client how to calculate caloric intake and caloric expenditure and how to explore forms of exercise that meet client's needs. Assist client to replace frequent unhealthy snacking with nutritious snacks. Teach dietary guidelines and food choices for Americans recommended by the U.S. Department of Agriculture, Center for Nutrition Policy and Promotion (April, 2012).

 Nursing Diagnosis: *Imbalanced Nutrition: risk for more than body requirements*

Teach parents to avoid overfeeding infants. Encourage proper formula dilution. Teach avoidance of empty caloric foods. Discourage use of food for rewarding behavior. Teach parents that childhood obesity has been shown to increase the risk of developing cardiovascular disease, prediabetes/diabetes, bone and joint disorders, sleep apnea and social/psychological problems such as decreased self-esteem. Encourage healthy lifestyle practices such as eating healthy and exercising daily to lower the risk of childhood obesity and developing the related chronic diseases.

The Dietary Guidelines for Americans (2012) recommends that children get at least 60 minutes of physical activity each day. Furthermore, parents should limit inactive forms of play such as television viewing and computer gaming.

 Nursing Diagnosis: *Imbalanced Nutrition: risk for less than body requirements*

- Teach parents to avoid restricting normal intake of fat. Teach that low-fat diets are dangerous to growing infants because

fat is essential to metabolism of some vitamins and other substances and to hormone production associated with growth and development. Educate parents regarding the nutritional daily guidelines for girls and boys for each age. The recommended daily intake of calories, protein, fruits, vegetables, grains, and dairy products vary according to age and size.

- Encourage parent and child to visit www.nourishinteractive.com or www.choosemyplate.gov/children-over-five.html for kid friendly interactive. Use MyPlate foods learning activities and nutrition information for children.

CHAPTER **10**

Assessing Skin, Hair, and Nails

Structure and Function Overview

SKIN

The skin is composed of three layers: the epidermis, dermis, and subcutaneous tissue (Fig. 10-1). The skin is a physical barrier that protects the underlying tissues and structures and plays a vital role in temperature maintenance, fluid and electrolyte balance, absorption, excretion, sensation, immunity, vitamin D synthesis, and individual identity related to appearance. The **sebaceous glands** are attached to hair follicles over most of the body, excluding the soles and palms, and secrete an oily substance called **sebum** that waterproofs the hair and skin. There are two types of **sweat glands**. The **eccrine glands**, located over the entire skin, secrete sweat and affect thermoregulation by evaporation of sweat from the skin surface. The **apocrine glands**, associated with hair follicles in the axillae, perineum, and areolae of

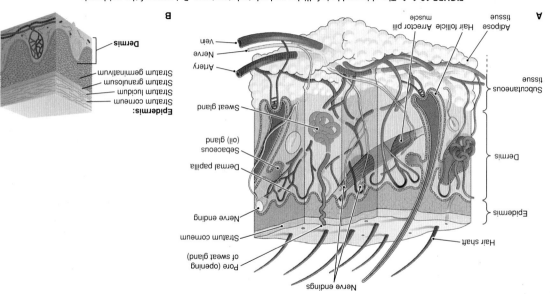

FIGURE 10-1 A: The skin and hair follicles and related structures. **B:** Layers of the epidermis.

the breasts, are small and nonfunctional until puberty when they secrete a milky sweat.

HAIR

Hair consists of layers of keratinized cells found over much of the body except for the lips, nipples, soles of the feet, palms of the hands, labia minora, and penis. There are two types of hair. **Vellus hair (peach fuzz)** is short, pale, and fine over much of the body and provides thermoregulation by wicking sweat away from the body. **Terminal hair** (particularly scalp and eyebrows) is longer, generally darker, and coarser than vellus hair and provides insulation and allows for self-expression. Nasal hair, auditory canal hair, eyelashes, and eyebrows filter dust and other airborne debris. Puberty initiates the growth of additional terminal hair in both sexes on the axillae, perineum, and legs. Hair color varies and is determined by the type and amount of pigment (melanin and pheomelanin) production.

NAILS

The nails, located on the distal phalanges of fingers and toes, are hard, transparent plates of keratinized epidermal cells that grow from a root underneath the skin fold called the cuticle (Fig. 10-2).

The **nail body** extends over the entire nail bed and has a pink tinge as a result of blood vessels underneath. The **lunula** is a crescent-shaped area located at the base of the nail. It is the visible aspect of the nail matrix. The nails protect the distal ends of the fingers and toes, enhance precise movement of the digits, and allow for an extended precision grip.

Nursing Assessment

COLLECTING SUBJECTIVE DATA

Focus Questions

Skin rashes, lesions, itching, dryness, oiliness, bruising, tingling, or numbness (location; onset; precipitating factors: stress, weather, drugs, exposure to allergens)? Methods of relief (e.g., medications, lotions, soaks)? Changes in skin color, lesions, bruising (onset, type of change)? Scalp lesions, itching, infections? Excessive or insufficient sweating or uncontrolled body odors? History of skin disorders (acne, dermatitis, cancer, ulcers, others)? Viruses (chicken pox, measles)? Sunburns or other burns? Surgical excision of skin lesions? Tattoos? Body piercings? Describe. Changes in texture, condition, and amount of hair? Changes in condition of nails and cuticles? Nail breaking, splitting? Cuticle

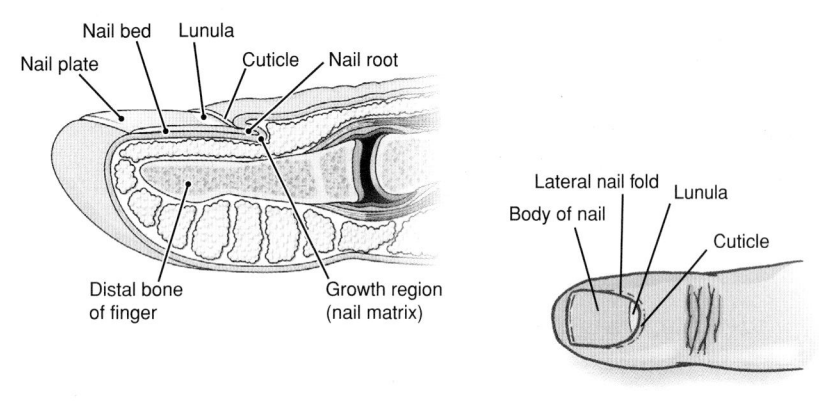

FIGURE 10-2 The nail and related structures.

inflammation? Artificial nails? Changes in body odor? Skin, hair, and nail care habits; bathing patterns; soaps and lotions used? Shampoo, hair spray, coloring, nail enamels used? Amount of sun/tanning exposure (types of oils and lotions used)? Exposure to chemicals?

Risk Factors

Risk for skin cancer related to repeated, intermittent sun exposure with sunburn beginning at early age; use of tanning booths; medical therapies (PUVA and radiation); genetic susceptibility; fair skinned, light eyes, hair; immunosuppression; human papilloma virus (HPV);

chemical exposure (tar, coal, arsenic, paraffin, some oils); age; actinic keratosis or change in mole; long-term skin irritation.

COLLECTING OBJECTIVE DATA

Equipment Needed

- Adequate lighting (natural daylight is best) or examination light
- Comfortable room temperature
- Gloves
- Penlight
- Magnifying glass
- Centimeter ruler
- Mirror for client's self-examination of skin

- Wood light
- Examination gown or drape
- Braden Scale to measure pressure sore risks
- Pressure Ulcer Scale for Healing (PUSH) tool to measure pressure ulcer healing

Physical Assessment

Review Figures 10-1 and 10-2 for a diagram of the skin and related structures and the nails. Expose the body part to be inspected by asking the client to remove clothing, jewelry, nail polish, makeup, wigs, toupees, or hairpieces and to put on a gown. Cleanse skin as needed. Provide privacy, comfortable temperature, and good lighting for skin inspection.

SKIN INSPECTION AND PALPATION		
ASSESSMENT PROCEDURE	**NORMAL FINDINGS**	**ABNORMAL FINDINGS**
Inspect the skin for the following: • Generalized color	• *In white skin:* Light to dark pink • *In dark skin:* Light to dark brown, olive	• *In white skin:* Extreme pallor, flushed, bluish (cyanosis). • *In dark skin:* Loss of red tones in pallor; ashen gray in cyanosis.

Continued on following page

SKIN INSPECTION AND PALPATION (Continued)

ASSESSMENT PROCEDURE	NORMAL FINDINGS	ABNORMAL FINDINGS
Note: Keep in mind that the amount of pigment in the skin accounts for the intensity of color as well as hue. Table 10-1 on p. 196 describes the six skin types.		Bluish-colored palms, soles, lips, nails, earlobes are seen with cyanosis. Cyanosis is seen in vasoconstriction, myocardial infarction, or pulmonary insufficiency. Pallor is seen in arterial insufficiency and anemia.
• Color variations in patches on the body	• *In white skin:* Sun-tanned areas, white patches (vitiligo)	• *In white skin:* Generalized pale yellow to pumpkin color (jaundice).
	• *In dark skin:* Lighter-colored palms, soles, nail beds, and lips; black/blue area over lower lumbar area (Mongolian spot); freckle-like pigmentation of nail beds and sclerae	• *In dark skin:* Yellow color may appear in sclerae, oral mucous membranes, hard and soft palates, palms, and soles.
		Increased pigmented areas; decreased pigmented areas; reddened, warm areas (erythema); black and blue marks (ecchymosis); tiny red spots (petechiae). Jaundice is often seen in liver or gallbladder disease, hemolysis, or anemia.
Palpate skin for the following:		
• Texture	• Smooth, soft	• Rough, thick, dry skin is seen in hypothyroidism.

ASSESSMENT PROCEDURE	NORMAL FINDINGS	ABNORMAL FINDINGS
• Temperature and moisture: feel with back of hand.	• Warm, dry	• Extremely cool or warm, wet, oily. Cold skin is seen in shock, hypotension, arterial insufficiency. Very warm skin is seen in fever and hyperthyroidism.
• Turgor: pinch up skin on sternum or under clavicle.	• Pinched-up skin returns immediately to original position.	• Pinched-up skin takes 30 seconds or longer to return to original position. Turgor is decreased in dehydration.
• Edema: press firmly for 5–10 seconds over tibia and ankle.	• No swelling, pitting, or edema	• Swollen, shallow to deep pitting, ascites. Generalized edema is seen in congestive heart failure or kidney disease. Unilateral, localized edema is seen in peripheral vascular problems such as venous stasis, obstruction, or lymphedema.
• Skin integrity: pay special attention to pressure point areas. Use Braden Scale (Box 10-1, p. 197) to determine the client's risk for skin breakdown.	• Skin intact, no reddened areas	• Skin breakdown: see Assessment Guide 10-1, p. 201, for staging of any pressure ulcer detected. See the PUSH tool (Box 10-2, p. 202) to document the degree of skin breakdown and to measure pressure ulcer healing over time.

Continued on following page

SKIN INSPECTION AND PALPATION (Continued)

ASSESSMENT PROCEDURE	NORMAL FINDINGS	ABNORMAL FINDINGS
If a skin lesion is detected, inspect and palpate for size, location, mobility, consistency, and pattern (circular, clustered, or straightlined).	Silver-pink stretch marks (striae), moles (nevi), freckles, birthmarks	Primary lesions arise from normal skin owing to disease or irritation (see Abnormal Findings 10-1, pp. 207–208). Secondary lesions arise from changes in primary lesions (see Abnormal Findings 10-2, p. 209). Vascular lesions may be seen with increased venous pressure, aging, liver disease, or pregnancy (see Abnormal Findings 10-3, p. 210). Skin cancer can manifest as either primary or secondary lesions.

TABLE 10-1 The Six Skin Types

Type	Description	Tanning Behavior	von Luschan Scale
I	Very light, "Celtic" type.	Often burns, occasionally tans.	1–5
II	Light, or light-skinned European.	Usually burns, sometimes tans.	6–10
III	Light intermediate, or dark-skinned European.	Rarely burns, usually tans.	11–15
IV	Dark intermediate, also "Mediterranean" or "olive skin."	Rarely burns, often tans.	16–21
V	Dark or "brown" type.	Naturally brown skin, sometimes darkens.	22–28
VI	Very dark, or "black" type.	Naturally black–brown skin.	29–36

Used with permission: Weller, R., Hunter, J., Savin, J., & Dahl, M. (2007). *Clinical dermatology* (4th ed.). Malden, Massachusetts: Blackwell Publishing.

(Continued on page 204)

BOX 10-1 BRADEN SCALE FOR PREDICTING PRESSURE SORE RISK

Patient's Name _____   Evaluator's Name _____   Date of Assessment _____

SENSORY PERCEPTION	1. Completely Limited	2. Very Limited	3. Slightly Limited	4. No Impairment			
Ability to respond meaningfully to pressure-related discomfort.	Unresponsive (does not moan, flinch, or grasp) to painful stimuli, due to diminished level of consciousness or sedation. OR Limited ability to feel pain over most of the body.	Responds only to painful stimuli. Cannot communicate discomfort except by moaning or restlessness. OR Has a sensory impairment that limits the ability to feel pain or discomfort over ½ of the body.	Responds to verbal commands, but cannot always communicate discomfort of the need to be turned. OR Has some sensory impairment that limits the ability to feel pain or discomfort in 1 or 2 extremities.	Responds to verbal commands. Has no sensory deficit that would limit the ability to feel or voice pain or discomfort.			

Continued on following page

BOX 10-1 BRADEN SCALE FOR PREDICTING PRESSURE SORE RISK (Continued)

MOISTURE	1. Constantly Moist	2. Very Moist	3. Occasionally Moist	4. Rarely Moist			
Degree to which skin is exposed to moisture.	Skin is kept moist almost constantly by perspiration, urine, etc. Dampness is detected every time the patient is moved or turned.	Skin is often, but not always moist. Linen must be changed at least once a shift.	Skin is occasionally moist, requiring an extra linen change approximately once a day.	Skin is usually dry. Linen only requires changing at routine intervals.			
ACTIVITY	**1. Bedfast**	**2. Chairfast**	**3. Walks Occasionally**	**4. Walks Frequently**			
Degree of physical activity.	Confined to bed.	Ability to walk severely limited or nonexistent. Cannot bear own weight and/or must be assisted into a chair or a wheelchair.	Walks occasionally during day, but for very short distances, with or without assistance. Spends majority of each shift in bed or chair.	Walks outside the room at least twice a day and inside the room at least once every 2 hours during waking hours.			

MOBILITY	1. Completely Immobile	2. Very Limited	3. Slightly Limited	4. No Limitation				
Ability to change and control body position.	Does not make even slight changes in body or extremity position without assistance.	Makes occasional slight changes in body or extremity position but unable to make frequent or significant changes independently.	Makes frequent though slight changes in body or extremity position independently.	Makes major and frequent changes in position without assistance.				
NUTRITION	**1. Very Poor**	**2. Probably Inadequate**	**3. Adequate**	**4. Excellent**				
Usual food intake pattern.	Never eats a complete meal. Rarely eats more than ⅓ of any food offered. Eats 2 servings or less of protein (meat or dairy products) per day. Takes fluids poorly. Does not take a liquid dietary supplement OR Is NPO and/or maintained on clear liquids or IVs for more than 5 days.	Rarely eats a complete meal and generally eats only about ½ of any food offered. Protein intake includes only 3 servings of meat or dairy products per day. Occasionally will take a dietary supplement OR Receives less than optimum amount of liquid diet or tube feeding.	Eats over half of most meals. Eats a total of 4 servings of protein (meat, dairy products) per day. Occasionally will refuse a meal, but will usually take a supplement when offered OR Is on a tube feeding or TPN regiment that probably meets most nutritional needs.	Eats most of every meal. Never refuses a meal. Usually eats a total of 4 or more servings of meat and dairy products. Occasionally eats between meals. Does not require supplementation.				

Continued on following page

BOX 10-1 BRADEN SCALE FOR PREDICTING PRESSURE SORE RISK (continued)

FRICTION & SHEAR	1. Problem	2. Potential Problem	3. No Apparent Problem			
	Requires moderate to maximum assistance in moving. Complete lifting without sliding against sheets is impossible. Frequently slides down in bed or chair, requiring frequent repositioning with maximum assistance. Spasticity, contractures, or agitation leads to almost constant friction.	Moves feebly or requires minimum assistance. During a move, the skin probably slides to some extent against sheets, chair, restraints, or other devices. Maintains relatively good position in chair or bed most of the time but occasionally slides down.	Moves in bed and in chair independently and has sufficient muscle strength to lift up completely during move. Maintains good position in bed or chair.			
Total Score						

ASSESSMENT GUIDE 10-1 Identification of Pressure Ulcer Stage

Suspected Deep Tissue Injury. Purple or maroon localized area of discolored intact skin or blood-filled blister due to damage of underlying soft tissue and/or shear. The area may be preceded by tissue that is painful, firm, mushy, boggy, warmer, or cooler as compared to adjacent tissue. Deep tissue injury may be difficult to detect in individuals with very dark skin tones. Evolution may include a thin blister over a dark wound bed. The wound may further evolve and become covered by eschar. Evolution may be rapid exposing additional layers of tissue even with optimal treatment.

Stage I. Intact skin with nonblanchable redness of a localized area usually over a bony prominence. Darkly pigmented skin may not have visible blanching; its color may differ from the surrounding area. The area may be painful, firm, soft, warmer, or cooler as compared to adjacent tissue. Stage I may be difficult to detect in individuals with dark skin tones.

Stage II. Partial thickness loss of dermis presenting as a shallow open ulcer with a red pink wound bed without slough. May also present as an intact or open/ruptured serum-filled blister. Presents as a shiny or dry shallow ulcer without slough or bruising; bruising indicates suspected deep tissue injury. This stage should not be used to describe skin tears, tape burns, perineal dermatitis, maceration, or excoriation.

Stage III. Full thickness tissue loss. Subcutaneous fat may be visible but bone, tendon, or muscle is not exposed. Slough may be present but does not obscure the depth of tissue loss. May include undermining and tunneling. The depth of a stage III pressure ulcer varies by anatomical location. The bridge of the nose, ear, occiput, and malleolus do not have subcutaneous tissue, and stage III ulcers can be shallow. In contrast, areas of significant adiposity can develop extremely deep stage III pressure ulcers. Bone/tendon is not visible or directly palpable.

Stage IV. Full thickness tissue loss with exposed bone, tendon, or muscle. Slough or eschar may be present on some parts of the wound bed. Often includes undermining and tunneling. The depth of a stage IV pressure ulcer varies by anatomical location (see stage III). Stage IV ulcers can extend into muscle and/or supporting structures (e.g., fascia, tendon, or joint capsule) making osteomyelitis possible. Exposed bone/tendon is visible or directly palpable.

Unstageable. Full thickness tissue loss in which the base of the ulcer is covered by slough (yellow, tan, gray, green, or brown) and/or eschar (tan, brown, or black) in the wound bed. Until enough slough and/or eschar is removed to expose the base of the wound, the true depth, and therefore stage, cannot be determined. Stable (dry, adherent, intact without erythema or fluctuance) eschar on the heels serves as "the body's natural (biologic) cover" and should not be removed.

Source: National Pressure Ulcer Advisory Panel, 2007. www.npuap.org/pr2.htm. *Copyrighted and used with permission.*

BOX 10-2   PUSH TOOL TO MEASURE PRESSURE ULCER HEALING

PUSH Tool 3.0

Patient Name _____ Patient ID# _____

Ulcer Location _____ Date _____

Directions: Observe and measure the pressure ulcer. Categorize the ulcer with respect to surface area, exudate, and the type of wound tissue. Record a sub-score for each of these ulcer characteristics. Add the sub-scores to obtain the total score. A comparison of total scores measured over time provides an indication of the improvement or deterioration in pressure ulcer healing.

LENGTH × WIDTH (in cm²)	0	1	2	3	4	5	Sub-score
	0	<0.3	0.3–0.6	0.7–1.0	1.1–2.0	2.1–3.0	
		6	7	8	9	10	
		3.1–4.0	4.1–8.0	8.1–12.0	12.1–24.0	>24.0	

EXUDATE AMOUNT	0 None	1 Light	2 Moderate	3 Heavy		Sub-score

TISSUE TYPE	0 Closed	1 Epithelial Tissue	2 Granulation Tissue	3 Slough	4 Necrotic Tissue	Sub-score

| | | | | | **TOTAL SCORE** | |

Length × Width: Measure the greatest length (head to toe) and the greatest width (side to side) using a centimeter ruler. Multiply these two measurements (length × width) to obtain an estimate of surface area in square centimeters (cm^2). Caveat: Do not guess! Always use a centimeter ruler and always use the same method each time the ulcer is measured.

Exudate Amount: Estimate the amount of exudate (drainage) present after removal of the dressing and before applying any topical agent to the ulcer. Estimate the exudate (drainage) as none, light, moderate, or heavy.

Tissue Type: This refers to the types of tissue that are present in the wound (ulcer) bed. Score as a "4" if there is any necrotic tissue present. Score as a "3" if there is any amount of slough present and necrotic tissue is absent. Score as a "2" if the wound is clean and contains granulation tissue. A superficial wound that is reepithelializing is scored as a "1." When the wound is closed, score as a "0."

4—Necrotic Tissue (Eschar): black, brown, or tan tissue that adheres firmly to the wound bed or ulcer edges and may be either firmer or softer than surrounding skin.

3—Slough: yellow or white tissue that adheres to the ulcer bed in strings or thick clumps, or is mucinous.

2—Granulation Tissue: pink or beefy red tissue with a shiny, moist, granular appearance.

1—Epithelial Tissue: for superficial ulcers, new pink or shiny tissue (skin) that grows in from the edges or as islands on the ulcer surface.

0—Closed/Resurfaced: the wound is completely covered with epithelium (new skin).

*Source: National Pressure Ulcer Advisory Panel. www.npuap.org/PDF/**push**3.pdf. Copyrighted and used with permission.*

HAIR INSPECTION AND PALPATION

ASSESSMENT PROCEDURE	NORMAL FINDINGS	ABNORMAL FINDINGS
Inspect and palpate hair for the following:		
• Color	• Varies	• Patchy gray areas are seen in nutritional deficiencies. Copper-red hair in an African American child may indicate severe malnutrition.
• Amount and distribution	• Vary	• Sudden loss of hair (alopecia) or increase in facial hair in females (hirsutism). Hirsutism is seen in Cushing syndrome; general hair loss seen in infections, nutritional deficiencies, hormonal disorders, some types of chemotherapy, or radiation therapy; patchy loss seen with scale infection and lupus erythematosus.
• Texture	• Fine to coarse, pliant	• Change in texture. Dull, dry hair is seen in hypothyroidism and malnutrition.
• Presence of parasites	• None	• Lice (body or head), eggs attached to hair shaft, usually accompanied by severe itching.

SCALP INSPECTION AND PALPATION

ASSESSMENT PROCEDURE	NORMAL FINDINGS	ABNORMAL FINDINGS
Inspect and palpate scalp for the following:		
• Symmetry	• Symmetrical	• Asymmetrical
• Texture	• Smooth, firm	• Bumpy, scaly, excoriated. Scaly, dry flakes are seen in dermatitis; gray scaly patches seen in fungal infections; dandruff seen with psoriasis.
• Lesions	• None	• Open or closed lesions

NAIL INSPECTION AND PALPATION

PROCEDURE	NORMAL FINDINGS	ABNORMAL FINDINGS
Inspect and palpate nails for the following:		
• Color	• Pink nail bed	• Pale or cyanotic nails are seen in hypoxia or anemia; yellow discoloration seen in fungal infections or psoriasis; splinter hemorrhages (vertical lines) seen in trauma; Beau lines (horizontal) seen in acute trauma; nail pitting seen in psoriasis (see Abnormal Findings 10-4, p. 211).
	In dark skin: may have small or large pigmented deposits, streaks, freckles	

Continued on following page

NAIL INSPECTION AND PALPATION (Continued)

PROCEDURE	NORMAL FINDINGS	ABNORMAL FINDINGS
• Shape	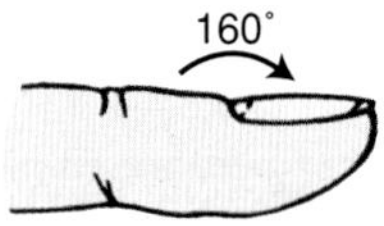 • Round nail with 160° nail base (see Fig. 10-3).	• Clubbing: 180° or more nail base is seen with hypoxia. Spoon nails occur with iron deficiency anemia (see Abnormal Findings 10-4, p. 211).

Normal angle

160°

FIGURE 10-3 Normal angle.

PROCEDURE	NORMAL FINDINGS	ABNORMAL FINDINGS
• Texture	• Nail is round, hard, immobile • Smooth, firm, and pink *In dark skin:* may be thick	• Thickened nails are seen with decreased circulation.
• Condition of nail bed		• Paronychia (inflamed nail head) indicates infection. Onycholysis (detached nail plate from nail bed) indicates infection or trauma (see Abnormal Findings 10-4).

ABNORMAL FINDINGS 10-1 Primary Skin Lesions

Nonpalpable Lesion
Macule: Flat and colored (Example: freckle, petechia, ecchymoses)

Palpable Lesions
Papule: Elevated and superficial (Example: wart)

Palpable Lesions With Fluid
Bulla, vesicle: Elevated and filled with fluid (Example: blister)

Cyst: Encapsulated, filled with fluid or semisolid mass (Example: epidermoid cyst)

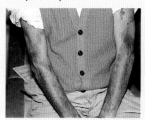 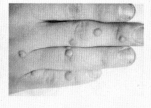 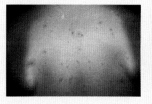 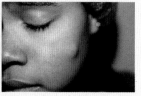

Continued on following page

ABNORMAL FINDINGS 10-1 Primary Skin Lesions (Continued)

Nodule, tumor: elevated and firm, has the dimension of depth (Example: lipoma)

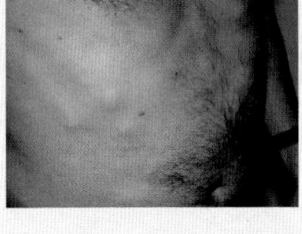

Wheal: localized edema (Example: insect bite)

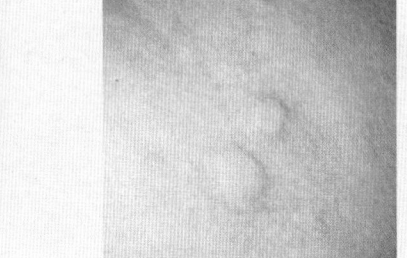

Pustule: elevated and filled with pus (Example: acne)

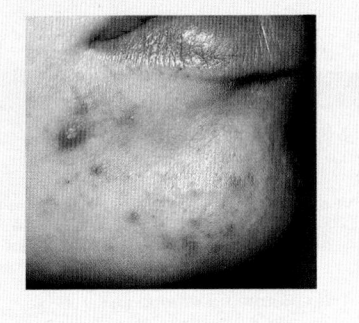

ABNORMAL FINDINGS | 10-2 | **Secondary Skin Lesions (Changes in Primary Skin Lesions)**

Ulcer: Skin surface loss, often bleeds

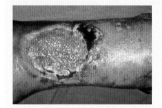

Atrophy: Thin, shiny, taut skin

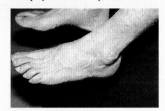

Crust: Dried pus or blood

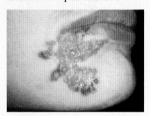

Lichenification: Thickened, roughened skin

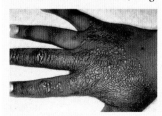

Scale: Thin, flaky skin

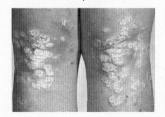

Keloid: Hypertrophied scar

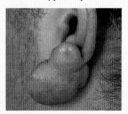

ABNORMAL FINDINGS 10-3 Vascular Lesions

Cherry angioma: Ruby red; flat or raised

Spider vein: Bluish; may have radiating legs; seen mostly on legs

Spider angioma: Bright red with radiating legs; pullulating seen on the center of lesion, or legs, or arms, and upper trunk; blanches when pressure is applied to the center.

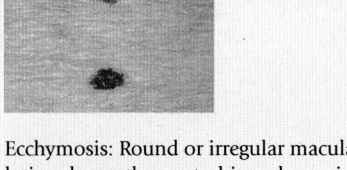

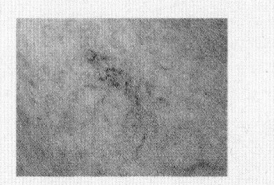

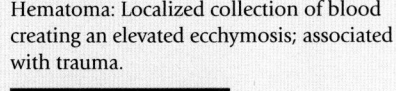

Ecchymosis: Round or irregular macular lesion; larger than petechia; color varies and changes black, yellow, and green.

Petechiae: Round red or purple macules

Hematoma: Localized collection of blood creating an elevated ecchymosis; associated with trauma.

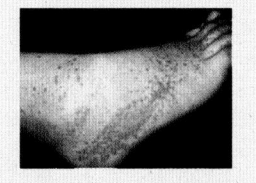

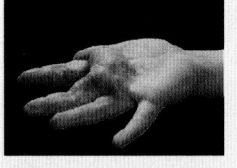

| ABNORMAL FINDINGS | 10-4 | Nail Abnormalities |

Splinter hemorrhages

Beau lines (acute illness)

Spoon nails (iron deficiency anemia)

Early clubbing (oxygen deficiency)

180

Late clubbing (oxygen deficiency)

>180

Paronychia (local infection)

PEDIATRIC VARIATIONS

Subjective Data: Focus Questions

Skin eruptions or rashes and relationship to any allergies (e.g., food, formula, type of diapers used, diaper creams, soaps, dust)? Bathing routines and soap used? Play injuries (cuts, abrasions, bruises)? Indicators of physical abuse (bruises)? Exposure to communicable diseases? Exposure to pets, stuffed animals? Eczema (onset, precipitating factors, treatment)? Acne (during adolescence; location: face, back, chest; onset; precipitating factors; treatment)? Excessive nail biting? Twirling of hair? History of communicable diseases?

Objective Data: Assessment Techniques

ASSESSMENT PROCEDURE	NORMAL FINDINGS	ABNORMAL FINDINGS
Inspect the following:		
• Skin color	• Infant's skin is lighter shade than parents'; Mongolian spot is a common hyperpigmentation variation in African Americans, Native Americans, Latin Americans, and Asians. Body piercing may be cultural or a fad. Excessive piercing or tattooing that is "homemade" may increase the risk for hepatitis B or HIV from infected needles.	• Yellow skin is seen in jaundice or with ingestion of too many yellow/orange vegetables in infants/toddlers. Bruising (purple, green, yellow) discoloration in the skin indicates injury to the skin tissue. If markings suggest imprint of hand/fingers, evaluate for physical abuse.
• Oiliness and acne	• Adolescents have increased sebaceous gland activity.	• Cystic acne, acne vulgaris
• Skin lesions	• None	• Crusted or ruptured vesicles are seen in impetigo. Pruritic macular–papular skin eruptions that become vesicular are seen in chicken pox. Pink to red macular–papular rash is seen in measles. Erythemic vesicular rash in linear formation may indicate contact dermatitis (poison ivy). Annular, raised erythemic lesion with central clearing indicates fungal infection

ASSESSMENT PROCEDURE	NORMAL FINDINGS	ABNORMAL FINDINGS
• Hand creases: assess dermatoglyphics by inspecting flexion creases in palm	• Three flexion creases present in palm (Fig. 10-4)	• More or fewer than three flexion creases with varied pattern in palm (e.g., one horizontal crease in palm [Simian crease]) (Fig. 10-5)
• Hair	• Lustrous, strong, elastic, shiny. Scalp clean and dry. No scaling, flaking.	Thick or flaky greasy yellow scales on scalp in young children, flakes in hair with yellow greasy scales on scalp, forehead eyebrows, ears indicate seborrhea (cradle cap). Small white nits in hair shaft (resembles a piece of rice) are eggs of head lice, Pediculosis capitis. Adult lice are tiny, brown bugs found in hair shaft.

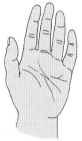

Normal creases

FIGURE 10-4 Normal creases.

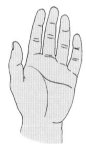

Simian creases

FIGURE 10-5 Simian creases.

GERIATRIC VARIATIONS

Skin

- Thinning epithelium
- Wrinkles, decreased turgor, and elasticity
- Dry, itchy skin due to decrease in activity of eccrine and seba-ceous glands
- Seborrheic or senile keratosis (tan to black macular–papular lesions on neck, chest, or back)
- Senile lentigines ("liver spots," or "age spots"—flat brown maculae on hands, arms, neck, face) (Fig. 10-6)

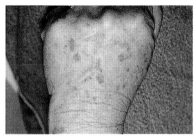

FIGURE 10-6 Senile lentigines are common on aging skin.

- Cherry angiomas (small, round, red elevated spots)
- Senile purpura (vivid purple patches)
- Acrochordons (soft, light-pink to brown skin tags)
- Prominent veins due to thinning epithelium

Hair

- Loss of pigment; fine, brittle texture
- Alopecia, especially in men; sparse body hair
- Coarse facial hair, especially in women
- Decreased axillary, pubic, and extremity hair

Nails

- Thickened, yellow, brittle nails
- Ingrown toenails

CULTURAL VARIATIONS

- Infants and newborns of African American, Native American, or Asian descent often have Mongolian spots, a blue-black or purple macular area on buttocks and sacrum; sometimes this pattern appears on the abdomen, thighs, or upper extremities.

- Dark-skinned clients tend to have lighter-colored palms, soles, nail beds, and lips. They may also have freckle-like pigmentation of nail beds and sclera. Nails may also be thick.
- Females of certain cultural groups shave or pluck pubic hair.
- Pallor is assessed in the dark-skinned client by observing the absence of underlying red tones. (Brown skin appears yellow-brown; black skin appears ashen-gray.)
- Erythema is detected by palpation of increased warmth of skin in dark-skinned clients.
- Cyanosis is detected in dark-skinned clients by observing the lips and tongue, which become ashen-gray.
- Inspect for petechiae in the oral mucosa or conjunctiva of the dark-skinned client, because they are difficult to see in dark-pigmented areas; also observe the sclerae, hard palate, palms, and soles for jaundice.
- Presence of body piercing may be a fad or a cultural norm.

POSSIBLE COLLABORATIVE PROBLEMS—RISK OF

Skin infections	Burns	Allergic reactions (skin)
Skin rashes	Graft rejection	Insect/animal bite
Skin lesions	Hemorrhage	

Teaching Tips for Selected Nursing Diagnoses

Nursing Diagnosis: *Readiness for enhanced self-health management related to desire to learn about ways to protect skin integrity*

Teach the client that regular exercise improves circulation and oxygenation of skin.

Encourage protective clothing and boots when walking in wooded areas.

Teach client to:
- Reduce sun exposure.
- Always use sunscreen (solar protection factor [SPF] 15 or higher) when sun exposure is anticipated.
- Wear long-sleeved shirts and wide-brimmed hats.
- Avoid sunburns.
- Avoid intermittent tanning.
- Understand the link between sun exposure and skin cancer and the accumulating effects of sun exposure on developing cancers.
- Carry out routine skin self-assessment (Box 10-3) and seek professional advice as soon as possible if anything unusual is detected.

BOX 10-3 SELF-ASSESSMENT: HOW TO EXAMINE YOUR OWN SKIN

Examine head and face using one or both mirrors. Use a blow dryer to inspect scalp.

With back to the mirror, use hand mirror to inspect back of neck, shoulders, upper arms, back, buttocks, legs.

Check hands, including nails. In full-length mirror, examine elbows, arms and underarms.

Sitting down, check legs and feet, including soles, heels, and nails. Use hand mirror to examine genitals.

Focus on neck, chest, torso. Women: check under breasts.

Nursing Diagnosis: *Ineffective Health Maintenance related to lack of hygienic care of skin, hair, and nails, and/or excessive piercing/tattooing performed with "homemade" materials*

Assess hair, nail, and skin care, and instruct the client on appropriate hygiene measures as necessary (e.g., use mild soap, lotion for dry skin; wash oily areas with warm soap and water three times a day).

Teach dangers of hepatitis B and HIV when using contaminated needles.

Nursing Diagnosis: *Risk for Impaired Skin Integrity related to prolonged sun exposure*

Caution the client against prolonged sun exposure or tanning lamp, and instruct that proper use of sunscreen agents can decrease the risk of skin pathologies. Teach the client to report a change in the size or appearance of a mole, nodule, pigmented area, new growth on the skin; to limit or avoid sun exposure between 10 AM and 4 PM, when the sun's ultraviolet rays are strongest; to use a sunscreen with an SPF of at least 15; to wear protective clothing and hats (American Cancer Society, 2013b).

Nursing Diagnosis: *Risk for Impaired Nail Integrity related to prolonged use of nail polish*

Caution the client of potential nail damage caused by prolonged use of nail polish.

 Nursing Diagnosis: *Risk for Impaired Skin Integrity: "diaper rash" related to parental knowledge deficit of skin care for diapered infant or child*

Inform parents of products available for treatment of rash and importance of frequent diaper changes and cleansing of skin with mild soap (e.g., Ivory or Dove). Teach parents to keep skin cool and dry, avoid restricting clothing, and allow air-drying for 15 to 20 minutes several times a day.

 Nursing Diagnosis: *Impaired Skin Integrity related to improper care of acne lesions*

Teach adolescents proper skin cleansing, using mild soaps such as cetaphil soap on face, good hand washing, and avoid picking lesions. Stress the importance of adequate rest, moderate exercise, and a balanced diet. Encourage hydration and avoiding foods, soaps, and creams that irritate skin.

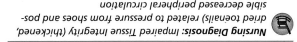

Nursing Diagnosis: *Risk for Impaired Skin Integrity related to immobility, decreased production of natural oils, and thinning skin*

Teach the client and family the benefits of turning of client, range-of-motion (ROM) exercises, massage, and cleaning of skin for reducing the risk of skin breakdown. Teach the family and client how to observe for reddened pressure areas. Encourage the use of lotions to replace skin oils. Massage skin with lotions.

Instruct the client to decrease the frequency of baths and use a humidifier during the cold seasons. Explain the effects of proper nutrition and adequate fluids on skin integrity.

Nursing Diagnosis: *Impaired Tissue Integrity (thickened, dried toenails) related to pressure from shoes and possible decreased peripheral circulation*

Instruct the client to soak nails 15 minutes in warm water before cutting. Use good scissors and lighting. Refer to podiatrist as necessary. Ascertain whether shoes fit correctly.

CHAPTER 11

Assessing Head and Neck

Structure and Function Overview

HEAD

The framework of the head is the skull, which can be divided into two subsections, the cranium and the face (Fig. 11-1). The cranium has eight bones that protect the brain and the major sensory organs: Frontal (1), parietal (2), temporal (2), occipital (1), ethmoid (1), and sphenoid (1). In adults, these bones are joined together by immovable sutures: the sagittal, coronal, squamosal, and lambdoid sutures. The face has 14 bones: Maxilla (2), zygomatic (cheek) (2), inferior conchae (2), nasal (2), lacrimal (2), palatine (2), vomer (1), and mandible (jaw) (1). The mandible is the only movable facial joint and joins the cranium at the temporal bone forming the temporomandibular joint (TMJ). Other important structures in the head are the temporal artery, the parotid glands, and the submandibular glands.

NECK

The structure of the neck is composed of muscles, ligaments, and the cervical vertebrae. Contained within the neck are the hyoid bone, several major blood vessels, the larynx, the trachea, and the thyroid gland (Fig. 11-2).

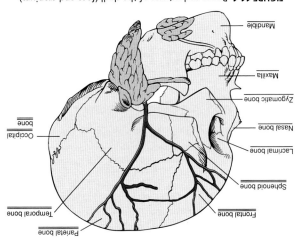

FIGURE 11-1 Bones and sutures of the skull (face and cranium).

Mandible

Maxilla

Zygomatic bone

Nasal bone

Lacrimal bone

Sphenoid bone

Frontal bone

Temporal bone

Parietal bone

Temporal bone

Occipital bone

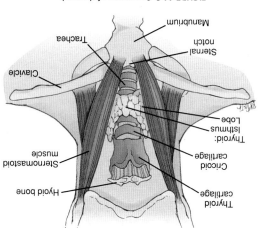

FIGURE 11-2 Structures of the neck.

Manubrium

Sternal notch

Trachea

Clavicle

Thyroid:
Isthmus
Lobe

Sternomastoid muscle

Cricoid cartilage

Hyoid bone

Thyroid cartilage

The thyroid gland is the largest endocrine gland in the body. The first upper tracheal ring, called the cricoid cartilage, has a small notch in it. The thyroid cartilage (Adam's apple) is larger and located just above the cricoid cartilage. The hyoid bone, which is attached to the tongue, lies above the thyroid cartilage and under the mandible (see Fig. 11-2).

MUSCLES AND LYMPH NODES

The sternomastoid muscle rotates and flexes the head, whereas the trapezius muscle extends the head and moves the shoulders (Fig. 11-3). The eleventh cranial nerve is responsible for muscle movement that permits shrugging of the shoulders by the trapezius muscles and turning the head against resistance by the sternomastoid muscles. These two major muscles also form two triangles that provide important landmarks for assessment. The anterior triangle is located under the mandible, anterior to the sternomastoid muscle. The posterior triangle is located between the trapezius and the sternomastoid muscles. The cervical vertebrae (C1 to C7) are located in the posterior neck and support the cranium. The vertebra prominens is C7, which can easily be palpated when the neck is flexed. Using C7 as a landmark will help you to locate other vertebrae. In addition, several lymph nodes are located in the head and the neck (see Fig. 11-8, p. 233).

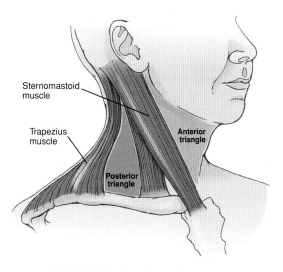

FIGURE 11-3 Neck muscles and landmarks.

Nursing Assessment

COLLECTING SUBJECTIVE DATA

Focus Questions

Lumps (onset, location, size, texture)? Limited movement of neck? Describe: Facial pain/neck pain/headaches (location, onset, duration, precipitating factors, relief)? See Box 11-1 for kinds and characteristics of headaches. Muscle tension, vertebral joint dysfunction, limited mobility of head and neck? Prior neck injuries (date, related to work, recreation, treatment)? Prior radiation therapy to head or neck? Prior thyroid surgery? Family history of head/neck cancer, migraines? Head and neck self-care: posture, use of helmet, seat belts, tobacco products. Use of caffeine and alcohol? Type of work and recreation in relation to posture and possible injuries?

Risk Factors

For head injury: age (newborn to 4 years old), high-risk sports, lack of protective devices (e.g., seatbelts, helmet), violence, falls (especially after age 65), excessive alcohol ingestion. For thyroid disease: radiation to upper body, family history. For lymphatic enlargement: immunosuppression, chronic disease, malnutrition.

COLLECTING OBJECTIVE DATA

Equipment Needed

- Clean gloves
- Small cup of water for client during thyroid exam
- Stethoscope

Physical Assessment

See Figures 11-1 to 11-3 for a review of the anatomy of the head and the neck.

Ask the client to remove any hats, hairpieces, wigs, hair ornaments, pins, rubber bands, jewelry, and head or neck scarves. Ask client to put on gown if a wearing clothing that covers the neck. Explain what you are doing through the exam to decrease client anxiety.

BOX 11-1 TYPES AND CHARACTERISTICS OF HEADACHES

SINUS HEADACHE

Character: Deep, constant, throbbing pain; pressure-like pain in one specific area of the face or the head (e.g., behind the eyes); face tender to the touch

Onset and precipitating factors: Occurs with or after a cold or acute sinusitis or acute febrile illness with purulent discharge from nose

Location: May occur in one area of the face or along the eyebrow ridge and below the cheek bone (see Figure below)

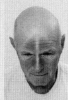

Sinus
headache

Duration: Lasts until associated condition is improved

Severity: May be moderately severe; not debilitating

Pattern: Pain worsens with sudden movements of the head, bending forward, lying down, in the morning (due to mucus collecting and draining all night), or with sudden temperature changes (going from warm room to cold)

Associated factors: Associated with other symptoms of sinusitis, such as nasal drainage and congestion, fever, and foul-smelling breath. Sinus headaches may be confused with tension headaches and migraines. Hutchinson (2007) advises, "Migraines also have forehead and facial pressure over the sinuses, nasal congestion, and runny nose. In the absence of fever, pus from your nose, alteration in smell or foul-smelling breath, you likely have a migraine headache."

Continued on following page

BOX 11-1 TYPES AND CHARACTERISTICS OF HEADACHES (Continued)

CLUSTER HEADACHE

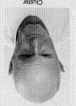

Cluster

Character: Stabbing pain; may be accompanied by tearing, eyelid drooping, reddened eye, or runny nose

Onset and precipitating factors: Has a sudden onset; may be precipitated by ingesting alcohol

Location: Localized in the eye and orbit and radiating to the facial and temporal regions

Duration: Typically occurs in the late evening or night

Severity: Intense

Pattern: Movement or walking back and forth may relieve the discomfort

Associated factors: Occurs more in young males

TENSION HEADACHE

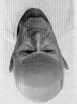

Tension

Character: Dull, tight, diffuse

Onset and precipitating factors: No prodromal stage, may occur with stress, anxiety, or depression

Location: Usually located in the frontal, temporal, or occipital region

Duration: Lasts for days, months, or years

Severity: Aching

Pattern: Symptomatic relief may be obtained by local heat, massage, analgesics, antidepressants, and muscle relaxants

Associated factors: Affects women more often than men

MIGRAINE HEADACHE

Character: Accompanied by nausea, vomiting, and sensitivity to noise or light

Onset and precipitating factors: May have prodromal stage (visual disturbances, vertigo, tinnitus, numbness, or tingling of fingers or toes); may be precipitated by emotional disturbances, anxiety, or ingestion of alcohol, cheese, chocolate, or other foods and substances to which the client is sensitive

Location: Located around eyes, temples, cheeks, or forehead; may affect only one side of the face

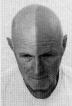

Migraine

Duration: Lasts up to 3 days

Severity: Throbbing, severe

Pattern: Rest may bring relief

Associated factors: Occurs more often in women

TUMOR-RELATED HEADACHE

Character: Aching, steady; neurologic and mental symptoms and nausea and vomiting may develop

Onset and precipitating factors: No prodromal stage; may be aggravated by coughing, sneezing, or sudden movements of the head

Location: Varies with location of tumor

Duration: Commonly occurs in the morning and lasts for several hours

Severity: Variable in intensity

Pattern: Usually subsides later in the day

Modified from Hutchinson, S. (2007). "Sinus headache" or migraine. Available at http://www.achenet.org/education/patients/SinusHeadacheorMigraine.asp; WebMD. (2009). Migraine & Headache Health Center: Sinus headaches. Available at http://www.webmd.com/migraines-headaches/guide/sinus-headaches; and University of Maryland (2011). Sinus headache. Available at http://www.umm.edu/altmed/articles/sinus-headache-000073.htm

SCALP, FACE, AND NECK INSPECTION AND PALPATION

ASSESSMENT PROCEDURE	NORMAL FINDINGS	ABNORMAL FINDINGS
Inspect and palpate the scalp for the following:		
• Size	• Varies, especially in accord with ethnicity. Usually the head is symmetric, round, erect, and in midline, and appropriately related to body size (normocephalic).	• Extremely large or small. Scalp is thick in acromegaly (increase in growth hormones); large, acorn-shaped in Paget disease.
• Shape	• Symmetrical and round. May vary, especially in accord with ethnicity.	• Asymmetrical
• Consistency	• Hard and smooth	• Bumpy or soft. Lumps or lesions are seen in cancer and trauma.
Observe the face for the following:		
• Symmetry	• Symmetrical	• Asymmetrical. Face is asymmetrical (drooping, weakness, or paralysis) with parotid gland enlargement or Bell palsy, mask-like face in Parkinson disease. Asymmetric orofacial movements may be from organic disease or neurologic problem; refer client for follow-up. Drooping, weakness, or

ASSESSMENT PROCEDURE	NORMAL FINDINGS	ABNORMAL FINDINGS
• Facial features	• Features vary • Symmetrical, centered head position	paralysis on one side of the face may occur with stroke (cerebrovascular accident [CVA]). "Sunken" face with depressed eyes and hollow cheeks is typical of cachexia (emaciation or wasting). Pale, swollen face may result from nephritic syndrome. • Distorted features: mask-like face in Parkinson disease; tightened, hard face in scleroderma; sunken, hollow face in cachexia; swollen face in nephrotic syndrome; moon shape with red cheeks, facial hair in Cushing syndrome. A moon-shaped face with reddened cheeks and increased facial hair may indicate Cushing syndrome.
Observe the **neck** for the following: • Appearance	• Symmetrical neck with head centered. No bulging masses or swollen enlarged lymph nodes.	• Asymmetrical head position, masses, or scars present. Swelling is seen in cancer, enlarged thyroid, or inflamed lymph nodes.

Continued on following page

SCALP, FACE, AND NECK INSPECTION AND PALPATION (Continued)

ASSESSMENT PROCEDURE	NORMAL FINDINGS	ABNORMAL FINDINGS
Palpate the temporal artery, located between the top of the ear and the eye (Fig. 11-4).	Temporal artery elastic and nontender.	Temporal artery is hard, thick, and tender with inflammation as seen with temporal arteritis.
• Movement	Smooth, controlled movements; range of motion (ROM) from upright position: • Flexion = 45° • Extension = 55° • Lateral abduction = 40° • Rotation = 70°	• Rigid, jerky movements; ROM less than normal values; pain on movement. Limited ROM, stiffness, and rigidity are seen with muscle spasms, inflammation, meningitis, cervical arthritis.

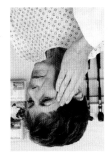

FIGURE 11-4 Palpating the temporal artery.

ASSESSMENT PROCEDURE	NORMAL FINDINGS	ABNORMAL FINDINGS
Palpate the temporomandibular joint (TMJ) by placing your index finger over the front of each ear as you ask the client to open mouth (Fig. 11-5).	No swelling, tenderness, or crepitation with movement. Mouth opens and closes fully (3–6 cm between upper and lower teeth). Lower jaw moves laterally 1–2 cm in each direction.	Limited ROM, swelling, tenderness, or crepitation may indicate TMJ syndrome.

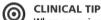 **CLINICAL TIP**
When assessing TMJ syndrome, be sure to explore the client's history of headaches, if any.

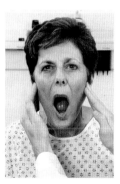

FIGURE 11-5 Palpating the TMJ.

Continued on following page

TRACHEA, THYROID, AND LYMPH NODE PALPATION

Palpate the trachea first, followed by observing and then palpation of the thyroid gland using the guidelines described below. After palpating the thyroid gland, palpate the cervical lymph nodes.

ASSESSMENT PROCEDURE	NORMAL FINDINGS	ABNORMAL FINDINGS
Palpate the **trachea** for position and landmarks (tracheal rings, cricoid, and thyroid cartilage) (see Fig. 11-2, p. 220, for location).	Midline position; symmetrical; landmarks identifiable	Asymmetrical position deviates from the midline with tumor, enlarged thyroid, aortic aneurysm, pneumothorax, atelectasis, or fibrosis.
Observe the movement of the thyroid cartilage. Ask the client to swallow a small sip of water.	The thyroid cartilage and the cricoid cartilage move upward symmetrically as the client swallows.	Asymmetric movement or generalized enlargement of the thyroid gland is considered abnormal.
Palpate the thyroid by standing behind the client and asking him to lower the chin to the chest and turn the neck slightly to the right. This will relax client's neck muscles. Place your thumbs on the nape of the client's neck with your other fingers on either side of the trachea below the cricoid cartilage.		

ASSESSMENT PROCEDURE	NORMAL FINDINGS	ABNORMAL FINDINGS
Use your left fingers to push the trachea to the right. Then use your right fingers to feel deeply in front of the sternomastoid muscle (Fig. 11-6). Repeat on the opposite side. You may offer the client a sip of water to assist with swallowing. Note the position, landmarks, and characteristics as you palpate.		

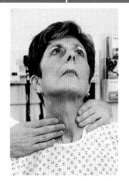

FIGURE 11-6 Palpating the thyroid.

• Position	• Usually not palpable. However, isthmus may be palpated in midline. Ability to see or palpate the thyroid varies considerably with client's thyroid size and body build.	• Deviates from the midline if obscured by masses or growths.

Continued on following page

TRACHEA, THYROID, AND LYMPH NODE PALPATION (Continued)

ASSESSMENT PROCEDURE	NORMAL FINDINGS	ABNORMAL FINDINGS
• Characteristics, landmarks	Glandular thyroid tissue may be felt rising underneath your fingers. Lobes should feel smooth, rubbery, firm, nontender, and free of nodules. The right lobe is often 25% larger than the left lobe.	• Enlarged lobes, irregular consistency, tender on palpation. Diffuse enlargement is seen in hyperthyroidism, Graves disease, or endemic goiter; rapid enlargement of a single nodule suggests malignancy. Diffuse enlargement of the thyroid gland
Auscultate the thyroid only if you find an enlarged thyroid gland during inspection or palpation. Place the bell of the stethoscope over the lateral lobes of the thyroid gland (Fig. 11-7). Ask the client to hold his breath (to obscure any tracheal breath sounds while you auscultate).	No bruits are auscultated.	A soft, blowing, swishing sound auscultated over the thyroid lobes is often heard in hyperthyroidism because of an increase in blood flow through the thyroid arteries.

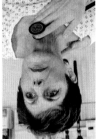

FIGURE 11-7 Auscultating for bruits over the thyroid gland.

ASSESSMENT PROCEDURE	NORMAL FINDINGS	ABNORMAL FINDINGS

Palpate the **cervical lymph nodes** (Fig. 11-8 for location) for the following:

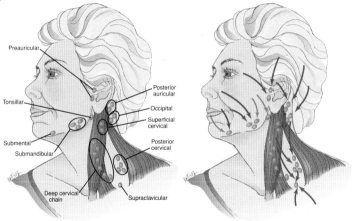

FIGURE 11-8 Left: Lymph nodes in the neck. **Right:** Direction of lymph flow. *Note:* Lymph nodes (represented by green dots) that are covered by hair may be palpated in the scalp under the hair.

Continued on following page

TRACHEA, THYROID, AND LYMPH NODE PALPATION (Continued)

ASSESSMENT PROCEDURE	NORMAL FINDINGS	ABNORMAL FINDINGS
• Size and shape	• Cervical lymph nodes are usually not palpable. If palpable, they should be 1 cm or less and round.	• Enlarged nodes with irregular borders. Enlarged nodes greater than 1 cm are seen in acute or chronic infection, autoimmune disorders, or metastatic disease; hard, fixed, enlarged, unilateral nodes seen in metastasis; tender, enlarged nodes seen in acute infections; enlarged occipital nodes seen in HIV infection.
• Delineation	• Discrete	• Confluent
• Mobility	• Mobile	• Fixed to tissue
• Consistency	• Soft	• Hard, firm
• Tenderness	• Nontender	• Client verbalizes pain on palpation.

🐎 PEDIATRIC VARIATIONS

ASSESSMENT PROCEDURE	NORMAL FINDINGS	ABNORMAL FINDINGS
Observe **head shape, size** (see Appendix 8 for head circumference norms), **and symmetry.**	Normocephalic and symmetrical, features appropriate for size. Head may have odd shape due to molding during birth.	Uneven molding, asymmetrical masses, enlarged head. Hydrocephalus is seen with increased cerebrospinal fluid. Microcephaly is a head circumference less than normal.

ASSESSMENT PROCEDURE	NORMAL FINDINGS	ABNORMAL FINDINGS
Observe **head control**.	Holds head erect in midline by 4 months; moves head up and down, side to side.	Resistance to movement (head lag after 6 months seen with cerebral injury).
Palpate **skull and fontanelles** very gently when infant is quiet in sitting position.	Smooth, fused except for fontanelles. Immediately following birth, edema crossing suture lines is normal (caput succedaneum). Edema not crossing the suture line indicates cephalohematoma.	Ecchymotic areas on scalp; loss of hair in spots; posterior fontanelle (triangular) open after 2 months of age, anterior fontanelle open after 12–18 months of age. Bulging fontanelle is seen in increased intracranial pressure; depressed fontanelles seen in dehydration or malnutrition; delayed fusion of fontanelles seen with hydrocephalus, Down syndrome, hypothyroidism, or rickets; third fontanel seen in Down syndrome; limited ROM seen in torticollis (wryneck).
Palpate the **neck** for lymph nodes.	Moderate number of small (>3 mm), shotty, firm lymph nodes in child (age 3–12 years).	Diffuse large lymph nodes, asymmetrical placement. Enlarging supraclavicular lymph nodes are seen with Hodgkin disease.

POSSIBLE COLLABORATIVE PROBLEMS—RISK OF

- Lymphedema
- Hypercalcemia
- Hypocalcemia

GERIATRIC VARIATIONS

- Lower face may shrink and the mouth may be drawn inward as a result of resorption of mandibular bone.
- Bones of face and nose are more angular in appearance.
- Facial wrinkles are prominent because subcutaneous fat decreases with age.
- Muscle atrophy and loss of fat cause shortening of neck.
- Strength of the pulsation of the temporal artery may be decreased.
- Cervical curvature may increase because of kyphosis of the spine.
- Fat may accumulate around the cervical vertebrae (especially in women) and is referred to as a "dowager's hump."
- Decreased flexion, extension, lateral bending, and rotation of the neck due to arthritis.
- Thyroid may feel more nodular or irregular because of fibrotic changes and may be felt lower in neck because of age-related structural changes.

Teaching Tips for Selected Nursing Diagnoses

Nursing Diagnosis: *Risk for Injury to Head and Neck related to poor posture*

Teach correct posture and body mechanics for sitting, lifting, and pushing.

Nursing Diagnosis: *Risk for Injury to Head and Neck related to not wearing protective devices (e.g., head gear during contact sports, seat belts, eye goggles)*

Teach risk reduction tips:
- Use safe driving techniques.
- Wear protective gear such as helmets and seat belts, especially when riding a bicycle or motorcycle.
- Avoid violent or potentially violent environments when possible.
- Modify one's residence to prevent falls.
- Avoid dangerous contact sports likely to cause brain injury; wear protective equipment when engaging in such activity.

Nursing Diagnosis: *Risk for Injury related to open fontanelles*

Teach parents normal development of fontanelles and how to protect infants from pressure and injury.

 Nursing Diagnosis: *Ineffective Health Maintenance related to a knowledge deficit on the effects of smokeless tobacco*

Teach that "dipping snuff" increases the risk of oral cancer, leukoplakia, receding gums, bone loss around roots of teeth, tooth loss, stained teeth, and bad breath (American Cancer Society, 2012e). Explain that this is *not* a healthy substitute for smoking cigarettes (Mayo Clinic, 2011).

 Nursing Diagnosis: *Risk for Injury to Teeth and Oral Mucous Membrane related to tongue piercing and wearing metal balls*

Teach risks of teeth chipping with tongue piercing. Explain that there is high risk of contacting hepatitis B virus and HIV when contaminated needles are used.

CHAPTER 12

Assessing Eyes

Structure and Function Overview

EXTERNAL STRUCTURES OF THE EYE

The *eyelids* (upper and lower) are two movable structures composed of skin and two types of muscle—striated and smooth (Fig. 12-1). The palpebral conjunctiva lines the inside of the eyelids, and the bulbar conjunctiva covers most of the anterior eye, merging with the cornea at the limbus.

The *lacrimal apparatus* consists of glands and ducts that serve to lubricate the eye (Fig. 12-2). The *lacrimal gland*, located in the upper outer corner of the orbital cavity just above the eye, is responsible for tear production. Tears are channeled into the *nasolacrimal sac*, through the *nasolacrimal duct*. They drain into the nasal meatus.

The *extraocular muscles* are the six muscles attached to the outer surface of each eyeball (Fig. 12-3).

INTERNAL STRUCTURES OF THE EYE

The eyeball is composed of three separate coats or layers (Fig. 12-4). The outermost layer consists of the *sclera* and *cornea*.

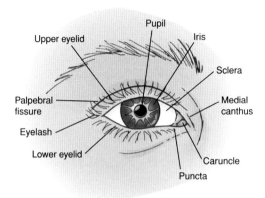

FIGURE 12-1 External structures of the eye.

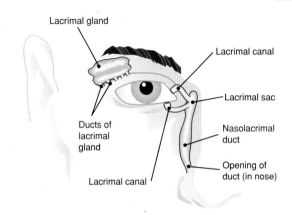

FIGURE 12-2 The lacrimal apparatus consists of tear (lacrimal) glands and ducts.

The *iris* is a circular disc of muscle that contains pigments that determine eye color. The central aperture of the iris is called the *pupil*.

The *lens* is a biconvex, transparent, avascular, encapsulated structure located immediately posterior to the iris.

The innermost layer, the *retina*, extends only to the ciliary body anteriorly and consists of numerous layers of nerve cells, including the cells commonly called rods and cones.

The *optic disc* is a cream-colored, circular area located on the retina toward the medial or nasal side of the eye (Fig. 12-5).

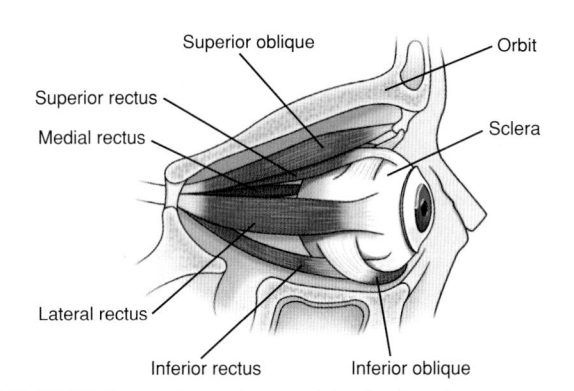

FIGURE 12-3 Extraocular muscles control the direction of eye movement.

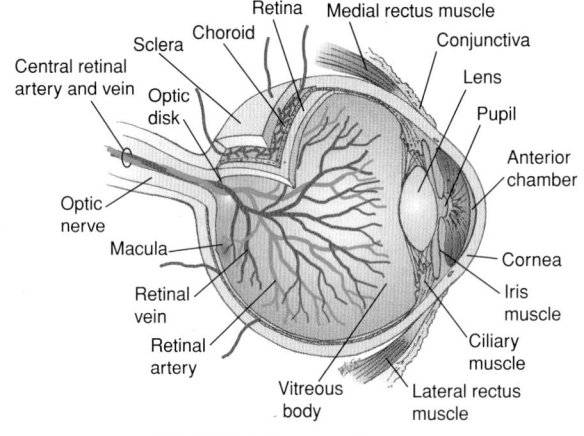

FIGURE 12-4 Anatomy of the eye.

A small circular area that appears slightly depressed is referred to as the *physiologic cup*.

The *retinal vessels* can be readily viewed with the aid of an ophthalmoscope. Four sets of *arterioles* and *venules* travel through the optic disc, bifurcate, and extend to the periphery of the fundus.

Vessels are dark red and grow progressively narrower as they extend out to the peripheral areas. A retinal depression known as the fovea centralis is located adjacent to the optic disc in the temporal section of the fundus (see Fig. 12-5). This area is surrounded by the macula, which appears darker than the rest of the fundus.

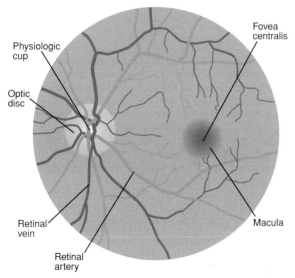

Physiologic cup

Optic disc

Retinal vein

Retinal artery

Fovea centralis

Macula

FIGURE 12-5 Normal ocular fundus.

VISION

A **visual field** refers to what a person sees with one eye. The visual field of each eye can be divided into four quadrants: Upper temporal, lower temporal, upper nasal, and lower nasal.

Visual perception occurs as light rays strike the retina, where they are transformed into nerve impulses, conducted to the brain through the optic nerve, and interpreted. In the eye, light must pass through transparent media (cornea, aqueous humor, lens, and vitreous body) before reaching the retina.

Visual Reflexes

The **pupillary light reflex** causes pupils to constrict when exposed to bright light. This can be seen as a *direct reflex*, in which constriction occurs in the eye exposed to the light, or as an *indirect or consensual reflex*, in which exposure to light in one eye results in constriction of the pupil in the opposite eye.

Accommodation is a functional reflex allowing the eyes to focus on near objects. This is accomplished through movement of the ciliary muscles causing an increase in the curvature of the lens, which is not visible. However, convergence of the eyes and constriction of the pupils can be seen.

Nursing Assessment

COLLECTING SUBJECTIVE DATA

Focus Questions

Recent changes in vision? (Spots? Floaters? Blind spots? Halos? Rings? Difficulty with night vision? Double vision? Blurred vision? Strabismus?) Use of Amsler grid? Eye pain? Redness or swelling? Eye discharge? Excessive watering or tearing? History of prior eye surgery? Trauma? Use of corrective glasses or contact lenses? Date of last eye exam? Eye care habits? (Use of sunglasses? Safety glasses? Work around chemicals, sparks, smokes, fumes, or dust?) Have visual changes affected work or ability to care for self? Typical 24-hour dietary recall? Use of vitamins or supplements (lutein, zeaxanthin, zinc, vitamin C, vitamin E, zinc and beta-carotene supplements)? Use of medications that may affect vision such as corticosteroids, lovastatin, pyridostigmine, quinidine, risperidone, and rifampin?

Risk Factors

Risk for glaucoma related to diabetes mellitus, myopia, age older than 75 years, hypothyroidism, eye injury or prolonged inflammation, prolonged steroid drop use, ethnic origin (African American, Mexican American, Asian American), or family history of glaucoma. Risk for cataracts related to increasing age, ultraviolet light exposure, excessive sunlight exposure, diabetes mellitus, hypertension, obesity, smoking, alcohol use, diet low in antioxidant vitamins, previous eye surgery, injury, prolonged inflammation, prolonged corticosteroid medication use in any form, exposure to ionizing radiation (e.g., x-rays), and family history.

COLLECTING OBJECTIVE DATA

Equipment Needed

- Eye chart (Snellen or handheld Rosenbaum)
- Near-vision chart or newsprint
- Amsler grid
- Cover card or occluder
- Penlight
- Ophthalmoscope (see Assessment Guide 12-1)
- Ruler
- Disposable gloves for eye drainage/exudate

Physical Assessment

Review Figures 12-1 to 12-5 for diagrams of the anatomy of the internal and external eye structures. Make sure the client is seated

ASSESSMENT GUIDE 12-1 Using the Ophthalmoscope

The examiner can rotate the lenses that are labeled with a negative or positive number. Red numbers indicate a negative diopter and are used for myopic (nearsighted) clients. Black numbers indicate a positive diopter and are used for hyperopic (farsighted) clients. The zero lens is used if neither the examiner nor the client has a refractive error.

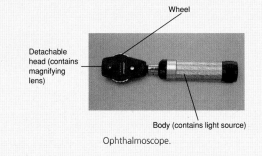

Wheel

Detachable head (contains magnifying lens)

Body (contains light source)

Ophthalmoscope.

1. Turn ophthalmoscope on and select the aperture with the large, round beam of white light.
2. Ask the client to remove glasses. Remove your glasses. Contact lenses can be left in the eyes of the client or examiner.
3. Ask the client to fix gaze on an object that is straight ahead and slightly upward.
4. Darken the room to allow pupils to dilate.
5. Hold the ophthalmoscope in your right hand with your index finger on the lens wheel and place the instrument to your right eye (braced between the eyebrow and the nose). Examine the client's right eye. Use your left hand and left eye to examine the client's left eye.
6. Begin about 25.4–38.1 cm (10–15 in) from the client at a 15° angle to the client's side.
7. Keep focused on the red reflex as you move in closer, and then rotate the diopter setting to see the optic disc.

comfortably in a well-lighted room that can be darkened for the ophthalmic examination. First, visual acuity, visual fields for peripheral vision, corneal light perception, eye alignment, extra-ocular muscle strength, and cranial nerve function are tested. Next, the external eye structures are assessed. Finally, the ophthalmic examination of internal eye structures is performed.

VISION TESTING

ASSESSMENT PROCEDURE	NORMAL FINDINGS	ABNORMAL FINDINGS
Check **visual acuity:**		
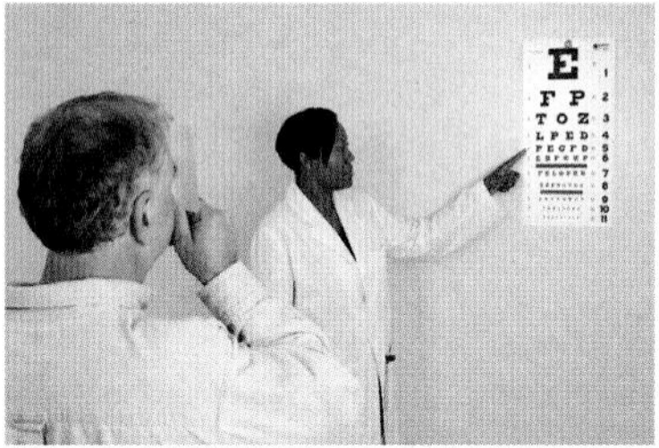 • Check **distance vision** with Snellen chart 609.6 cm (20 ft) from client (Fig. 12-6).	• 20/20 OD and OS with no hesitation, frowning, or squinting.	• Any letters missed on 20/20 line or above; client reads chart by leaning forward, with head tilted or squinting. *Myopia,* impaired far vision, occurs when second number is larger than first number (e.g., 20/40).
FIGURE 12-6 Checking distance vision.		
• Check **near vision** with newspaper approximately 35.6 cm (14 in) from client's head.	• Client reads print at 35.6 cm (14 in) without difficulty.	• Client reads print by holding it closer or farther away than 35.6 cm (14 in). *Presbyopia,* impaired near vision, is seen when client moves reading material farther away to read owing to decreased accommodation of lenses.

ASSESSMENT PROCEDURE	NORMAL FINDINGS	ABNORMAL FINDINGS
• Check **vision with Amsler chart** posted at eye level with client wearing their glasses, using bottom portion to view chart if they wear bifocals. Ask client to stand 30.5–35.6 cm (12–14 in) away from covering one eye. They should look at the center dot. Clients over the age of 45 years or with a family history of retinal problems, such as macular degeneration, should have eyes checked periodically (AMDF, 2012).	• No distortions, graying, blurring, or blank spots seen by client. No changes from prior baseline with Amsler chart as noted previously by primary health care provider.	• Mark areas of distortion, graying, blurring, or blank spots seen by client on his or her chart and notify the primary care provider. If client has already developed a baseline with distortions that their primary care provider is aware of, then report any changes from their baseline to their primary care provider.
• Check **peripheral vision** (Fig. 12-7): Face client at a distance of 61.0–91.4 cm (2–3 ft); client and examiner look directly ahead and cover eye directly opposite each other. Extend your arm and bring in one to two fingers and ask client if they see one or two fingers. Repeat this in all four visual fields (inferior, superior, nasal, and temporal)	• Client and examiner report seeing object at the same time as it approaches from the periphery.	• With reduced peripheral vision, client does not report seeing object at the same time as the examiner.

Continued on following page

ASSESSMENT PROCEDURE	NORMAL FINDINGS	ABNORMAL FINDINGS
FIGURE 12-7 Checking peripheral vision.		

EXTRAOCULAR MUSCLE FUNCTION TESTING

• Check **corneal light reflex** by asking the client to look straight ahead and then shining light toward facial midline.	• Reflections of light noted at same location on both eyes	• Light reflections noted at different areas on both eyes occur with deviation in alignment of eyes due to muscle weakness or paralysis (see Abnormal Findings 12-1 on page 257). • *Strabismus* is constant malalignment of eyes. • *Tropia* is a specific type of misalignment; *esotropia* is an inward turn of the eye, and *exotropia* is an outward turn of the eye.

ASSESSMENT PROCEDURE	NORMAL FINDINGS	ABNORMAL FINDINGS
• Check for **abnormal eye movement** using cover/uncover test (Fig. 12-8). This test detects deviation in alignment or strength and slight deviations in eye movement by interrupting the fusion reflex that normally keeps the eyes parallel. Ask client to look straight ahead, covering one eye with a cover card, and observe uncovered eye for movement. Now remove the cover card and observe the previously covered eye for any movement. Repeat the test on the opposite eye.	• Uncovered eye does not move when opposite eye is covered. • Covered eye does not move as cover is removed. 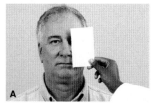 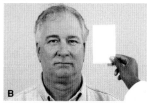 **FIGURE 12-8** Performing the cover/uncover test.	• Uncovered eye moves to focus when the opposite eye is covered. Covered eye moves to focus when cover is removed. These findings are seen with eye muscle weakness and deviation in alignment of eyes. • *Phoria* is a term used to describe misalignment that occurs only when fusion reflex is blocked (see Abnormal Findings 12-1 on pages 258 and 259).

Continued on following page

EXTRAOCULAR MUSCLE FUNCTION TESTING (Continued)

ASSESSMENT PROCEDURE	NORMAL FINDINGS	ABNORMAL FINDINGS
• Check extraocular movements by performing the position test (Fig. 12-9): Ask client to focus on an object that you are holding. Instruct the client to follow its movement through the six cardinal fields of gaze. Observe the client's eye movements.	• Both eyes move in a smooth, coordinated manner in all directions.	• Jerky eye movements (nystagmus) are seen with inner ear disorders, multiple sclerosis, brain lesions, or narcotics use; failure to follow object with one or both eyes indicate muscle weakness or cranial nerve dysfunction.

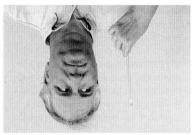

FIGURE 12-9 Checking extraocular movements.

EXTERNAL EYE STRUCTURES

ASSESSMENT PROCEDURE	NORMAL FINDINGS	ABNORMAL FINDINGS
Inspect **eyelids and lashes** (see Fig. 12-1 on page 239) for the following: • Position and appearance	• Lid margins moist and pink; lashes short, evenly spaced, and curled outward; lower margins at bottom edge of iris; upper margins of lid cover approximately 2 mm of iris.	Crusting, scales; lashes absent or curled inward; edema or xanthelasma present; itching; ulcerative lesions; asymmetry of lids; weak muscles. See Abnormal Findings 12-2 for illustrations of the following: • *Ectropion:* Lower lids turn outward • *Chalazion:* Inflammation of meibomian glands • *Hordeolum:* Stye or inflammation of glands in lid • *Entropion:* Lower lids turn inward • *Blepharitis:* Waxy, white scales (seborrheic) or inflammation of hair follicles (*Staphylococcus*) • *Ptosis:* Drooping of lids; seen with oculomotor nerve damage, myasthenia gravis. Protrusion of eyeballs with retracted lids seen with hyperthyroidism

Continued on following page

EXTERNAL EYE STRUCTURES (Continued)

ASSESSMENT PROCEDURE	NORMAL FINDINGS	ABNORMAL FINDINGS
• Inspect **conjunctiva** (bulbar and palpebral) and **sclera** for clarity and appearance by asking the client to keep the head still while looking up, down, and to either side. An object may be moved up, down, and to either side to guide the client's eye movements (Fig. 12-10).	• Blinking symmetrical, involuntary, at approximately 15 blinks/min	• Asymmetrical blink, incomplete closure, rapid blinking
• Blinking	• Bulbar conjunctiva is clear with tiny vessels visible; palpebral conjunctiva is pink with no discharge; sclera is blue-white.	• Lesions, nodules, discharge, crusting, or foreign body present. Marked redness of the conjunctiva is seen with conjunctivitis (see Abnormal Findings 12-2 on pages 258 and 259). Sclera with petechiae; marked jaundice.

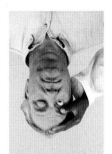

FIGURE 12-10 Inspecting the conjunctiva.

ASSESSMENT PROCEDURE	NORMAL FINDINGS	ABNORMAL FINDINGS
• Inspect **cornea** (using oblique lighting) for appearance.	• Transparent, smooth, moist	• Lesions, opacities, irregular light reflections, or foreign body present. Rough or dry cornea is seen with trauma or allergic responses.
Inspect **iris and pupil** for the following: • Shape	• Round	• Irregular. Miosis is constricted, fixed pupils; mydriasis (see Abnormal Findings 12-2 on pages 258 and 259).
• Color (iris) • Equality	• Uniform color • Equal in size (3–5 mm). • An inequality in pupil size of less than 0.5 mm occurs in 20% of clients. This condition, called anisocoria, is normal.	• Inconsistent color • Unequal; if the difference in pupil size (anisocoria) changes throughout pupillary response tests, the inequality of size is abnormal (see Abnormal Findings 12-2 on pages 258 and 259).
Test **pupillary reaction to light** by performing the following tests: Check **direct pupil response** by asking the client to look straight ahead and approaching each eye from the client's side with a penlight (Fig. 12-11). Observe the pupillary reaction.	• Illuminated pupils constrict.	• Illuminated pupils fail to constrict.

Continued on following page

EXTERNAL EYE STRUCTURES (Continued)

ASSESSMENT PROCEDURE	NORMAL FINDINGS	ABNORMAL FINDINGS
Check **consensual pupil response** by asking the client to look straight ahead and approaching each eye from the client's side with a penlight. Observe the pupillary reaction in the opposite eye.	• Pupil opposite the one illuminated constricts simultaneously.	• Pupil opposite the one illuminated fails to constrict; monocular blindness is seen when light directed to blind eye results in no response in either pupil.
Check **accommodation** (Fig. 12-12): Ask client to stare at an object 91.4–122 cm (3–4 ft) away, and move object in toward client's nose.	• Pupils converge and constrict as object moves in toward the nose; pupil responses are uniform.	• Pupils do not converge or constrict. Pupil responses are unequal.

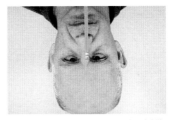

FIGURE 12-12 Checking accommodation of pupils.

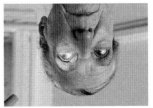

FIGURE 12-11 Observe the pupils with a pen-light or similar device, test pupillary reaction to light (Photo by B. Proud).

ASSESSMENT PROCEDURE	NORMAL FINDINGS	ABNORMAL FINDINGS
Inspect **lens** for clarity.	• Clear	• Cloudy; opacities are seen with cataracts.
Inspect and palpate **lacrimal apparatus** (Fig. 12-13) for the following:		

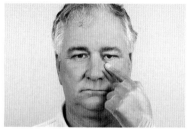

FIGURE 12-13 Palpating the lacrimal apparatus.

• Appearance	• Puncta (small elevations on the nasal side of the upper and lower lids), mucosa pink	• Puncta markedly reddened and edematous with infection, blockage, or inflammation
• Response to pressure applied at nasal side of lower orbital rim	• No tenderness or discharge noted when pressure is applied	• Fluid or purulent discharge expressed with pain on palpation with duct blockage

OPHTHALMIC EXAMINATION OF INTERNAL EYE STRUCTURES

ASSESSMENT PROCEDURE	NORMAL FINDINGS	ABNORMAL FINDINGS
(See Assessment Guide 12-1 Guidelines for Using the Ophthalmoscope.) • Inspect **red reflex** for shape and color (Fig. 12-14).	• Red reflex is round, bright, with red-orange glow	• Red reflex has decreased color or abnormal shape; dark spots are seen with cataracts. • Nuclear cataracts appear gray when seen with a flashlight; they appear as a black spot against the red reflex when seen through an ophthalmoscope.

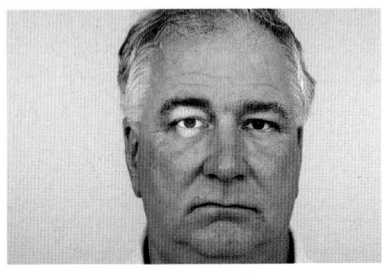

FIGURE 12-14 Inspecting the red reflex.

ASSESSMENT PROCEDURE	NORMAL FINDINGS	ABNORMAL FINDINGS
Inspect **optic disc** (see Fig. 12-5) for the following: • Shape 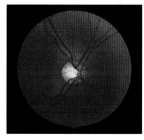	• Round or slightly oval disc with sharply defined margins (Fig. 12-15) **FIGURE 12-15** Normal ocular fundus (also called the optic disc).	• Irregularly shaped disc, blurred margins. A swollen disc with blurred margins is papilledema and is seen with hypertension or increased intracranial pressure (see Abnormal Findings 12-3 on page 260). Optic atrophy is a white-colored disc without vessels and is seen with the death of optic nerves.
• Color • Size • Physiologic cup	• Creamy pink (lighter than retina) • Approximately 1.5 mm size, symmetrical in both eyes • Small area is noted as paler than disc located just temporal of center of disc; occupies $^4/_{10}$–$^5/_{10}$ of the diameter of the disc.	• Pallor of entire disc or one section • Size of disc not equal in both eyes • Cup location and size are not symmetrical in both eyes; cup occupies more than $^5/_{10}$ diameter of the disc. • Enlarged physiologic cup seen in glaucoma (see Abnormal Findings 12-3 on page 260)

Continued on following page

OPHTHALMIC EXAMINATION OF INTERNAL EYE STRUCTURES (Continued)

ASSESSMENT PROCEDURE	NORMAL FINDINGS	ABNORMAL FINDINGS
Inspect **retinal vessels** for the following:		
• Appearance	• *Arteries:* Light red and smaller than veins • *Veins:* Darker in color and larger than arteries	• Arteries less than ³/₅ size of veins; arteries pale • Arterioles widen and have copper color in hypertension; with long-standing hypertension arterioles have silver color. • Vessels irregular in shape and uneven in distribution, narrowing of underlying vessels at crossings of arteries and veins; abnormal arteriovenous crossings are seen with hypertension and arteriosclerosis. • Pallor of the fundus, soft or hard exudates (cotton–wool patches) seen in hypertension; red spots or streaks may be microaneurysms or hemorrhages (see Abnormal Findings 12-3).
• Distribution	• Vessels regular in shape and decreasing in size as they branch and move toward the periphery; crossing of arteries and veins show no changes in the diameter of the underlying vessel.	
• Inspect **retinal background** for appearance	• Fine texture with pink, uniform color	
• Inspect **macula** for appearance	• Darker than the remainder of retina; fovea seen as a tiny bright light in the center of macula.	• Abnormalities in color of vessels; lesions present. Clumped pigment is seen with detached retinas or injuries.

ABNORMAL FINDINGS **12-1** **Extraocular Muscle Function**

CORNEAL LIGHT REFLEX TEST ABNORMALITIES

Strabismus (or Tropia)

A constant malalignment of the eye axis, strabismus is defined according to the direction toward which the eye drifts and may cause amblyopia.

Esotropia (eye turns inward).

Exotropia (eye turns outward)

COVER/UNCOVER TEST ABNORMALITIES

Phoria (Mild Weakness)

Noticeable only with the cover test, phoria is less likely to cause amblyopia than strabismus. **Esophoria is an inward drift and exophoria an outward drift of the eye.**

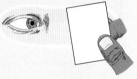

The uncovered eye is weaker; when the stronger eye is covered, the weaker eye moves to refocus.

Once the eye is uncovered, it will quickly move back to re-establish fixation.

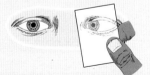

When the weaker eye is covered, it will drift to a relaxed position.

ABNORMAL FINDINGS 12-2 External Eye Examination: Deviations from Normal

Ectropion

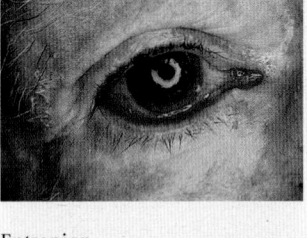

Chalazion

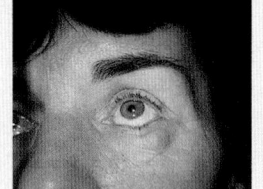

Hordeolum (stye)

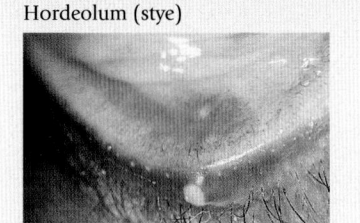

Entropion

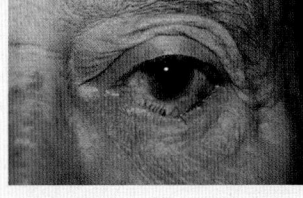

Blepharitis

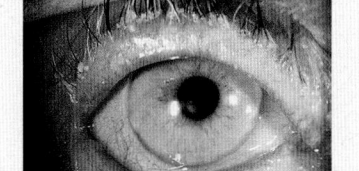

Ptosis

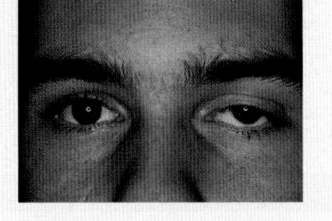

ABNORMAL FINDINGS 12-2 External Eye Examination: Deviations from Normal (Continued)

Conjunctivitis

(© 1995 Dr. P. Marazzi/Science Photo Library/ CMSP)

Cataracts

Miosis

Anisocoria

Mydriasis

| ABNORMAL FINDINGS | 12-3 | **Ophthalmoscope Examination: Deviations from Normal** |

| Papilledema | Glaucomatous cupping | Cotton–wool patches | Retinal hemorrhage |

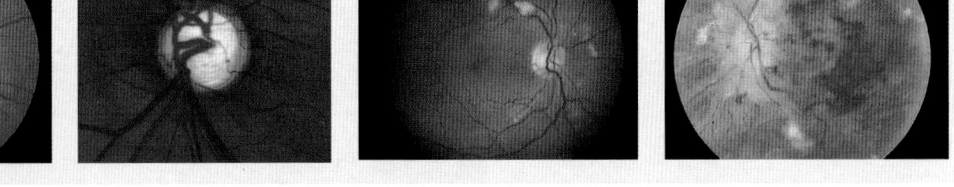

Source for Glaucomatous cupping: Tasman, W., & Jaeger, E. (Eds.). (2001). The Wills Eye Hospital atlas of clinical ophthalmology (2nd ed.). Philadelphia: Lippincott Williams & Wilkins.

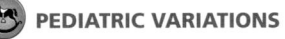 **PEDIATRIC VARIATIONS**

Explain procedure to decrease child's fear when room is darkened.

Assess cranial nerves III and IV (oculomotor and abducens) by evaluating extraocular muscle function in children by assess-ing the six cardinal positions of gaze. Test young children by having them follow a toy or an interesting object.

In older children, evaluate eye muscle strength by performing the Hirschberg test and the cover/uncover test.

ASSESSMENT PROCEDURE	NORMAL FINDINGS	ABNORMAL FINDINGS
Inspect **placement of light** on cornea (Hirschberg test).	• Light falls symmetrically within each pupil. *Note: Pseudostrabismus is considered normal in young children. The pupils will appear at the inner canthus due to the epicanthic fold.*	• Asymmetrical location of light reflection on pupil signals strabismus. The absence of the red reflex may indicate the presence of cataracts.
Measure **inner canthal distance**.	• Average distance 3 cm (1.2 in)	• Wide-set eyes, upward slant, and thick epicanthal folds may suggest Down syndrome.
Assess **palpebral slant**. FIGURE 12-16 Outer canthus is in alignment with the tip of the pinna (Photo by B. Proud).	• Outer canthus aligns with tips of pinna (except in Asian children) (Fig 12-16).	• Presence of upward slant in non-Asians • Upper lid that lies above iris ("setting-sun" sign) suggests hydrocephalus. • Black and white speckling of iris (Brushfield spots) seen in Down syndrome.

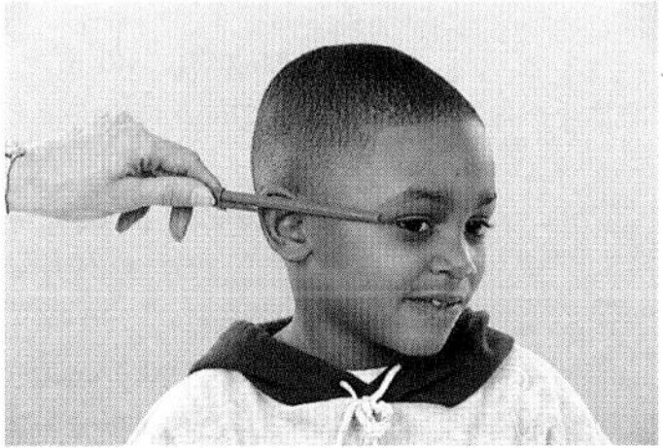

Continued on following page

ASSESSMENT PROCEDURE	NORMAL FINDINGS	ABNORMAL FINDINGS
Observe **placement of lids**.	• With eye open, lids lie between upper iris and pupil.	
• Inspect **iris**.	• Color varies from brown to green to blue.	
• Inspect **lacrimal apparatus**.	• Lacrimal meatus not present until 3 months of age	
• Perform **visual acuity tests**. Use E chart for preschoolers.	• Children can differentiate colors by the age of 5 years.	• A one-line difference indicates visual impairment and should be referred; may be due to congenital defects, chronic disease, or refractive errors.

OLDER ADULT VARIATIONS

Vision examination reveals the following:
- Presbyopia (decreased near vision due to decreased elasticity of lens) common in clients older than 45 years
- Poorer night vision and decreased tolerance to glare
- Decreased peripheral vision
- Difficulty in differentiating blues from greens

External eye examination reveals the following:
- Dry eyes due to decreased tear production
- Drooping eyelids (senile ptosis)
- Entropion and ectropion common in the older adult
- Conjunctiva thins and becomes yellowish
- Clouding of lens (cataracts)
- Yellowish nodules on bulbar conjunctiva (pinguecula) common
- White ring around iris (arcus senilis)—does not affect vision
- Slowed pupillary response and slowed accommodation

Ophthalmic examination reveals the following:
- Pale, narrowed arterioles

CULTURAL VARIATIONS

- Asians and members of some other groups may have common variation of epicanthal folds or narrowed palpebral fissures.
- Dark-skinned clients may have sclera with yellow or pigmented freckles.

POSSIBLE COLLABORATIVE PROBLEMS—RISK OF

Visual changes	Glaucoma
Eye infections	Impaired functioning of lacrimal apparatus
Cataracts	Corneal abrasions

Teaching Tips for Selected Nursing Diagnoses

Nursing Diagnosis: *Ineffective Health Maintenance related to lack of knowledge of necessity for eye examinations.*

Teach clients that a thorough eye examination every 2 years is recommended for healthy clients without risk factors between 18 and 60 years of age; annually for age 61 and older (AOA, 2006–2012). Clients at risk for eye problems should be examined annually or as recommended by their physician. Patients at risk include those:

- With diabetes, hypertension, or a family history of ocular disease (e.g., glaucoma, macular degeneration)
- Working in occupations that are highly demanding visually or eye hazardous
- Taking prescription or nonprescription drugs with ocular side effects
- Wearing contact lenses
- Who have had eye surgery
- With other health concerns or conditions

See Table 12-1 on page 264 for guidelines for clients with risk factors.

Nursing Diagnosis: *Ineffective Health Maintenance related to inadequate knowledge of eye infection care.*

Instruct client on proper administration of eye drops and ointments. Discuss proper cleansing from inner to outer canthus and changing of cleansing cloth to prevent cross-contamination (from eye to eye).

TABLE 12-1 Comprehensive Medical Eye Evaluation for Patients With Diabetes Mellitus or Risk Factors for Glaucoma

Condition/Risk Factor	Frequency of Evaluation*	
Diabetes Mellitus	Recommended Time of First Examination	Recommended Follow-up*
Type 1[1]	5 years after onset	Yearly
Type 2[2]	At time of diagnosis	Yearly
Prior to pregnancy[3-5] (Type 1 or 2)	Prior to conception and early in the first trimester	See Diabetic Retinopathy PPP[6] for interval recommendations based on findings at first examination

Condition/Risk Factor		
Risk Factors for Glaucoma[7-12]	Frequency of Evaluation*	
Age 65 or older	Every 6–12 months	
Age 55–64	Every 1–2 years	
Age 40–54	Every 1–3 years	

American Academy of Ophthalmology. (2010). *Comprehensive adult medical eye examination: Preferred practice guidelines.* Available at http://one.aao.org/CE/
PracticeGuidelines/PPP_Content.aspx?cid=64e9df91-dd10-4317-8142-6a87eee7f517.

IOP, intraocular pressure; NPDR, nonproliferative diabetic retinopathy.

*The ophthalmologist's assessment of degree of risk or abnormal findings may dictate more frequent follow-up examinations.

TABLE 12-1 **Comprehensive Medical Eye Evaluation for Patients With Diabetes Mellitus or Risk Factors for Glaucoma** (Continued)

References

[1]Klein R, Klein BE, Moss SE, et al. The Wisconsin epidemiologic study of diabetic retinopathy. II. Prevalence and risk of diabetic retinopathy when age at diagnosis is less than 30 years. *Arch Ophthalmol* 1984;102:520–6. [II+]

[2]Klein R, Klein BE, Moss SE, et al. The Wisconsin epidemiologic study of diabetic retinopathy. III. Prevalence and risk of diabetic retinopathy when age at diagnosis is 30 or more years. *Arch Ophthalmol* 1984;102:527–32. [II+]

[3]Klein BE, Moss SE, Klein R. Effect of pregnancy on progression of diabetic retinopathy. *Diabetes Care* 1990;13:34–40. [II+]

[4]Chew EY, Mills JL, Metzger BE, et al. Metabolic control and progression of retinopathy. The Diabetes in Early Pregnancy Study. *Diabetes Care* 1995;18:631–7. [II+]

[5]Diabetes Control and Complications Trial Research Group. Effect of pregnancy on microvascular complications in the Diabetes Control and Complications Trial. *Diabetes Care* 2000;23:1084–91. [II+]

[6]American Academy of Ophthalmology Retina Panel. *Preferred Practice Pattern Guidelines, Diabetic Retinopathy.* San Francisco, CA: American Academy of Ophthalmology; 2008. Available at www.aao.org/ppp.

[7]Friedman DS, Wolfs RC, O'Colmain BJ, et al. Prevalence of open-angle glaucoma among adults in the United States. *Arch Ophthalmol* 2004;122:532–8. [II++]

[8]Gordon MO, Beiser JA, Brandt JD, et al. The Ocular Hypertension Treatment Study: baseline factors that predict the onset of primary open-angle glaucoma. *Arch Ophthalmol* 2002;120:714–20; discussion 829–30. [I+]

[9]Kass MA, Gordon MO, Gao F, et al. Ocular Hypertension Treatment Study Group. Delaying treatment of ocular hypertension: the Ocular Hypertension Treatment Study. *Arch Ophthalmol* 2010;128:276–87. [I+]

[10]Kass MA, Heuer DK, Higginbotham EJ, et al. The Ocular Hypertension Treatment Study: a randomized trial determines that topical ocular hypotensive medication delays or prevents the onset of primary open-angle glaucoma. *Arch Ophthalmol* 2002;120:701–13; discussion 829–30. [I+]

[11]Quigley HA, West SK, Rodriguez J, et al. The prevalence of glaucoma in a population-based study of Hispanic subjects: Proyecto VER. *Arch Ophthalmol* 2001;119:1819–26. [II+]

[12]Varma R, Ying-Lai M, Francis BA, et al. Los Angeles Latino Eye Study Group. Prevalence of open-angle glaucoma and ocular hypertension in Latinos: the Los Angeles Latino Eye Study. *Ophthalmology* 2004;111:1439–48. [II+]

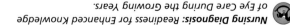

Nursing Diagnosis: *Readiness for Enhanced Knowledge of Eye Care During the Growing Years.*

Teach parents the following schedule for eye examinations:

Recommended Examination Frequency for the Pediatric Patient

Patient Age	Examination Interval	
	Asymptomatic/ Risk Free	At Risk
Birth to 24 months	At 6 months of age	By 6 months of age or as recommended
2–5 years	At 3 years of age	At 3 years of age or as recommended
6–18 years	Before first grade and every 2 years thereafter	Annually or as recommended

Children considered at risk for the development of eye and vision problems may need additional testing or more frequent re-evaluation. Factors placing an infant, toddler, or child at significant risk for visual impairment include (AOA, 2006–2012) the following:

- Prematurity, low birth weight, oxygen at birth, grade III or IV intraventricular hemorrhage
- Family history of retinoblastoma, congenital cataracts, or metabolic or genetic disease
- Infection of mother during pregnancy (e.g., rubella, toxoplasmosis, venereal disease, herpes, cytomegalovirus, or AIDS)
- Difficult or assisted labor, which may be associated with fetal distress or low Apgar scores
- High refractive error
- Strabismus
- Anisometropia
- Known or suspected central nervous system dysfunction evidenced by developmental delays

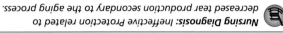

Nursing Diagnosis: *Ineffective Protection related to decreased tear production secondary to the aging process.*

Instruct client on the use of artificial tears as necessary.

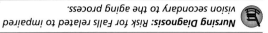

Nursing Diagnosis: *Risk for Falls related to impaired vision secondary to the aging process.*

Explore visual aids for independent living to assist client with visual loss (magnifying glasses, audio tapes, CDs, large-print books, special glasses for viewing television, large-numbered phones, large-print checks, cane).

Encourage further evaluation, if necessary. Instruct family to keep furniture in same place and to provide better lighting. Provide the following eye care guidelines: Adults aged 65 years or older with no risk factors should have an ophthalmologic eye examination every 1 to 2 years. To promote this goal, the National Eye Care Project is a nationwide outreach program sponsored by the American Academy of Ophthalmology as a public service. It is designed to help the disadvantaged elderly obtain medical eye care. The toll-free phone number is 1–800–222-EYES. To be eligible, a person must be a US citizen or legal resident, age 65 years or older, who does not have access to an ophthalmologist he or she may have seen in the past.

Instruct clients to wear sunglasses and hats in the sun. This is important because even on bright cloudy days, ultraviolet light can penetrate clouds. Squinting does not eliminate ultraviolet light entering the eye.

Explain that adults with diabetes mellitus should have an ophthalmologic eye examination at the time of diagnosis and yearly thereafter. Abnormal findings may require more frequent examinations.

Following are eye disorders commonly seen in older clients. Discuss symptoms of each with the client.

- Presbyopia (difficulty reading printed material)
- Floaters (moving specks or clouded vision)
- Cataracts (painless blurring of vision, glare or light sensitivity, poor night vision, double vision in one eye, needing brighter light to read, fading or yellowing of colors)
- Glaucoma (symptoms of glaucoma are not noticeable until damage has already occurred. Early diagnosis and treatment are keys to preventing blindness). Tonometry is used to measure pressure within the eye. Normal eye pressures range from 10 to 21 millimeters of mercury (mm Hg). Eye pressures greater than 22 mm Hg increases one's risk for developing glaucoma. However, people with normal eye pressure may develop **glaucoma** (AOA, 2011).
- Macular degeneration (words on a page look blurred in the center; straight lines look distorted, especially toward the center; a dark or empty area appears in the center of vision; colors look dim). Refer the client to the Macular Degeneration Partnership website http://www.amd.org/living-with-amd/resources-and-tools/31-amsler-grid.html to download the Amsler grid with directions to use to test for any visual changes.

CHAPTER 13

Assessing Ears

Structure and Function Overview

EXTERNAL STRUCTURES OF THE EAR

The external ear is composed of the auricle or pinna and the external auditory canal (Fig. 13-1). A translucent, pearly gray, concave membrane, the tympanic membrane (TM), or eardrum, serves as a partition stretched across the inner end of the auditory canal, separating it from the middle ear.

The distinct landmarks (Fig. 13-2) of the TM include the following:

- Handle and short process of the malleus
- Umbo
- Cone of light
- Pars flaccida
- Pars tensa

The middle ear, or tympanic cavity, is a small, air-filled chamber in the temporal bone. It is separated from the external ear by the eardrum and from the inner ear by a bony partition containing two openings, the round and oval windows. The middle ear contains three auditory ossides: The malleus, the incus, and the stapes (see Fig. 13-1).

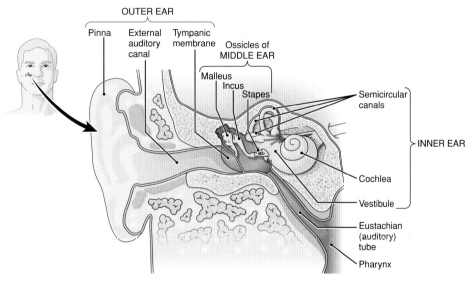

FIGURE 13-1 The ear. Structures in the outer, middle, and inner divisions are shown.

The inner ear, or labyrinth, is fluid filled and is made up of the bony labyrinth and an inner membranous labyrinth. The bony labyrinth has three parts: The cochlea, the vestibule, and the semicircular canals.

HEARING

The ears serve as sensory organs for hearing. Sound vibrations travelling through air are collected by and funneled through the external ear and cause the eardrum to vibrate. Sound waves are then transmitted through auditory ossicles as the vibration of the eardrum causes the malleus, the incus, and then the stapes to vibrate. As the stapes vibrates at the oval window, the sound waves are passed to the fluid in the inner ear. The movement of this fluid stimulates the hair cells of the spiral organ of Corti and initiates the nerve impulses that travel to the brain by way of the acoustic nerve.

Sounds waves are transmitted through

- the external and middle ear and referred to as "**Conductive hearing**." Conductive hearing loss is related to dysfunction of the external or middle ear (e.g., impacted ear wax, otitis

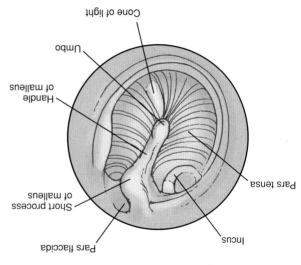

FIGURE 13-2 Right tympanic membrane.

Labels: Cone of light, Umbo, Handle of malleus, Short process of malleus, Pars flaccida, Incus, Pars tensa

media, foreign object, perforated eardrum, middle ear drainage, otosclerosis).

- the inner ear and referred to as **"Sensorineural hearing"** (or perceptive hearing). Sensorineural hearing loss is related to dysfunction of the inner ear (i.e., organ of Corti, cranial nerve VIII, temporal lobe of the brain).
- the skull bones also serve to augment usual sound waves through air, bone, and finally fluid. This pathway is less efficient than the conductive or sensorineural pathway.

Nursing Assessment

COLLECTING SUBJECTIVE DATA

Collecting subjective data consists of asking the client focus questions and assessing for risk factors.

Focus Questions

Recent changes in hearing? All or some sounds affected? Ear drainage? Type? Ear pain? Occurrence? Relief? Associated factors such as sore throat, sinus infection, or gum/teeth problems? Ringing or cracking in ears (tinnitus)? Dizziness, unbalanced, or spinning (vertigo)? Loss of high-frequency sounds? History of prior ear surgery? Trauma? Ear infections? Swimmer's ear? Sudden deafness? Use of ototoxic medications? Prolonged exposure to loud noises? Last hearing examination?

Risk Factors

Risk for hearing loss related to genetic predisposition, congenital anomalies, otitis media, fluid in inner ear, loud noises (especially prolonged exposure or short exposure to more than 110 dB), ototoxic medications, aging (presbycusis), trauma to eardrum, otosclerosis, viral inner ear infections, impacted cerumen, hypoxia during birth, or neonatal jaundice.

COLLECTING OBJECTIVE DATA

Equipment Needed

- Otoscope with good batteries (pneumatic bulb device for young children) (Assessment Guide 13-1)
- Tuning fork (512 and 1024 Hz)

ASSESSMENT GUIDE 13-1 Using an Otoscope to Inspect the External Canal and the Tympanic Membrane

1. Ask clients to sit comfortably with the back straight and the head tilted slightly away from you toward their opposite shoulder.

2. Choose the largest speculum that fits comfortably into the ear canal (usually 5 mm in the adult) and attach it to the otoscope. Hold otoscope in your dominant hand and turn the otoscope light to "on."

3. Use thumb and fingers of your opposite hand to grasp client's auricle firmly but gently. Pull out, up, and back to straighten the external auditory canal. Do not alter this position during the examination.

4. Grasp the otoscope handle between your thumb and fingers. Hold otoscope up or down, whichever is comfortable for you. If you hold the otoscope down, steady your hand holding the otoscope against the client's head or face.

5. Insert the speculum gently down and forward into the ear canal (approximately 1.27 cm [0.5 in]). Be careful not to touch the inner portion of the sensitive canal wall.

6. Position your eye against the lens.

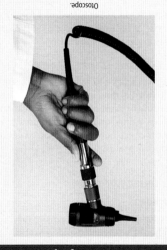

Otoscope.

Physical Assessment

Review Figures 13-1 to 13-2 for the anatomy of the external, middle, and inner ear.

Make sure the client is seated comfortably in such a way that you can easily visualize both ears. First examine the external ear, then examine the ear canal and TM with the otoscope, and finally assess hearing function.

ASSESSMENT PROCEDURE	NORMAL FINDINGS	ABNORMAL FINDINGS
Inspect **external ear** (Fig. 13-3) for the following: 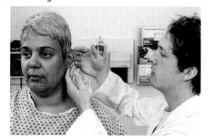 **FIGURE 13-3** Inspecting the external ear.		
• Size and shape	• Ears of equal size and similar appearance	• Ears of unequal size or configuration (smaller than 4 cm or larger than 10 cm)

Continued on following page

ASSESSMENT PROCEDURE	NORMAL FINDINGS	ABNORMAL FINDINGS
• Position	• Alignment of pinna with corner of eye and within 10° angle of vertical position	• Pinna positioned below a line from corner of eye, or unequal alignment. Malaligned or low-set ears are seen with chromosomal defects or genitourinary disorders.
• Lesions and discolorations	Skin smooth and without nodules; pink color	• Erythema, edema, nodules, or areas of discoloration. Postauricular cysts are seen with blocked sebaceous glands; ulcerated crusted nodules may be malignant; pale-blue color seen in frostbite.
Palpate external ear (see Fig. 13-3)	Nontender auricle, tragus	Painful auricle or tragus associated with otitis externa or postauricular cyst. Tenderness behind ear is associated with otitis media.
Palpate mastoid process for the following:		
• Tenderness	• No tenderness or pain when palpated	• Pain on palpation of mastoid process with mastoiditis
• Temperature	• Warm	• Erythema
• Edema	• Mastoid process easily palpated	• Actual process difficult to palpate; ear displaced outward owing to edema

ASSESSMENT PROCEDURE	NORMAL FINDINGS	ABNORMAL FINDINGS
Inspect **auditory canal** using otoscope (see Assessment Guide 13-1) for the following:		
• Cerumen	• *Color:* Black, dark red, gray, or brown • *Consistency:* Waxy, flaky, soft, or hard • *Odor:* None	• Impacted cerumen (obstructs visualization of membrane); bloody purulent discharge is seen in otitis media with perforated eardrum; foul-smelling discharge associated with otitis externa or impacted foreign body (see Abnormal Findings 13-1 on page 278).
• Appearance	• Canal walls pink and uniform with TM visible	• Lesions, foreign body, erythema, or edema present in canal. Red, swollen canals are seen with otitis media; polyps or nonmalignant nodular swellings can block the view of the eardrum (see Abnormal Findings 13-1 on page 278).
• Tenderness	• Little or no discomfort on manipulation of pinna; inner two thirds of canal very tender if touched with speculum	• Moderate-to-severe pain when pinna is moved or otoscope speculum is inserted
Inspect **TM**, using otoscope (see Assessment Guide 13-1), for the following:		
• Color	• Little or no discomfort on manipulation of pinna; inner two thirds of canal very tender if touched with speculum	• Dull appearance: Blue (blood) or pink/red (inflammation). Red, bulging TM is seen with acute otitis media (see Abnormal Findings 13-2); yellow, bulging TM seen with serous otitis media; blue or dark color seen in trauma when there is blood behind the TM.

Continued on following page

ASSESSMENT PROCEDURE	NORMAL FINDINGS	ABNORMAL FINDINGS
• Consistency	• Intact; may show movement when swallowing	• *Perforations, scarring,* or immobility. White spots are seen with scarring of the TM (see Abnormal Findings 13-2 on page 279).
• Landmarks (see Fig. 13-2 on page 270)	• Cone of light, umbo, handle of malleus, and short process of malleus visualized	• Retracted TM accentuates landmarks; bulging TM partially occludes landmarks. Prominent landmarks indicate TM retraction due to negative pressure from obstructed eustachian tube, whereas obscured landmarks indicate thickened TM due to chronic otitis media.
Assess **auditory function** for the following:		
• Gross hearing ability: Whisper words 2.6–5.1 cm (1–2 ft) behind client; hold watch 2.5–5.1 cm (1–2 in) from client's ear.	• Client is able to hear whispered words from 2.6–5.1 cm (1–2 ft); able to hear watch tick from 2.5–5.1 cm (1–2 in).	• Client is unable to hear whispered words or watch tick; unequal response.
• Lateralization of sound—Weber test: Place activated tuning fork on center top of client's head (Fig. 13-4A).	• Vibration heard equally in both ears.	• Vibratory sound lateralized to poor ear in conductive loss and to good ear in sensorineural loss.

ASSESSMENT PROCEDURE	NORMAL FINDINGS	ABNORMAL FINDINGS
• Comparison of air conduction (AC) to bone conduction (BC)—Rinne test: Place tuning fork on mastoid process until no longer heard, and then move it to front of ear (Fig. 13-4B,C).	• AC ≥ BC (AC is twice as long as BC)	• BC ≥ AC: BC heard longer than or equal to AC in conductive loss; AC longer than, but not twice as long as, BC in sensorineural loss

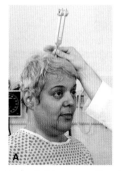 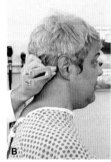 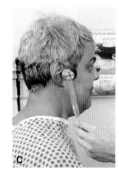

FIGURE 13-4 Using a tuning fork to assess auditory function. **A:** Weber test. **B:** Rinne test: Bone conduction. **C:** Rinne test: Air conduction.

Continued on following page

ASSESSMENT PROCEDURE	NORMAL FINDINGS	ABNORMAL FINDINGS
Perform **Romberg test for equilibrium** by having client stand with feet together first with eyes open, then with eyes closed (put your arms around client to prevent fall).	Client stands straight with minimal swaying.	Client sways and moves feet apart to prevent fall—may indicate vestibular disorder.

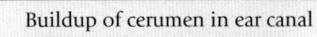

ABNORMAL FINDINGS   13-1   **Abnormal External Ear Findings**

Otitis externa

Buildup of cerumen in ear canal

Polyp

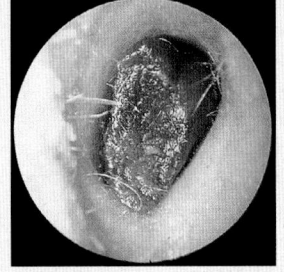

(© 1992 Science Photo Library/CMSP)

ABNORMAL FINDINGS **13-2** **Abnormal Tympanic Membrane Findings**

Acute otitis media

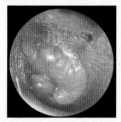

Perforated tympanic membrane

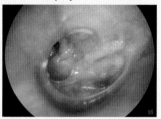

(© 1992 Science Photo Library/CMSP)

Scarred tympanic membrane

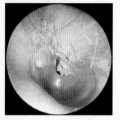

 PEDIATRIC VARIATIONS

- Impacted cerumen in the canal may impede visual examination of TM. Careful removal of wax with a curette may be performed.
- Irrigation of the external ear may also be attempted to remove cerumen with warm water. Never use hot or cold water.
- Scarring may be visible in children with a history of tympanostomy tubes.

- The TM should appear pink, shiny, and translucent allowing visualization of the bony landmarks. If child has been crying then the TM may appear red.
- Assess the TM for mobility by compressing a pneumatic insufflator bulb with a small puff of air. The healthy membrane should be mobile. Immobility of the TM may be caused by fluid or pus accumulation behind the TM, perforation of the TM, scarring or the presence of tympanostomy tubes.

PROCEDURE	NORMAL FINDINGS	ABNORMAL FINDINGS
Observe for placement and alignment of pinna.	Pinna slightly crosses the horizontal line (Fig. 13-5A), extends slightly forward from skull symmetrically.	Pinna falls below horizontal line (Fig. 13-5B); low ears with vertical alignment greater than 10° angle suggests mental retardation or congenital syndrome; abnormal shape indicates renal pathology.

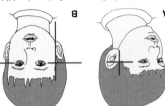

FIGURE 13-5 Placement and alignment of pinna in children. A: Normal.
B: Low-set ears with alignment greater than 10° angle.

Observe inner canal.

Note: For otoscope examination of infants and young children, restraint may be necessary to accomplish a safe, effe e ffe e assessment. In infants and young children, perform the otoscope examination last in the assessment because this part of the examination is often distressing to children in this age group.

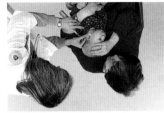

FIGURE 13-6 Infant being restrained in the upright position. (Photo by B. Proud).

PROCEDURE	NORMAL FINDINGS	ABNORMAL FINDINGS
Child younger than 3 years. Restrain; pull pinna downward and backward. *Children older than 3 years.* Pull pinna upward and backward.		
Inspect **TM** using otoscope with pneumatic device.	TM moves with introduction of air.	TM does not move with introduction of air.

GERIATRIC VARIATIONS

- Elongated lobule with linear wrinkles.
- Tuft of wire-like hair may be present at entrance of ear canal.
- More cerumen buildup; drier; harder cerumen due to rigid cilia in ear canal.
- Perception of consonants (Z, T, F, G) and high-frequency sounds (S, Sh, Ph, K) decreases.
- Dull, retracted TM—may be cloudy with more prominent landmarks owing to normal aging process.
- Diminished hearing acuity (presbycusis).

CULTURAL VARIATIONS

- Consistency and color of earwax varies. Dry, gray, flaky wax is usual in Asians and Native Americans. Wetter, light-honey to orange to dark-brown wax is most common in African Americans and Caucasians.

POSSIBLE COLLABORATIVE PROBLEMS—RISK OF

- Otitis media: Acute, chronic, serous otitis externa
- Perforated TM
- Hearing impairment

Teaching Tips for Selected Nursing Diagnoses

Nursing Diagnosis: Risk for Disordered Perception (auditory) related to working in loud, noisy environment.

Teach client to wear a protective hearing device when in an environment with loud noises (e.g., loud music, loud engines, aircraft, explosives, or firearms).

Teach client to recognize hearing loss by using the self-assessment tool in Box 13-1 to determine the need to seek medical evaluation if hearing loss is suspected.

Nursing Diagnosis: Risk for Injury related to decreased auditory perception.

Teach safety measures (e.g., burglar alarms, lights on telephone and alarms, phone designed for hearing impaired). Explore availability of resources for hearing aids, and refer client to reading materials or sign language learning if appropriate. Encourage client to ask others to repeat what is not heard.

Nursing Diagnosis: Readiness for Enhanced Self-health Management related to statements of desire to learn safe ear care.

Teach client to cleanse ears with damp cloth and to avoid use of cotton-tipped applicators for cleaning internal auditory canal. Encourage use of sunscreen on external ear. Teach client to shake head to remove water in ear and to dry ear after swimming to prevent swimmer's ear.

Nursing Diagnosis: Risk for Injury related to attempts to insert foreign objects in ear.

Teach parents and child (as appropriate for age) dangers of insertion of foreign objects in ear. Teach parents to avoid toys with small, removable parts. Also, teach parents to avoid putting infant to bed with bottle filled with formula, juices, or sugar water, because this can settle in the oral pharynx and provide medium for bacterial growth and cause middle ear infections. Encourage yearly ear screening with physical examination during growing years.

Nursing Diagnosis: Disordered Perception (auditory) related to aging process.

Advise caregivers and family to speak clearly, and allow client to see your lips. Speak within distance of 91.4–122 cm (3–6 ft).

BOX 13-1 TEN WAYS TO RECOGNIZE HEARING LOSS

The following questions will help you determine if you need to have your hearing evaluated by a medical professional:

Do you have a problem hearing over the telephone?	Yes ☐	No ☐
Do you have trouble following the conversation when two or more people are talking at the same time?	Yes ☐	No ☐
Do people complain that you turn the TV volume up too high?	Yes ☐	No ☐
Do you have to strain to understand conversation?	Yes ☐	No ☐
Do you have trouble hearing in a noisy background?	Yes ☐	No ☐
Do you find yourself asking people to repeat themselves?	Yes ☐	No ☐
Do many people you talk to seem to mumble (or not speak clearly)?	Yes ☐	No ☐
Do you misunderstand what others are saying and respond inappropriately?	Yes ☐	No ☐
Do you have trouble understanding the speech of women and children?	Yes ☐	No ☐
Do people get annoyed because you misunderstand what they say?	Yes ☐	No ☐

If you answered "yes" to three or more of these questions, you may want to see an otolaryngologist (an ear, nose, and throat specialist) or an audiologist for a hearing evaluation.

The material on this page is for general information only and is not intended for diagnostic or treatment purposes. A doctor or other health care professional must be consulted for diagnostic information and advice regarding treatment.

Excerpt from NIH Publication No. 01-4913

For more information, contact the **NIDCD Information Clearinghouse**.

The NIDCD Information Clearinghouse is a service of the National Institute on Deafness and Other Communication Disorders (NIDCD), National Institutes of Health (NIH), U.S. Department of Health and Human Services (HHS).

CHAPTER 14

Assessing Mouth, Throat, Nose, and Sinuses

Structure and Function Overview

The mouth or oral cavity is formed by the lips, cheeks, hard and soft palates, uvula, and the tongue and its muscles (Fig. 14-1). Contained within the mouth are the tongue, teeth, gums, and openings of the salivary glands (parotid, submandibular, and sublingual). The gums (gingiva) are covered by mucous membrane and normally hold 32 permanent teeth in the adult (Fig. 14-2).

Three pairs of salivary glands secrete saliva (watery, serous fluid containing salts, mucus, and salivary amylase) into the mouth (Fig. 14-3): The submandibular glands and the sublingual glands. The throat (pharynx), located behind the mouth and nose, serves as a muscular passage for food and air (see Fig. 14-4). The upper part of the throat is the nasopharynx. Below the nasopharynx lies the oropharynx, and below the oropharynx lies the laryngopharynx.

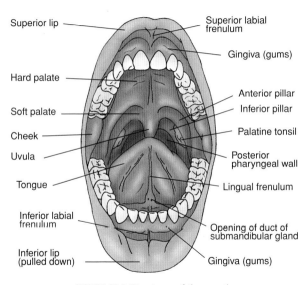

FIGURE 14-1 Structures of the mouth.

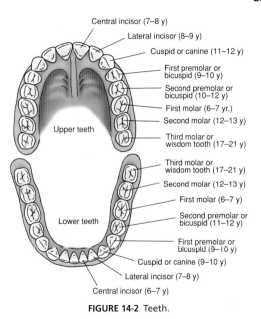

FIGURE 14-2 Teeth.

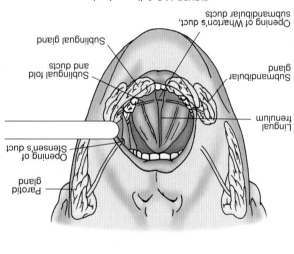

FIGURE 14-3 Salivary glands.

Sublingual gland

Sublingual fold and ducts

Opening of Wharton's duct, submandibular ducts

Submandibular gland

Lingual frenulum

Opening of Stensen's duct

Parotid gland

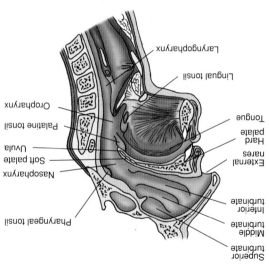

FIGURE 14-4 Nasal cavity and throat structures.

Laryngopharynx

Lingual tonsil

Oropharynx

Palatine tonsil

Uvula

Soft palate

Nasopharynx

Pharyngeal tonsil

Superior turbinate

Middle turbinate

Inferior turbinate

External nares

Hard palate

Tongue

The nose is composed of bone and cartilage covered with skin and an internal nasal cavity, lined with mucous membrane. The **external nose** consists of a bridge (upper portion), tip, and two oval openings called **nares**. The **nasal cavity** (Fig. 14-4) is located between the roof of the mouth and the cranium separated into halves by the nasal septum. The front of the nasal **septum** contains the Kiesselbach's area, a rich supply of blood vessels.

The superior, middle, and inferior **turbinates (conchae)** are bony lobes that project from the nasal cavity increase the surface area that is exposed to incoming air (see Fig. 14-4). As the person inspires air, nasal hairs (vibrissae) filter large particles from the air. Ciliated mucosal cells then capture and propel debris toward the throat, where it is swallowed. A meatus underlies each turbinate and receives drainage from the **paranasal sinuses** and the **nasolacrimal duct.**

Four pairs of **paranasal sinuses** (frontal, maxillary, ethmoidal, and sphenoidal) are located in the skull. The paranasal sinuses are lined with ciliated mucous membrane that traps debris and propels it toward the outside. The **frontal sinuses** (above the eyes) and the **maxillary sinuses** (in the upper jaw) are accessible to examiner whereas the **ethmoidal and sphenoidal sinuses** are smaller, located deeper in the skull, and not accessible for direct examination.

Nursing Assessment

COLLECTING SUBJECTIVE DATA

Focus Questions

Prior dental problems? Dentures? Lip or oral lesions? Redness or swelling (location, occurrence, relief)? Sore throat? Dysphagia? Hoarseness? History of mouth, nose, or throat cancer in family? Smoking or use of smokeless tobacco? Dental care practices? Brushing, flossing, dental checkups? Teeth grinding? History of braces? Nosebleeds? Change in ability to smell? Nasal drainage and character of drainage? Seasonal or other allergies? Use of nose sprays or allergy medications? Difficulty breathing through nostrils? Sinus pain? Past sinus infections (frequency)? Past oral, nasal, or sinus surgery? Trauma? Headaches located in sinus areas? Postnasal drip?

Risk Factors

Risk for oropharyngeal cancer related to smoking or use of smokeless tobacco; family history; alcoholism or heavy alcohol use; working with wood, nickel refining, or textile fibers; infection with certain human papillomavirus (HPV); poor oral hygiene; poor diet/nutrition (low in fruits, vegetables, vitamin A deficiency); and chewing betel nuts containing a mild stimulant that is popular in Asia.

COLLECTING OBJECTIVE DATA

Equipment Needed

- Penlight
- Tongue blade

ASSESSMENT GUIDE 14-1 Using Otoscope with Wide-tipped Attachment

- Use nondominant hand to stabilize and gently tilt the client's head back.
- Insert the short wide tip of the otoscope into the client's nostril without touching the sensitive nasal septum.
- Slowly direct the otoscope back and up.
- View the nasal mucosa, nasal septum, the inferior and middle turbinates, and the nasal passage (the narrow space between the septum and the turbinates).

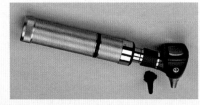

Otoscope with wide-tipped attachment.

- 4- × 4-inch gauze pad
- Clean gloves
- Nasal speculum or short, wide-tipped speculum attached to head of otoscope (Assessment Guide 14-1)

Physical Assessment

Review Figures 14-1 to 14-4 for diagrams of the mouth, oropharynx, and nose.

ASSESSMENT PROCEDURE	NORMAL FINDINGS	ABNORMAL FINDINGS
Mouth		
Inspect **mouth** for symmetry and alignment while asking client to open and close mouth (Fig. 14-5).	Lips and surrounding tissue relatively symmetrical in net position and with smiling. No lesions, swelling, drooping.	Asymmetrical mouth may indicate neurologic condition (e.g., Bell palsy, stroke), tumors, infections, or dental abnormalities or poorly fitting dentures.
	Upper teeth resting on top of lower teeth with upper incisors slightly overriding lower ones	Malocclusion of teeth, separation of individual teeth, or protrusion of upper or lower incisors
Wearing gloves, inspect and palpate **lips** for the following (Fig. 14-6): • Color	• *In white skin:* Pink • *In dark skin:* May have bluish hue or freckle-like pigmentation	• Cyanotic, pale lips in shock or anemia; reddish in ketoacidosis or carbon monoxide poisoning

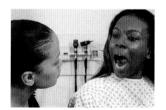

FIGURE 14-5 Inspecting the open mouth.

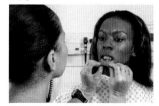

FIGURE 14-6 Palpating the lips.

Continued on following page

ASSESSMENT PROCEDURE	NORMAL FINDINGS	ABNORMAL FINDINGS
• Consistency	• Moist, smooth with no lesions	• Dry, cracked; nodules, fissures, or lesions present; cheilosis (cracking in the corners) seen in riboflavin deficiencies; broken vesicles with crusting in herpes simplex type I; scaly nodular lesions or ulcers occur with lip carcinoma (see Abnormal Findings 14-1 on page 299)
Note: Ask client to remove any dentures or dental appliances before continuing examination. Wearing gloves, inspect and palpate **buccal mucosa** for the following (Fig. 14-7):		
• Color	• Pink (increased pigmentation often noted in dark-skinned clients)	• Pale, cyanotic, or reddened mucosa

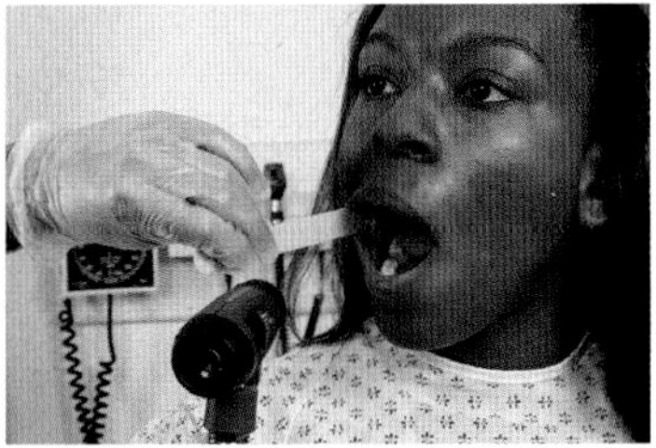

FIGURE 14-7 Inspecting the buccal mucosa.

ASSESSMENT PROCEDURE	NORMAL FINDINGS	ABNORMAL FINDINGS
	• Smooth, moist, without lesions	• Ulcers, dry mucosa, bleeding, or white patches are present. Thick, elevated white patches (leukoplakia) that do not scrape off are precancerous; white, curdy patches that scrape off and bleed indicate thrush; red spots over red mucosa (Koplik spots) indicate measles. Canker sores (painful vesicles that erupt) are seen with allergies and stress (see Abnormal Findings 14-1 on page 299).
• Landmarks	• Parotid duct (Stensen's duct) openings are seen as small papillae located near upper second molar	• Elevated, markedly reddened area near upper second molar
Wearing gloves, retract client's lips to inspect and palpate **gums** for the following:		
• Color	• Pink	• Pale, markedly reddened. Swollen gums that bleed are seen with gingivitis; recessed red gums with tooth loss seen with periodontitis (see Abnormal Findings 14-1); bluish black gum line present in lead poisoning.
• Consistency	• Moist, clearly defined margins	• Dry, edema, ulcers, bleeding, white patches, tenderness

Continued on following page

ASSESSMENT PROCEDURE	NORMAL FINDINGS	ABNORMAL FINDINGS
Wearing gloves, inspect and palpate **teeth** for the following:		
• Number (see Fig. 14-2)	• 32 teeth	• Missing teeth
• Position and condition	• Stable fixation, smooth surfaces, and edges	• Loose or broken teeth, jagged edges, dental caries
• Color	• Pearly white and shiny	• Darkened, brown, or chalky white discoloration. Teeth may be yellow-brown in clients who use excessive coffee, tea, tobacco, or fluoride. Chalky white area is seen with beginning cavity.
Inspect protruded **tongue** for the following:		
• Color, symmetry, and texture	• Pink, moist, papillae present; symmetrical appearance; midline fissures present	• Dry; nodules, ulcers present; papillae or fissures absent; asymmetrical. Deep fissures are seen in dehydration; black hairy tongue with use of some antibiotics; smooth, red, shiny tongue seen in niacin or vitamin B_{12} deficiency (see Abnormal Findings 14-1 on page 299)
	Common variations: Fissured, geographic tongue (Fig. 14-8)	

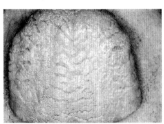

FIGURE 14-8 Fissured, geographic tongue.
(Courtesy of Dr. Michael Bennett.)

ASSESSMENT PROCEDURE	NORMAL FINDINGS	ABNORMAL FINDINGS
• Movement • Color	• Smooth • Pink	• Jerky or unilateral movement • Markedly reddened; white patches; pale
Inspect **ventral surface of the tongue and mouth floor** for the following: • Color, consistency, lesions	• Smooth, shiny, pink, or slightly pale with visible veins and no lesions. Slightly pale	• Markedly reddened, cyanotic, or extreme pallor, lesions
• Landmarks	• Submandibular duct openings (Wharton's ducts) are located on both sides of the frenulum. Tongue is free of lesions or increased redness; frenulum is centered (see Fig. 14-3).	• Lesions, ulcers, nodules, or hypertrophied duct openings are present on either side of the frenulum.
*Inspect and palpate **sides of tongue** for color and lesions (Fig. 14-9).*	Pink, smooth, moist; no lesions	White or reddened areas, ulcerations, or indurations present. Leukoplakia indicates precancerous lesions; may see canker sores (see Abnormal Findings 14-1).
*Inspect **hard and soft palate** (see Fig. 14-4) for the following:* • Color • Consistency	• Hard palate: Pale *Soft palate:* Pink *Hard palate:* Firm with irregular transverse rugae	• Extreme pallor, white patches, or markedly reddened areas

Continued on following page

ASSESSMENT PROCEDURE	NORMAL FINDINGS	ABNORMAL FINDINGS
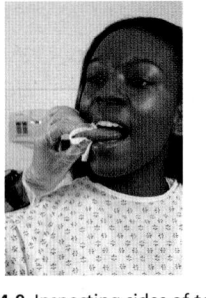 FIGURE 14-9 Inspecting sides of tongue.	*Common variation:* Palatine torus (bony protuberance) on hard palate (Fig. 14-10) *Soft palate:* Spongy texture with symmetrical elevation or phonation 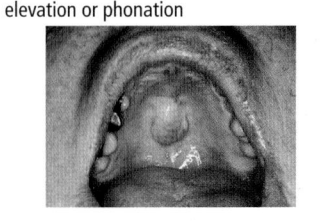 FIGURE 14-10 Torus palatinus.	• Softened tissue over hard palate; lesions present; absence of elevation; soft palate asymmetrical elevation with phonation. Thick, white plaques are seen in *Candida* infection; deep, purple lesions may indicate Kaposi sarcoma (see Abnormal Findings 14-1).
Throat		
Inspect **oropharynx** (see Fig. 14-11) for the following: • Color	• Pink	• Markedly reddened with exudate seen in pharyngitis; yellow mucus seen with postnasal sinus drainage.

ASSESSMENT PROCEDURE	NORMAL FINDINGS	ABNORMAL FINDINGS
• Landmarks 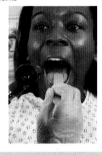	• Tonsillar pillars symmetrical; tonsils present (unless surgically removed) and without exudate; uvula at midline and rises on phonation	• Enlarged tonsils (tonsils are red, enlarged, and covered with exudate in tonsillitis); see tonsillitis grading scale in Abnormal Findings 14-2 on page 300; asymmetrical; uvula deviates from midline; edema, ulcers, lesions.

FIGURE 14-11 Inspecting oropharynx.

Nose

Inspect and palpate the **external nose**. Note nasal color, shape, consistency, and tenderness.	Color same as the rest of the face; smooth and symmetrical structure; no tenderness.	Nasal tenderness on palpation accompanies a local infection.
Check patency of air flow through the nostrils by occluding one nostril at a time and asking client to sniff.	Client is able to sniff through each nostril while other is occluded.	Client cannot sniff through a nostril that is occluded, nor can he or she sniff or blow air through the nostrils. May be a sign of swelling, rhinitis, or an obstructing foreign object.

Continued on following page

ASSESSMENT PROCEDURE	NORMAL FINDINGS	ABNORMAL FINDINGS
Inspect the internal nose using an otoscope with a short, wide-tipped attachment (or you can also use a nasal speculum and penlight) (Fig. 14-12). See Assessment Guide 14-1 on page 288.	Nasal mucosa dark pink, moist, and free of exudate. Nasal septum intact and free of ulcers or perforations. Turbinates dark pink, moist, and free of lesions (Fig. 14-13A).	Nasal mucosa swollen and pale pink or bluish gray in clients with allergies. Nasal mucosa red and swollen with upper respiratory infection. Exudate seen with infections. Purulent nasal discharge seen with acute bacterial rhinosinusitis. Bleeding (epistaxis) or crusting may be noted on lower anterior part of nasal septum with local irritation. Ulcers of the nasal mucosa or a perforated septum may be seen with the use of cocaine, trauma, chronic infection, or chronic nose picking. Small, pale, round, firm overgrowths or masses on mucosa (polyps) seen in clients with chronic allergies.

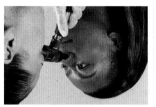

FIGURE 14-12 Inspecting the internal nose.

Note: The superior turbinate will not be visible from this point of view.

A deviated septum may appear to be an over-growth of tissue. This is a normal finding as long as breathing is not obstructed (Fig. 14-13B).

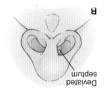

FIGURE 14-13 A: Normal internal nose. **B:** Deviated septum.

ASSESSMENT PROCEDURE	NORMAL FINDINGS	ABNORMAL FINDINGS
Sinuses		

Palpate the **sinuses.** When an infection is suspected, the nurse can examine the sinuses through palpation, percussion, and transillumination.

Palpate the **frontal sinuses** by using your thumbs to press up on the brow on each side of nose (Fig. 14-14A).

Palpate the **maxillary sinuses** by pressing with thumbs up on the maxillary sinuses (Fig. 14-14B).

Frontal and maxillary sinuses are nontender to palpation, and no crepitus is evident.

Frontal or maxillary sinuses are tender to palpation in clients with allergies or acute bacterial rhinosinusitis. If the client has a large amount of exudate, you may feel crepitus upon palpation over the maxillary sinuses.

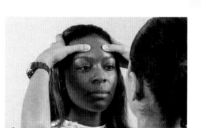 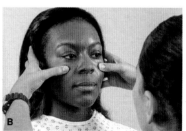

FIGURE 14-14 A: Palpating frontal sinuses. **B:** Palpating maxillary sinuses.

Continued on following page

ASSESSMENT PROCEDURE	NORMAL FINDINGS	ABNORMAL FINDINGS
Percuss the **sinuses**. Lightly tap (percuss) over the frontal sinuses and over the maxillary sinuses for tenderness.	The sinuses are not tender on percussion.	The frontal and maxillary sinuses are tender upon percussion in clients with allergies or sinus infection.
Transillumination		
Transilluminate the sinuses if sinus tenderness is present to detect the presence of fluid or pus. Transilluminate the frontal sinuses by holding light source snugly under the eyebrows. Use other hand to shield the light. Repeat for other frontal sinus. Transilluminate the maxillary sinuses by holding light over maxillary sinus and asking the client to open his or her mouth. Repeat for the other side.	A red glow transilluminates the frontal sinuses. This indicates a normal, air-filled sinus. A red glow transilluminates the maxillary sinuses. The red glow will be seen on the hard palate.	Absence of a red glow usually indicates a sinus filled with fluid or pus. Absence of a red glow usually indicates a sinus filled with fluid, pus, or thick mucus (from chronic sinusitis).

ABNORMAL FINDINGS **14-1** **Mouth and Throat Abnormalities**

Herpes simplex type I

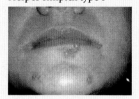

Carcinoma of lip

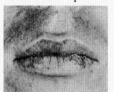

Canker sore

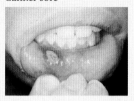

Receding gums (periodontitis).

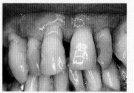

(Courtesy of Dr. Michael Bennett.)

Black hairy tongue.

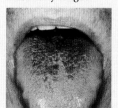

(Courtesy of Dr. Michael Bennett.)

Leukoplakia (ventral surface)

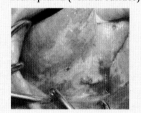

Candida albicans infection (thrush).

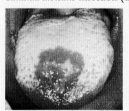

ABNORMAL FINDINGS | 14-2 | Detecting and Grading Tonsillitis

In a client who has both tonsils and a sore throat, tonsillitis can be identified and ranked with a grading scale from 1 to 4 as follows:

1. Tonsils are visible.
2. Tonsils are midway between tonsillar pillars and uvula.
3. Tonsils touch the uvula.
4. Tonsils touch each other.

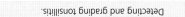

Detecting and grading tonsillitis.

PEDIATRIC VARIATIONS

Questions to ask the parents when collecting subjective data include the following.

- Number of teeth, time of eruptions?
- Thumb sucking, use of pacifier (type)?
- Sore throats?
- Use of bottle?
- Fluoridated water?

When collecting objective data note the following.

- Observe for eruption of deciduous teeth (Fig. 14-15).
- Observe for eruption of permanent teeth (see Fig. 14-2 on page 285).
- Inspect dental caries; may be due to bottle caries syndrome.
- **Note:** *A sucking pad inside upper lip of infant may be apparent due to sucking friction.*
- Tonsils reach adult size by the age of 6 years and continue to grow. By the age of 10 to 12 years, they are twice the adult size. By the end of adolescence they begin to atrophy back to normal adult size.

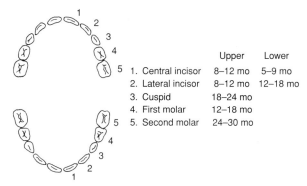

	Upper	Lower
1. Central incisor	8–12 mo	5–9 mo
2. Lateral incisor	8–12 mo	12–18 mo
3. Cuspid	18–24 mo	
4. First molar	12–18 mo	
5. Second molar	24–30 mo	

FIGURE 14-15 Timetable for eruption of deciduous teeth.

 GERIATRIC VARIATIONS

- Worn teeth, abraded enamel, and yellowing teeth
- Gums recede and undergo fibrotic changes.
- Poor fitting dentures may cause facial asymmetry and poor eating habits.
- Oral mucosa is drier owing to decreased production of saliva.

- Tongue may be fissured and have varicose veins on ventral surface.
- Decreased taste sensations due to a decrease in number of taste buds.
- Decreased sense of smell due to progressive atrophy of olfactory bulbs.

 CULTURAL VARIATIONS

- Dark-skinned clients may have lips with bluish hue or freckle-like pigmentation.
- Some groups have reduced teeth number; Australian aborigines have four extra molars.
- Dark-skinned clients may have dark pigment or freckling on side or ventral surface of tongue and floor of mouth; hard and soft palate may also be darkly pigmented.
- Females and groups such as Eskimos, Native Americans, and Asians are more likely to have a torus palatinus, a normal variation where there is a bony protuberance in the midline of the hard palate.
- Lip pits are seen in the crease between upper and lower lips in about 20% of African Americans and in some Asians and Caucasians.

Teaching Tips for Selected Nursing Diagnoses and Collaborative Problems

Nursing Diagnosis: Impaired Oral Mucous Membrane related to inadequate mouth care

Instruct client on proper brushing and flossing. (Client should brush teeth at least twice a day and floss once a day to remove plaque from under gum line and sides of teeth.)

Recommend a toothbrush with soft, rounded or polished bristles, to be replaced every 3 to 4 months or sooner when frayed.

POSSIBLE COLLABORATIVE PROBLEMS—RISK OF

- Stomatitis
- Gingivitis
- Oral lesions
- Periodontal (gum) disease (periodontitis)
- Nosebleed

- Some groups (especially Asians) may have mandibular torus (lump) on inner mandible near second premolar.
- Native Americans and Asians may have a split uvula.

---

in addition to an "American Dental Association—accepted" fluoride toothpaste and mouth rinse. Explain the role of fluoride in decreasing tooth decay. Refer to dentist for fluoride protection advice if client's water supply is not fluoridated. Explain the significance of a well-balanced diet in decreasing tooth decay and periodontal (gum) disease. Dry mouth can cause problems with oral health. Refer to dentist or physician for possible recommendation of artificial saliva or fluoride mouth rinse.

Collaborative Problem: Risk for Complication: Periodontal (gum) disease

Teach client warning signs:

- Gums that bleed with brushing
- Red, swollen, tender gums or gums that pull away from teeth
- Pus between teeth and gums
- Loose or separating teeth
- Change in position of teeth or denture fit
- Persistent bad breath

Teach prevention:

- Brush twice daily with soft toothbrush and fluoride toothpaste, and floss every day

- Replace toothbrush every 3 to 4 months, or sooner if bristles are frayed
- Eat a balanced diet and limit between-meal snacks
- Schedule regular dental visits (American Dental Association, 2012).

Collaborative Problem: *Risk for Complication: Oral cancer*

Teach client warning signs:
- Sore in mouth that does not heal
- White scaly patches in mouth
- Swelling or lumps in mouth/in throat/on lips
- Numbness or pain in mouth/in throat/on lips
- Repeated bleeding in mouth
- Difficulty chewing, swallowing, speaking, or moving tongue or jaw
- Change in bite

Teach client to:
- Stop smoking
- Limit alcohol consumption
- Eat a healthy, balanced diet, while limiting unhealthy snacks between meals

Teach client that there is no safe tobacco use:
- Spit tobacco (chewing tobacco) leads to gum inflammation, tooth loss, and oral cancer.
- Cigar smoking leads to mouth, throat, and lung cancer Healthy People 2020 (2013d).

Nursing Diagnosis: *Ineffective Health Maintenance related to a lack of information regarding over-the-counter nasal medications*

Instruct client on use, proper dosage, and effects of overuse of nasal sprays.

Collaborative Problem: *Risk for Complication: Nosebleed*

Instruct client to apply pressure for 5 minutes while breathing through mouth and leaning forward. Caution against blowing nose for several hours afterward. Refer as necessary.

 Nursing Diagnosis: *Impaired Dentition related to lack of proper mouth care*

Instruct parents not to put child to bed with a bottle filled with formula, milk, juices, or sugar water, because these liquids pool around teeth and promote tooth decay. Use only water in bottles when putting child to bed, to prevent so-called baby bottle tooth decay. Teach the importance of fluoride in drinking water and proper nutrition to prevent decay. Fluoride drops are recommended for infants and fluoride tablets for children up through the age of 14 years if adequate fluoride is not in water. Refer child who sucks thumb past years of age to the dentist. Explain the benefits of using a small, cool spoon rubbed over gums or using teething rings during teething period. Instruct parents to start brushing the child's teeth with eruption of first tooth. Begin flossing when primary teeth have erupted (2 to 2½ years). Teach parents to brush and floss child's teeth until child can be taught to do this alone (approximately at the age of 7 years for brushing and at the age of 10 years for flossing). Encourage a dental exam by a dentist when the child is between 6 and 12 months of age.

Nursing Diagnosis: *Risk for injury to teeth related to developmental age and play activities*

In case of broken or knocked-out tooth, instruct parents to rinse the tooth in cool water (do not scrub it); when possible, insert back in socket and hold in place. If this cannot be done, put tooth in cup of milk or water, or wrap it in wet cloth and take the child to dentist at once for possible replacement. Recommend use of mouth guards to prevent injuries in contact sports.

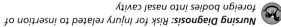

Nursing Diagnosis: *Risk for injury related to insertion of foreign bodies into nasal cavity*

Caution and give instructions to parents about child's interest in inserting objects into body openings such as the nose. Instruct on common objects to remove from child's reach.

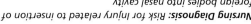

Nursing Diagnosis: *Imbalanced Nutrition: Less Than Body Requirements related to decreased appetite secondary to decreased senses of taste and smell*

Explore food preferences with client and use visual appeal of food to enhance appetite.

CHAPTER 15

Assessing Thorax and Lungs

Structure and Function Overview

THORAX

The term *thorax* identifies the portion of the body extending from the base of the neck superiorly to the level of the diaphragm inferiorly. This thoracic cage is constructed of the sternum, 12 pairs of ribs, 12 thoracic vertebrae, muscles, and cartilage. The thorax consists of the anterior thoracic cage (Fig. 15-1) and the posterior thoracic cage (Fig. 15-2).

The sternum, or breastbone, lies in the center of the chest anteriorly and is divided into three parts: The manubrium,

the body, and the xiphoid process. The clavicles (collar bones) extend from the manubrium to the acromion of the scapula. The manubrium connects laterally with the clavicles and the first two pairs of ribs. A U-shaped indentation located on the superior border of the manubrium is an important landmark known as the *suprasternal notch*. A few centimeters below the suprasternal notch, a bony ridge can be palpated at the point where the manubrium articulates with the body of the sternum. This landmark is referred to as the *sternal angle* (or angle of Louis).

Ribs (7 to 10) connect to the cartilages of the pair lying superior to them rather than to the sternum (see Fig. 15-1). This configuration forms an angle between the right and left costal margins meeting at the level of the xiphoid process, referred to as the *costal angle*.

Each pair of ribs articulates with its respective thoracic vertebra. The spinous process of the seventh cervical vertebra (C7), also called the *vertebra prominens*, can be easily felt with the client's neck flexed. The lower tip of each scapula is at the level of the seventh or eighth rib when the client's arms are at his or her side (see Fig. 15-2).

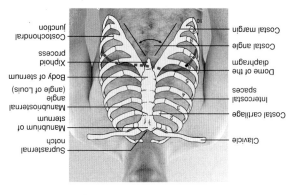

FIGURE 15-1 Anterior thoracic cage.

To describe a location around the circumference of the chest wall, imaginary lines running vertically on the chest wall are used. On the anterior chest, these lines are known as the *midsternal line* and the *right and left midclavicular lines* (Fig. 15-3A).

The posterior thorax includes the vertebral (or spinal) line and the right and left scapular lines, which extend through the

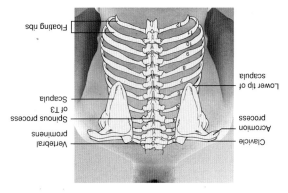

FIGURE 15-2 Posterior thoracic cage.

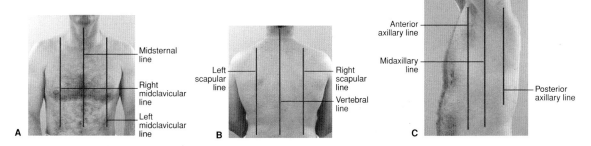

FIGURE 15-3 A: Anterior vertical lines, imaginary landmarks. **B:** Posterior vertical lines, imaginary landmarks. **C:** Lateral vertical lines, imaginary landmarks.

inferior angle of the scapulae when the arms are at the client's side (Fig. 15-3B).

The lateral aspect of the thorax is divided into three parallel lines. The *midaxillary line* runs from the apex of the axillae to the level of the twelfth rib. The *anterior axillary line* extends from the anterior axillary fold along the anterolateral aspect of the thorax, whereas the *posterior axillary line* runs from the posterior axillary fold down the posterolateral aspect of the chest wall (Fig. 15-3C).

THORACIC CAVITY

The thoracic cavity consists of the mediastinum and the lungs.

The lungs are two cone-shaped, elastic structures suspended within the thoracic cavity. The *apex* of each lung extends slightly above the clavicle, whereas the *base* is at the level of the diaphragm. At the point of the midclavicular line on the anterior surface of the thorax, the lung extends to approximately the sixth rib. Laterally, lung tissue reaches the level of the eighth rib, and, posteriorly, the lung base is at about the tenth rib (Fig. 15-4).

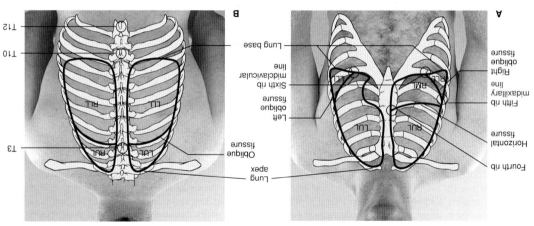

FIGURE 15-4 **A:** Anterior view of lung position. **B:** Posterior view of lung position. (*continued*)

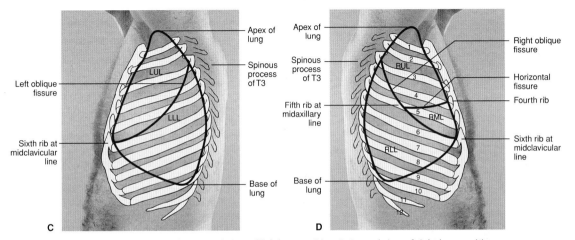

FIGURE 15-4 (*Continued*) **C:** Lateral view of left lung position. **D:** Lateral view of right lung position.

The thoracic cavity is lined by a thin, double-layered serous membrane collectively referred to as the pleura (Fig. 15-5). The *parietal pleura* lines the chest cavity, whereas the *visceral pleura* covers the external surfaces of the lungs. The *pleural space* lies between the two pleural layers. In the healthy adult, the lubricating serous fluid between the layers allows movement of the visceral layer over the parietal layer during ventilation without friction.

The trachea lies anterior to the esophagus and is approximately 10 to 12 cm long in an adult (see Fig. 15-5). At the level of the sternal angle, the trachea bifurcates into the right and left main bronchi.

Inspired air travels through the trachea into the main bronchi and continues through the system as the bronchi repeatedly bifurcate into smaller passageways known as *bronchioles*. Eventually, the bronchioles terminate at the alveolar ducts, and air is channeled into the alveolar sacs, which contain the alveoli (see Fig. 15-5).

MECHANICS OF BREATHING

The purpose of respiration is to maintain an adequate oxygen level by providing oxygen and eliminating carbon dioxide. Ventilation is the mechanical act of breathing accomplished by expansion of

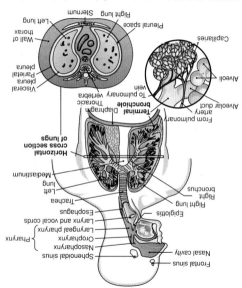

FIGURE 15-5 Major structures of the respiratory system.

Frontal sinus
Sphenoidal sinus
Nasal cavity
Pharynx
Nasopharynx
Oropharynx
Laryngeal pharynx
Larynx and vocal cords
Epiglottis
Esophagus
Trachea
Right bronchus
Left bronchus
Right lung
Left lung
Mediastinum
Horizontal cross section of lungs
Terminal bronchiole
Alveolar duct
From pulmonary artery
To pulmonary vein
Alveoli
Capillaries
Diaphragm
Thoracic vertebra
Visceral pleura
Parietal pleura
Wall of thorax
Left lung
Pleural space
Right lung
Sternum

the chest, both vertically and horizontally. Vertical expansion is accomplished through contraction of the diaphragm. Horizontal expansion occurs as the intercostal muscles lift the sternum and elevate the ribs, resulting in an increase in anterior–posterior diameter. As the chest cavity enlarges, a slight negative pressure is created in the lungs causing air to flow into the lungs called **inspiration. Expiration** is mostly passive occurring as the intercostal muscles and the diaphragm relax. As the diaphragm relaxes, it assumes a domed shape, decreasing the chest cavity size and creating a positive pressure, forcing air out of the lungs.

Nursing Assessment

COLLECTING SUBJECTIVE DATA

Focus Questions

Difficulty breathing? Timing? Associated factors? Precipitating factors? Relieving factors? Difficulty breathing when sleeping? Use of more than one pillow to sleep? Do you snore? Coughing (productive, nonproductive)? Sputum (type, amount, color)? Allergies? Dyspnea or shortness of breath (at rest or on exertion)? Chest pain? Location, timing? Associated factors? Precipitating factors? Relieving factors? History of asthma, bronchitis, emphysema, tuberculosis? Exposure to environmental inhalants (chemicals, fumes)? History of smoking (amount and length of time)? Efforts to quit?

Risk Factors

Risk for respiratory disease related to smoking, immobilization or sedentary lifestyle, aging, environmental exposures, and morbid obesity; risk for lung cancer related to cigarette smoking and genetic predisposition, asbestos, or radon exposure.

COLLECTING OBJECTIVE DATA

Equipment Needed

- Examination gown and drape
- Gloves and mask if indicated
- Stethoscope
- Tape measure with centimeters
- Marking pen
- Light source

Physical Assessment

Review Figures 15-1 to 15-5 for anatomy of the thorax and lungs. Expose anterior, posterior, and lateral chest with patient in sitting position. Locate landmarks (see Fig. 15-3, p. 307). Drape anterior chest and use finger pads or palms to palpate posterior chest. Have client fold arms across anterior chest and lean forward to increase area of lungs. First palpate, percuss, and auscultate the posterior lungs and thorax while the client is sitting. Then palpate, percuss, and auscultate lateral lungs and thorax while the client is in the supine position.

INSPECTION

ASSESSMENT PROCEDURE	NORMAL FINDINGS	ABNORMAL FINDINGS
Inspect anterior, posterior, and lateral thorax for the following:		
• Color	• Pink	• Pallor, cyanosis
• Intercostal spaces	• Even and relaxed	• Bulging, retracting
• Chest symmetry	• Equal	• Unequal
• Rib slope	• <90° downward	• Horizontal or ≥90°
• Respiration patterns (rate, rhythm, depth)	• Even, 14–20 per minute, unlabored	• Uneven, labored, <12 per minute or >20 per minute, shallow, deep. See Abnormal Findings 15-1, pp. 320–321 for altered respiration patterns.
• Anterior–posterior to lateral diameter	• 1:2 ratio (Fig. 15-6)	• >1:2 ratio (barrel chest seen in emphysema; Fig. 15-7) or <1:2 ratio
• Shape and position of sternum	• Level with ribs	• Depressed or projecting
• Position of trachea	• Midline	• Deviated to one side
• Chest expansion	• 7.6 cm (3 in) with deep inspiration	• <7.6 cm (3 in) with deep inspiration. Decreased chest excursion is seen with chronic obstructive pulmonary disease.

ASSESSMENT PROCEDURE	NORMAL FINDINGS	ABNORMAL FINDINGS

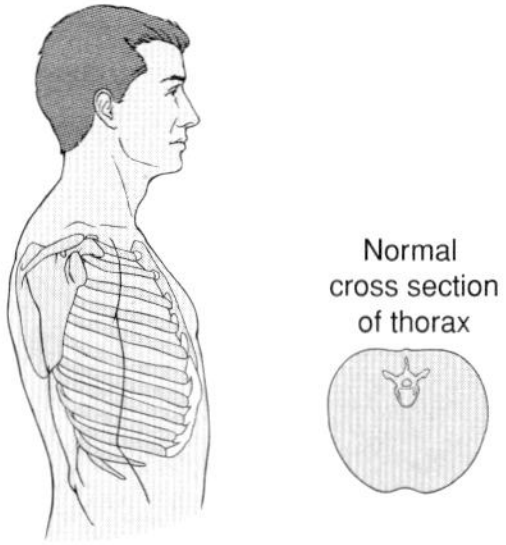

FIGURE 15-6 Cross section of thorax.

Normal cross section of thorax

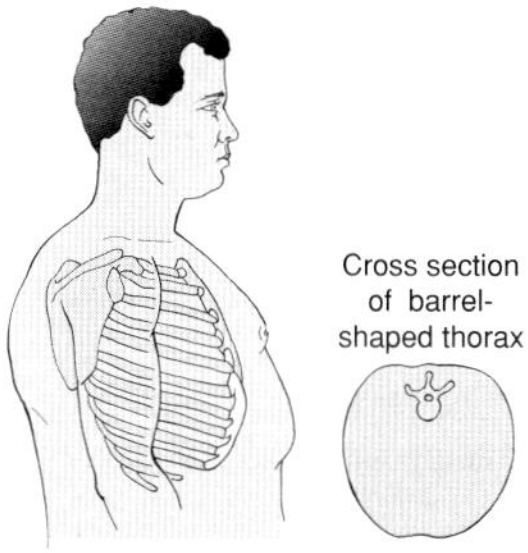

FIGURE 15-7 Cross section of barrel-shaped thorax.

Cross section of barrel-shaped thorax

PALPATION

Palpate thorax at three levels for the following:

• Sensation	• No pain or tenderness	• Pain, tenderness. Pain over thorax is seen with inflamed fibrous connective tissue; pain over intercostal area is seen with inflamed pleura.
• Vocal fremitus as client says "99"	• Vibration decreased over periphery of lungs and increased over major airways	• Vibration increased over lung with consolidation; vibration decreased over airway with obstruction, pleural effusion, or pneumothorax

Continued on following page

PALPATION (Continued)

ASSESSMENT PROCEDURE	NORMAL FINDINGS	ABNORMAL FINDINGS
Palpate thorax for thoracic expansion by the following methods:	5.08–7.62 cm (2–3 in) symmetrical thoracic expansion	Less than 5.08–7.62 cm (2–3 in) thoracic expansion; asymmetrical expansion seen with atelectasis or pneumonia.
• Place hands on posterior thorax at level of tenth vertebra. Gently press skin between thumbs and have client take deep breath. Observe thumb movement (Fig. 15-8A).	• Symmetrical expansion (thumbs move apart equal distance in both directions)	• Asymmetrical expansion (thumb movement apart is unequal)
• Anteriorly, press skin together at lower sternum and have client take deep breath. Observe thumb movement (Fig. 15-8B).	• Symmetrical expansion (thumbs move apart equal distance in both directions)	• Asymmetrical expansion (thumb movement apart is unequal)

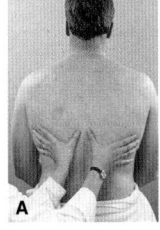
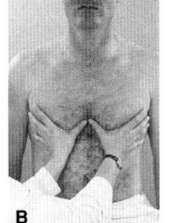

A   **B**

FIGURE 15-8 Palpation of thoracic expansion. **A:** Posterior. **B:** Anterior (Photo by B. Proud).

PERCUSSION

ASSESSMENT PROCEDURE	NORMAL FINDINGS	ABNORMAL FINDINGS
Use mediate percussion over shoulder apices and intercostal spaces. Compare both for symmetry of percussion notes, while moving from apex to base of lungs as illustrated (see Fig. 15-9).		
Percuss over shoulder apices and at posterior, anterior, and lateral intercostal spaces as illustrated (see Fig. 15-9A,B). See Figure 15-4 to determine which lung areas are being percussed.	Resonance (Fig. 15-9C,D)	Hyperresonance is heard over emphysematous lungs; dullness heard over solid masses or fluid, (e.g., in lobar pneumonia, pleural effusion, or tumor).

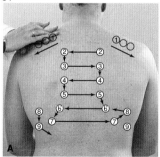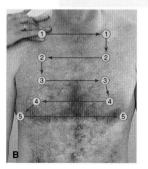

FIGURE 15-9 Intercostal landmarks for percussion and auscultation of thorax. **A:** Posterior. **B:** Anterior. (*continued*)

Continued on following page

PERCUSSION (Continued)

ASSESSMENT PROCEDURE	NORMAL FINDINGS	ABNORMAL FINDINGS
Percuss for posterior diaphragmatic excursions bilaterally, as illustrated (Fig. 15-10).	Diaphragm descends 3–6 cm from T10 (with full expiration held) to T12 (with full inspiration held).	Diaphragm descends <3 cm owing to atelectasis of lower lobes, emphysema, ascites, or tumors.

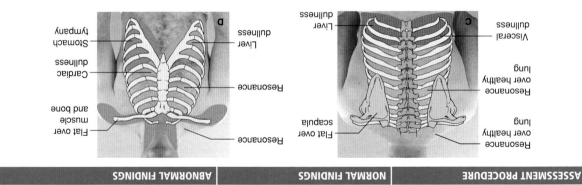

FIGURE 15-9 (Continued) **C:** Normal percussive notes (posterior). **D:** Normal percussive notes (anterior).

Labels for C:
- Visceral dullness
- Liver
- Resonance over healthy lung
- Flat over scapula
- Resonance over healthy lung

Labels for D:
- Liver dullness
- Stomach tympany
- Cardiac dullness
- Resonance
- Flat over muscle and bone
- Resonance

ASSESSMENT PROCEDURE	NORMAL FINDINGS	ABNORMAL FINDINGS

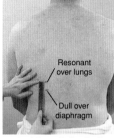

FIGURE 15-10 Percussing bilaterally for diaphragmatic excursions.

AUSCULTATION

Using diaphragm of stethoscope, exert firm pressure over intercostal space. Instruct client to take slow, deep breaths through the mouth. Listen for two full breaths and compare symmetrical sides of thorax while moving stethoscope from apex to base of lungs.

Continued on following page

AUSCULTATION (Continued)

ASSESSMENT PROCEDURE	NORMAL FINDINGS	ABNORMAL FINDINGS
Auscultate breath sounds over the following: • Trachea 	• Bronchial (loud, tubular) breath sounds heard over trachea; expiration longer than inspiration; short silence between inspiration and expiration. Bronchial breath sounds	• Bronchial sounds heard over lung periphery.
• Large-stem bronchi 	• Bronchovesicular breath sounds heard over mainstem bronchi: Below clavicles and between scapulae (inspiratory phase equal to expiratory phase). Bronchovesicular breath sounds	• Bronchovesicular breath sounds heard over lung periphery.

ASSESSMENT PROCEDURE	NORMAL FINDINGS	ABNORMAL FINDINGS
• Lung periphery	• Vesicular (low, soft, breezy) breath sounds heard over lung periphery (inspiration longer than expiration).	• Decreased breath sounds with obstruction, pleural thickening, pleural effusion, or pneumothorax.
Auscultate breath sounds for adventitious sounds (crackles, wheezes). If an abnormal sound is heard, ask client to cough. Note if adventitious sound is still present or if it cleared with cough.	Lungs clear to auscultation on inspiration and expiration.	Crackles, wheezes, and pleural friction rubs are described in Abnormal Findings 15-2, pp. 322–323.
Auscultate for altered voice sounds over lung periphery where any previous lung abnormality is noted.		
• Bronchophony (client says "99" while examiner auscultates).	• Sounds muffled and indistinct	• Sounds loud and clear over consolidation from pneumonia, atelectasis, or tumor.
• Whispered pectoriloquy (client whispers "one, two, three" while examiner auscultates).	• Sounds muffled, faint, and indistinct	• Sounds loud and clear over areas of consolidation.
• Egophony (client says "ee" while examiner auscultates).	• Sounds like muffled long "e"	• Sounds like "ay" over areas of consolidation or compression.

ABNORMAL FINDINGS	**15-1**	**Altered Respiration Patterns**

Type	Description	Pattern	Clinical Indication
Tachypnea	>24 per minute and shallow		May be a normal response to fever, anxiety, or exercise.
			Can occur with respiratory insufficiency, alkalosis, pneumonia, or pleurisy.
Bradypnea	<10 per minute and regular		May be normal in well-conditioned athletes
			Can occur with medication-induced depression of the respiratory center, diabetic coma, or neurologic damage.
Hyperventilation	Increased rate and increased depth		Usually occurs with extreme exercise, fear, or anxiety
			Kussmaul's respiration is a type of hyperventilation associated with diabetic ketoacidosis. Other causes of hyperventilation include disorders of the central nervous system, an overdose of the drug salicylate, or severe anxiety.

ABNORMAL FINDINGS	15-1	Altered Respiration Patterns (Continued)

Type	*Description*	*Pattern*	*Clinical Indication*
Hypoventilation	Decreased rate, decreased depth, irregular pattern		Usually associated with overdose of narcotics or anesthetics
Cheyne–Stokes respiration	Regular pattern characterized by alternating periods of deep, rapid breathing followed by periods of apnea		May result from severe congestive heart failure, drug overdose, incre ased intracranial pressure, or renal failure May be noted in older adults during sleep, not related to any disease process
Biot's respiration	Irregular pattern characterized by varying depth and rate of respirations followed by periods of apnea		May be seen with meningitis or severe brain damage.

ABNORMAL FINDINGS 15-2 Adventitious Breath Sounds

Abnormal Sound	Characteristics	Source	Associated Conditions
Discontinuous sounds Crackles (fine) 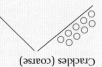	High-pitched, short, popping sounds heard during inspiration and not cleared with coughing; sounds are discontinuous and can be simulated by rolling a strand of hair between your fingers near your ear.	Inhaled air suddenly opens the small deflated air passages that are coated and sticky with exudate.	Crackles occurring late in inspiration are associated with restrictive diseases such as pneumonia and congestive heart failure. Crackles occurring early in inspiration are associated with obstructive disorders such as bronchitis, asthma, or emphysema.
Crackles (coarse) 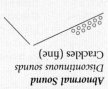	Low-pitched, bubbling, moist sounds that may persist from early inspiration to early expiration; also described as softly separating Velcro.	Inhaled air comes into contact with secretions in the large bronchi and trachea.	May indicate pneumonia, pulmonary edema, and pulmonary fibrosis. "Velcro rales" of pulmonary fibrosis are heard louder and closer to stethoscope, usually do not change location, and are more common in clients with long-term COPD.

ABNORMAL FINDINGS	15-2	Adventitious Breath Sounds (Continued)

Abnormal Sound	Characteristics	Source	Associated Conditions
Continuous sounds Pleural friction rub 	Low-pitched, dry, grating sound; sound is much like crackles, only more superficial and occurring during both inspiration and expiration.	Sound is the result of rubbing of two inflamed pleural surfaces.	Pleuritis
Wheeze (sibilant) 	High-pitched, musical sounds heard primarily during expiration but may also be heard on inspiration.	Air passes through constricted passages (caused by swelling, secretions, or tumor).	Sibilant wheezes are often heard in cases of acute asthma or chronic emphysema.
Wheeze (sonorous) 	Low-pitched snoring or moaning sounds heard primarily during expiration but may be heard throughout the respiratory cycle. These wheezes may clear with coughing.	Same as sibilant wheeze. The pitch of the wheeze cannot be correlated to the size of the passageway that generates it.	Sonorous wheezes are often heard in cases of bronchitis or single obstructions and snoring before an episode of sleep apnea. *Stridor* is a harsh honking wheeze with severe broncholaryngospasm, such as occurs with croup.

PEDIATRIC VARIATIONS

Questions to ask the parents when collecting *subjective data* include the following.

- History of wheezing, asthma, or other breathing problems?
- Exposure to passive smoke?
- Occurrence of sudden infant death syndrome (SIDS) in family?
- Frequent colds or congestion?

When collecting *objective data* note the following.

Inspection

In infants, anteroposterior (AP) diameter is equal to transverse diameter (1:1)—shape is nearly circular. By the age of 5 to 6 years, the AP diameter reaches that of the adult 1:2 or 1:7 ratio. Chest wall is thin with bony and cartilaginous rib cage is soft and pliant.

Respirations should be unlabored and quiet; rate varies according to age (Table 15-1).

Infants and children are diaphragmatic breathers (with inspiration and expiration the chest and abdominal walls will rise and fall together).

Infants have irregular respiratory patterns. As the infant gets older, the infant will develop a regular rhythm. Use of accessory

Auscultation

Use the bell or small diaphragm to localize findings, especially in infants and young children. Breath sounds will be louder and harsher owing to close proximity to origin of sounds from

Percussion

In infants and young children, findings are normally hyperresonant throughout because of thinness of chest wall. Any decrease in resonance is equal to dullness in the adult.

muscles, nasal flaring, and grunting is not normal in the infant or child.

TABLE 15-1 Respiratory Rates in Children

Age	Respiratory Rate (breaths/minute)
Newborn	30–60
Early childhood	20–40
Late childhood	15–25
Age 15 years and older	14–20

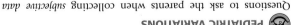
Adapted from Bickley, L.S. (2012). *Bates' guide to physical examination and history taking* (11th ed.). Philadelphia: Lippincott Williams & Wilkins.

thin chest wall. Adventitious lung sounds are not normal in the infant or child. Excessive secretions in the nose and pharynx may transmit noise to this area when auscultating the lungs. Attempt to clear this by having the child cough, clear the throat, or have the nurse suction the child to clear excessive secretions in the upper airway. Repeat auscultation of the lungs following this.

 GERIATRIC VARIATIONS

- Increase in normal respiratory rate (16 to 25 per minute)
- Loss of elasticity, fewer functional capillaries, and loss of lung resiliency
- Decreased ability to cough effectively due to weaker muscles and rigid thoracic wall
- Accentuated dorsal curve (kyphosis) of thoracic spine
- Sternum and ribs may be more prominent owing to loss of subcutaneous fat
- Decreased thoracic expansion due to calcification of costal cartilages and loss of the accessory musculature
- Increased diaphragmatic breathing due to anatomic changes
- Hyperresonance of thorax due to age-related emphysemic changes
- Decreased breath sounds and increased retention of mucus due to decreased pulmonary function

- Increased AP diameter (up to 5:7 AP-to-transverse diameter ratio) due to loss of resiliency and loss of skeletal muscle strength

 CULTURAL VARIATIONS

- Thoracic cavity size varies among cultural groups. The tendency is for Caucasians to have larger thoraxes than blacks, Asians, and Native Americans.
- Cyanosis in dark-skinned people does not necessarily appear as bluish skin, but may appear as dullness or lifelessness of the perioral, conjunctival, and nail bed areas.

POSSIBLE COLLABORATIVE PROBLEMS—RISK OF

- Respiratory insufficiency/failure
- Pneumonia
- Pulmonary edema
- Airway obstruction/atelectasis
- Laryngeal edema
- Pleural effusion
- Atelectasis
- Asthma
- Chronic obstructive pulmonary disease

- Oxygen toxicity
- Carbon dioxide toxicity
- Pneumothorax
- Respiratory acidosis
- Respiratory alkalosis
- Tracheal necrosis
- Tracheobronchial constriction

Teaching Tips for Selected Nursing Diagnoses

Nursing Diagnosis: Readiness for Enhanced Self-Health Management (Respiratory)

Encourage client to participate in a daily exercise program and to eat a healthy, low-cholesterol diet with adequate vitamin E and lutein. Provide client with information on the risks of second-hand smoke and how to decrease one's exposure. The Indoor Air Quality Information Hotline provides free information (phone 1-800-438-4318). Encourage client not to start smoking and to limit exposure to air pollution and dangerous substances.

Nursing Diagnosis: Ineffective Airway Clearance related to shallow coughing and thickened mucus

Instruct client on effective deep breathing and coughing. Encourage liquid intake of 2 to 3 quarts/day. Caution client to use protective measures to prevent spread of infections.

Nursing Diagnosis: Impaired Gas Exchange related to chronic lung tissue damage

Teach client diaphragmatic and pursed-lip breathing.

Nursing Diagnosis: Ineffective Airway Clearance related to chronic allergy

Provide literature on environmental control. Assess whether client has equipment to deal with emergencies (e.g., asthma inhaler, adrenaline kit). If allergy is produced by unknown food, assist client with keeping a diary of allergy attacks to determine cause.

Nursing Diagnosis: Ineffective Breathing Pattern: Hyperventilation related to hypoxia and lack of knowledge of controlled breathing techniques

Teach client how to become aware of breathing patterns and how to assess what aggravates hyperventilation (e.g., fatigue, stress). Teach controlled breathing techniques.

Nursing Diagnosis: Impaired Gas Exchange related to smoking and/or frequent exposure to air pollution or dangerous substances

Explain effects of smoking and how it is a primary risk factor for lung cancer. Assess client's desire to quit and refer to community agencies for self-help on smoking cessation programs. Discuss alternate methods of coping.

Wear mask if job requires exposure to dangerous inhalants.

Nursing Diagnosis: *Impaired Airway Clearance related to bronchospasm and increased pulmonary secretions*

Postural drainage and percussion may be used with children of various ages. Teach parents safety measures when using vaporizers. Teach alternate ways of humidifying air. For example, have parent run hot water in shower and close bathroom door. Sit with child in this room for approximately 10 minutes to liquefy secretions by steam (child must not be left alone in room). For spastic, croupy cough, night time exposure to cold air outdoors is beneficial.

If child has asthma: The number of asthma attacks should decrease over time as the child gets older. Assist parents with letting the child have more independence and avoiding overprotection. However, the child and parent must understand that an asthma attack can be an emergent situation if not controlled in a timely manner. Teach family how to decrease allergens (e.g., dust) in home by using smooth surfaces that are easy to clean.

Nursing Diagnosis: *Impaired Gas Exchange related to poor muscle tone and decreased ability to remove secretions*

Teach client the importance of mobility and exercise to maintain adequate respiratory hygiene. Encourage client to discuss consideration of the flu shot with the physician.

CHAPTER 16

Assessing Breasts and Lymphatic System

Structure and Function

The breasts are paired mammary glands that lie over the muscles of the anterior chest wall, anterior to the pectoralis major and serratus anterior muscles (Fig. 16-1). The male and female breasts are similar until puberty, when female breast tissue enlarges in response to hormones.

For assessment purposes, the breasts are divided into *four quadrants* by drawing horizontal and vertical imaginary lines that intersect at the nipple (Fig. 16-2).

The skin of the breasts is smooth and varies in color. The nipple contains the tiny openings of the *lactiferous ducts*. The areola surrounds the nipple and contains elevated sebaceous glands (*Montgomery glands*).

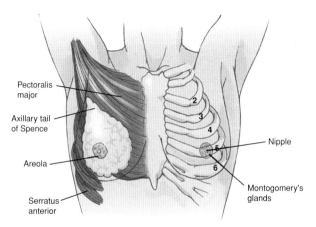

FIGURE 16-1 Anatomic breast landmarks and their position in the thorax.

Female breasts consist of three types of tissue: glandular, fibrous, and fatty (adipose; Fig. 16-3). The amount of glandular, fibrous, and fatty tissue varies according to various factors including the client's age, body build, nutritional status, hormonal cycle, and whether she is pregnant or lactating.

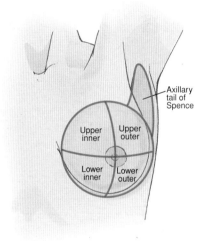

FIGURE 16-2 Breast quadrants. The upper outer quadrant is the area most targeted by breast cancer.

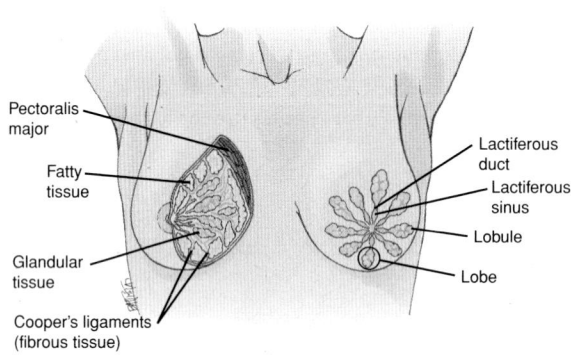

Pectoralis major

Fatty tissue

Glandular tissue

Cooper's ligaments (fibrous tissue)

Lactiferous duct

Lactiferous sinus

Lobule

Lobe

FIGURE 16-3 Internal anatomy of the breast.

The major *axillary lymph nodes* consist of the *anterior* (pectoral), *posterior* (subscapular), *lateral* (brachial), *central* (mid-axillary), *supraclavicular,* and *infraclavicular* nodes (Fig. 16-4).

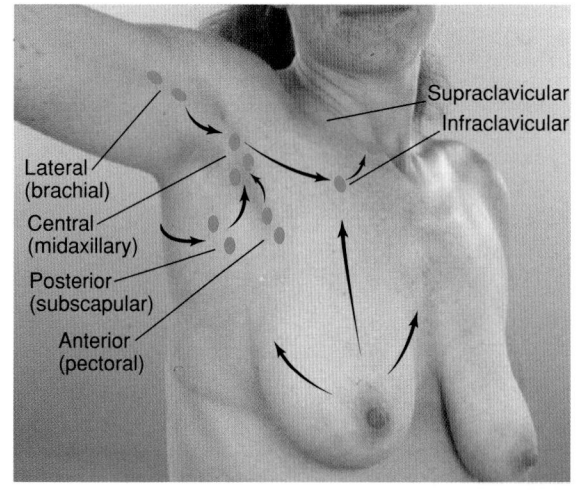

Supraclavicular

Infraclavicular

Lateral (brachial)

Central (midaxillary)

Posterior (subscapular)

Anterior (pectoral)

FIGURE 16-4 The lymph nodes drain impurities from the breasts (arrows show direction).

Nursing Assessment

COLLECTING SUBJECTIVE DATA

Focus Questions

Any lumps or lesions (location, size) or swelling in breasts? Change in size or firmness? Redness, warmth, or dimpling of breasts? Tenderness? Pain? Timing in menstrual cycle? Change in position of nipple or nipple discharge? Age of menstruation? Birth to children and age? Previous breast surgeries? History of breast cancer in family? Self-care: Breast self-examination (frequency and time performed)? Use of hormones, birth control, or antidepressants? Exposure to radiation, benzene, or asbestos? Use of alcohol, caffeine? Diet and daily exercise routine? Last breast exam? Last mammogram?

Risk Factors

Risk for breast cancer related to increasing age, personal history of breast cancer, family history of breast cancer, early menarche and late menopause, no natural children, first child after age 30 years, no history of breastfeeding, excessive weight (especially weight gain as an adult), higher education and socioeconomic status, regular alcohol intake (two to five drinks daily), previous breast irradiation, hormone replacement with progesterone, no or poor breast self-examination, poor screening, lack of adequate physical activity (45 to 60 minutes at least 5 days per week).

COLLECTING OBJECTIVE DATA

Equipment Needed

- Centimeter ruler
- Small pillow
- Breast self-examination guide to give to client (see Box 16-1)
- Gloves and slide for specimen if nipple discharge is present

Physical Assessment

Review Figures 16-1 to 16-4 (pp. 329–330) for anatomy of the breasts and regional lymphatics.

Keep in mind that the breast exam may evoke fear, anxiety, or embarrassment that may influence the client's ability to discuss the condition of the breasts and BSE. Men with gynecomastia may be embarrassed to have what they consider a "female condition." Explain the steps and purpose of the examination. Warm your hands. Remember it is important to carefully perform the breast examination on male as well as female clients.

BOX 16-1 SELF ASSESSMENT: BREAST AWARENESS AND SELF-EXAMINATION

Women should be told about the benefits and limitations of breast self-exam (BSE) in their twenties. They should become familiar with the way their breasts feel and report any new breast changes to a health professional. Changes do not necessarily indicate cancer.

A woman can notice changes by feeling her breasts occasionally (breast awareness), or by choosing to use the guidelines below to examine her breasts on a regular basis. Her examination technique should be reviewed periodically with a health care provider. It is best to examine her breasts when they are not tender or swollen. Women with breast implants may have the surgeon identify the implant edges. Pregnant or breastfeeding women may also choose to examine their breasts regularly. It is acceptable for women to choose not to do BSE or to only occasionally perform it. If women choose not to do BSE, they still need to become familiar with the normal look and feel of their breasts, and report any changes to their health care provider immediately.

How to examine your breasts

- Lie down with your right arm behind your head. Lying down spreads the breast tissue evenly over the chest wall, making it easier to feel.

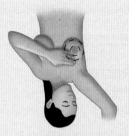

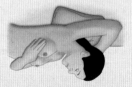

- Use the three middle finger pads of your left hand to feel for any right breast lumps, using overlapping small (dime-sized) circular motions to feel breast tissue.

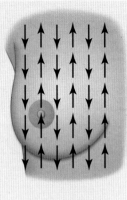

- Use light pressure to feel the tissue closest to the skin; medium pressure to feel deeper; and firm pressure to feel the tissue close to the chest and ribs. Use each pressure level to feel breast tissue before moving on to the next area. You may feel a firm ridge in the lower curve of each breast, which is normal. Tell your doctor if you feel anything else out of the ordinary. Move in an up-and-down pattern, starting at an imaginary line drawn straight down your side from the underarm. Move across the breast to the middle of the chest bone (sternum or breastbone). Check the entire breast area, going to your ribs and up to your neck or collar bone (clavicle).

- The up-and-down vertical pattern is most effective for covering the entire breast.

- Examine your left breast by putting your left arm behind your head and using your right-hand finger pads to do the exam.

- Next, stand in front of a mirror and press your hands firmly down on your hips (this contracts chest wall muscles and emphasizes any breast changes). At the same time look at your breasts for changes in size, shape, or contour. Note any dimpling, redness, or scaliness of the nipple or breast skin.

- Examine both underarms while sitting up or standing, with your arm slightly raised. Do not raise your arm straight up, because it will tighten the breast tissue, making it difficult to examine.

Based on American Cancer Society (2012). How to perform a breast self-exam. Available at http://www.cancer.org. This information is different from previous recommendations and represents an extensive review of the medical literature and input from an expert advisory group. There is evidence that the lying-down position, the area felt, the pattern of coverage of the breast, and the use of different amounts of pressure increase a woman's ability to find abnormal areas (American Cancer Society, 2012).

INSPECTION

Inspect the breasts with the client in a sitting position with arms at sides, arms overhead, hands pressed on hips, palms pressed together, and arms extended straight ahead as client leans forward (Fig. 16-5). Also inspect the areolae and nipples.

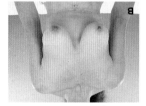

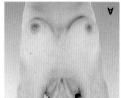

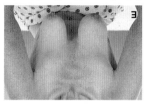

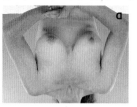

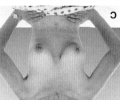

FIGURE 16-5 A: Arms over head. B: Arms at side. C: Arms pressed on hips. D: Hands pressed together. E: Leaning forward, arms extended.

ASSESSMENT PROCEDURE	NORMAL FINDINGS	ABNORMAL FINDINGS
Observe **breasts** for the following.		
• Size and symmetry	• Relatively equal with slight variation	• Recent change to unequal size. Recent increase in size of one breast may indicate inflammation or abnormal growth.
• Shape	• Round and pendulous	• Retraction or dimpling may be due to fibrosis and may indicate a malignant tumor.
• Color	• Pink; striae with age and pregnancy	• Redness, inflammation, blue hue, increased venous engorgement.
• Skin surface	• Smooth	• Retraction, dimpling, enlarged pores, "*peau d'orange*" (seen in metastatic breast disease due to edema from blocked lymphatic drainage), edema, lumps, lesions, rashes, ulcers.
Observe **areolae and nipples** for the following.		
• Size	• Relatively the same, slight variation	• Large variation
• Color	• Pink to dark brown (varies with skin and hair color)	• Inflamed

Continued on following page

INSPECTION (Continued)

ASSESSMENT PROCEDURE	NORMAL FINDINGS	ABNORMAL FINDINGS
• Shape	• Round, oval, everted	• Inversion, if it occurs after maturation or changes with movement. Recent retraction of previously everted nipple suggests malignancy.
• Discharge	• None; clear yellow 2 days after childbirth	• Foul, purulent, sanguineous drainage. Any spontaneous discharge needs to be referred for further evaluation.
• Texture	• Small Montgomery tubercles present	• Lesions, rashes, ulcers. Peau d'orange skin is seen with carcinoma. Red, scaly, crusty areas are indicative of Paget disease (see Abnormal Findings 16-1).

PALPATION

Use the flat pads of three fingers to compress tissue against breast wall gently. Then have patient lie down and place arm of side being examined overhead with small pillow under upper back. Palpate in circular motion starting at the 12-o'clock position and moving in concentric rings inward to areola and nipple (Fig. 16-6A). Bimanual palpation may be used in large-breasted clients. A wedge (Fig. 16-6B) or vertical (Fig. 16-6C) pattern may be used if preferred.

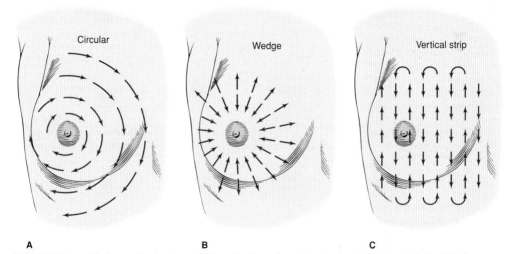

A   **B**   **C**

FIGURE 16-6 Patterns for breast palpation. Arrows indicate direction and areas for palpation. **A:** Circular or clockwise. **B:** Wedge. **C:** Vertical strip.

Continued on following page

PALPATION (Continued)

ASSESSMENT PROCEDURE	NORMAL FINDINGS	ABNORMAL FINDINGS
Palpate **breasts** for the following.		
• Temperature	• Warm	• Erythema; heat indicates inflammation if client is not lactating or has not just given birth.
• Elasticity	• Elastic	• Lumpy
• Tenderness	• Nontender; slightly tender (tenderness and fullness may occur before menses)	• Painful
• Masses (note size, shape, mobility, consistency, and location according to quadrant; see Fig. 16-2, p. 329).	• Bilateral firm inframammary transverse ridge at base of breasts	• Masses or nodules. Malignant tumors are most often found in upper outer quadrant of breast and are usually unilateral with irregular, poorly delineated borders; hard; nontender; and fixed to underlying tissues. *Fibroadenomas* (benign) are usually 1–5 cm, round or oval, mobile, firm, solid, elastic, nontender, and single or multiple in one or both breasts. *Fibrocystic disease* (benign) consists of bilateral, multiple, firm, regular, rubbery, mobile nodules with well-demarcated borders (see Abnormal Findings 16-1, p. 341).

ASSESSMENT PROCEDURE	NORMAL FINDINGS	ABNORMAL FINDINGS
Palpate **nipple** gently for discharge (Fig. 16-7).	None; clear yellow 2 days after childbirth.	Unilateral serous, serosanguineous, clear, yellow, dark red. Discharge may be seen in endocrine disorders and with some medications, such as antihypertensives, antidepressants, and estrogen. Discharge from one breast may indicate benign intraductal papilloma, fibrocystic disease, or breast cancer.

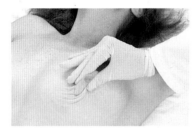

FIGURE 16-7 Palpating nipples for masses and discharge.

ASSESSMENT PROCEDURE	NORMAL FINDINGS	ABNORMAL FINDINGS
Palpate **lymph nodes** in the following areas. Supraclavicular, subclavian, intermediate, brachial, scapular, mammary, internal mammary (see Fig. 16-4, p. 330).	None palpable (<1 cm)	Palpable lymph nodes (>1 cm)

MALE VARIATIONS

Inspect and palpate breast with client seated, arms at sides. Palpate lymph nodes. No swelling, ulcerations, or nodules should be noted. Flat disk of undeveloped breast tissue under nipple is normally palpated. Soft fatty tissue enlargement seen in obesity.

Gynecomastia (Fig. 16-8) and a smooth, firm movable disk of glandular tissue may be seen in one breast during puberty for short time and may be seen in hormonal imbalances (disease or medication induced) and drug abuse. Irregular, hard nodules are seen in malignancy.

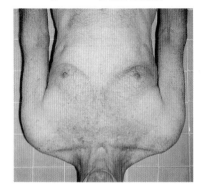

FIGURE 16-8 Gynecomastia.

Orange peel (peau d'orange) appearance of the breast · Retracted breast tissue · Tumor

Continued on following page

ABNORMAL FINDINGS **16-1** **Breast Abnormalities** (Continued)

Fibroadenoma   Benign breast disease (fibrocystic breast disease)

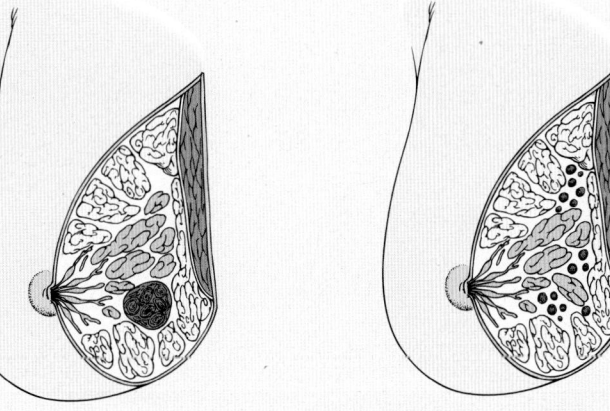

PEDIATRIC VARIATIONS

Subjective Data

Age of menarche? Asymmetrical breast growth? Girls prior to puberty: Pain or discomfort? Boys during adolescence: Abnormal increase in size?

Objective Data

See normal breast development in Chapter 23, Table 23-1 on page 537, which varies with age. Adolescent breast development is usually seen between age 10 and 13 years and takes about 3 years for full development.

 ## Geriatric Variations

- Breasts pendulous, atrophied, and less firm owing to a decrease in estrogen levels.
- May have smaller, flatter nipples that are less erectile on stimulation. Nipples may retract, but will evert with gentle pressure.
- Breasts may feel more granular with more fibrotic tissue.

 CULTURAL VARIATIONS

In the United States, white women are at greater risk for diagnosis of breast cancer, but black women are at greater risk for dying of breast cancer. Askenazi (Eastern European origin) Jewish women are most likely to have the genetic predisposition for the BRCA1 or BRCA2 gene that is associated with breast cancer.

POSSIBLE COLLABORATIVE PROBLEMS—RISK OF

- Infection (abscess)
- Hematoma
- Fibrocystic disease
- Breast cancer

Teaching Tips for Selected Nursing Diagnoses

Nursing Diagnosis: Deficient Knowledge related to inability to describe process for breast self-examination

- Teach women about the benefits and limitations of BSE beginning at age 20. Emphasize the importance of reporting any new breast symptoms to a health professional. It is acceptable for women to choose not to do BSE or do it irregularly. If a woman chooses to do BSE, instruct on proper BSE technique (see Appendix 9), allowing time for questions and review of technique (American Cancer Society, 2012a). The best time for BSE is right after menstruation or between the fourth and seventh day of the cycle if the cycle is regular. If the client is on cyclic estrogen therapy, she should examine her breasts on the last day that the medicine is not being taken. It is important for women to know their breasts and to report any breast changes promptly to their health care providers. Remember that most of the time breast changes are not cancer, but it is important to detect breast cancer early for effective treatment. Women who have had a breast lumpectomy, augmentation, or breast reconstruction may also perform BSE. Some women may choose not to do BSE even if knowledgeable of the benefits and limitations. This choice needs to be accepted by the examiner.

- Reinforce the following American Cancer Society, 2012a, examinations.
  - Breast clinical examination for women age 20 to 39 years as part of the periodic health examination, preferably at least every 3 years.
  - Breast clinical examination for women after age 40 every year as part of a periodic health examination. (The ACS recommends women be told about the benefits, limitations, and potential harms linked with mammograms before beginning annual mammograms).
  - Women at moderate to high risk for breast cancer should talk to their health care provider about adding MRI (especially for high risk) along with mammogram yearly.
  - Advise that cancer of the breast can be treated and often cured if detected early.
  - Encourage breastfeeding, exercise, and maintaining a healthy body weight.
    (American Cancer Society: Cancer prevention and early detection facts and figures, 2013a.)

CHAPTER 17

Assessing Heart and Neck Vessels

Structure and Function Overview

HEART AND GREAT VESSELS

The heart is a hollow, muscular, four-chambered organ located in the middle of the thoracic cavity between the lungs in the space called the *mediastinum*. It is about the size of a clenched fist and weighs approximately 255 g (9 oz) in women and 309 g (10.9 oz) in men. The heart extends vertically from the second to the fifth intercostal space (ICS) and horizontally from the right edge of the sternum to the left midclavicular line (MCL). The heart can be described as an inverted cone. The upper portion, near the second ICS, is the base, and the lower portion, near the fifth ICS and the left MCL, is the apex. The anterior chest area that overlies the heart and great vessels is called the *precordium* (Fig. 17-1).

The large veins and arteries leading directly to and away from the heart are referred to as the *great vessels*. The *superior and inferior venae cavae* return blood to the right atrium from the upper and lower torso, respectively. The *pulmonary artery* exits the right ventricle, bifurcates, and carries blood to the lungs. The *pulmonary veins* (two from each lung) return oxygenated blood to the

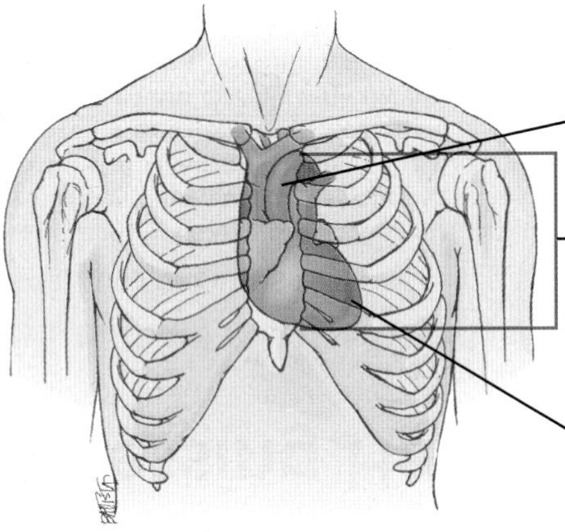

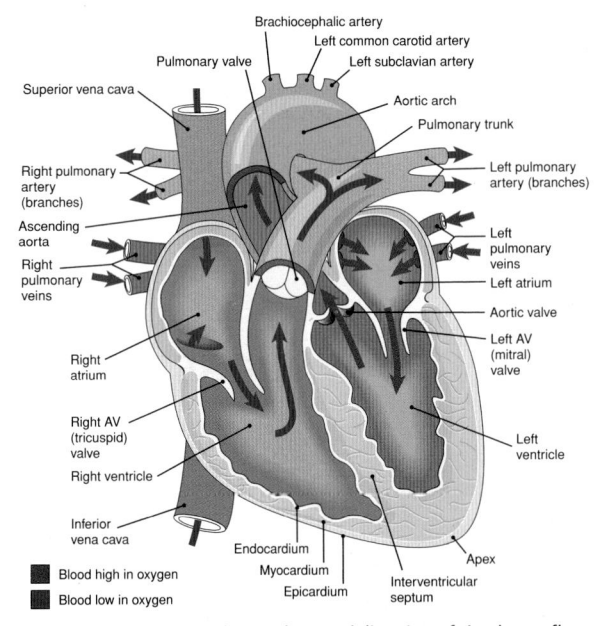

FIGURE 17-1 The heart and major blood vessels lie centrally in the chest behind the protective sternum.

left atrium. The *aorta* transports oxygenated blood from the left ventricle to the body (Fig. 17-2).

The heart coverings and walls consist of a *pericardium* (a tough, inextensible, loose-fitting, fibroserous sac that attaches

FIGURE 17-2 Heart chambers, valves, and direction of circulatory flow.

to the great vessels and surrounds the heart); the *parietal pericardium* (a serous which secretes a small amount of pericardial fluid that allows for smooth, friction-free movement of the heart); the *epicardium* (a serous membrane that covers the outer surface of the heart); the *myocardium* (the thickest layer of the heart made up of contractile cardiac muscle cells); and the *endocardium* (a thin layer of endothelial tissue that forms the innermost layer of the heart and is continuous with the endothelial lining of blood vessels).

The heart consists of four chambers or cavities: two upper chambers, the *right and left atria,* and two lower chambers, the *right and left ventricles.* One-way valves that direct the flow of blood through the heart protect the entrance and exit of each ventricle. The *atrioventricular* (AV) valves are located at the entrance into the ventricles. There are two AV valves: the tricuspid valve and the bicuspid, which is also called the *mitral valve.* The tricuspid valve is composed of three cusps or flaps and is located between the right atrium and the right ventricle; the bicuspid (mitral) valve is composed of two cusps or flaps and is located between the left atrium and the left ventricle.

Open AV valves allow blood to flow from the atria into the ventricles. However, as the ventricles begin to contract, the AV valves snap shut, preventing the regurgitation of blood into the atria.

The *semilunar valves* are located at the exit of each ventricle at the beginning of the great vessels. Each valve has three cusps or flaps that look like half-moons, hence the name "semilunar." There are two semilunar valves: the pulmonic valve is located at the entrance of the pulmonary artery as it exits the right ventricle, and the aortic valve is located at the beginning of the ascending aorta as it exits the left ventricle (see Fig. 17-2).

ELECTRICAL CONDUCTION SYSTEM OF THE HEART

Cardiac muscle cells have a unique inherent ability to spontaneously generate electrical impulses and conduct them through the heart. The generation and conduction of electrical impulses by specialized sections of the myocardium regulate the events associated with the filling and emptying of the cardiac chambers. The process is called the *cardiac cycle.* The *sinoatrial (SA) node,* located on the posterior wall of the right atrium, generates impulses (at a rate of 60 to 100 per minute) that cause the atria to contract simultaneously, sending blood into the ventricles. The current, initiated by the SA node, is conducted across the atria to the *AV node* located in the lower interatrial septum. The AV node slightly delays incoming electrical impulses from the atria then relays the impulse to the AV bundle (bundle of His) in the upper interventricular septum. The electrical impulse then travels down the right and left bundle branches and the *Purkinje fibers* in the myocardium of both ventricles, causing them to contract almost simultaneously. Although the SA node functions as the "pacemaker of the heart," this activity shifts to other areas of the conduction system, such as the *Bundle of His* (with an inherent discharge of 40 to 60 per minute), if the SA node cannot function.

PRODUCTION OF HEART SOUNDS

Heart sounds are produced by valve closure. The opening of valves is silent. Normal heart sounds, characterized as "lub dub" (S_1 and S_2), and, occasionally, extra heart sounds and murmurs can be auscultated with a stethoscope over the precordium, the area of the anterior chest overlying the heart and great vessels.

The first heart sound (S_1) is the result of closure of the AV valves—the mitral and tricuspid valves. S_1 correlates with the beginning of systole (Fig. 17-3). If heard as two sounds, the first component represents mitral valve closure (M_1) and the second component represents tricuspid closure (T_1).

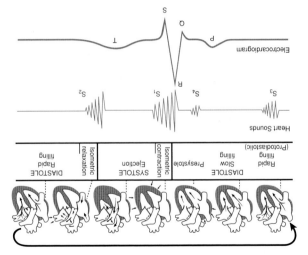

FIGURE 17-3 The cardiac cycle consists of filling and ejection. Heart sounds S_2, S_3, and S_4 are associated with diastole, whereas S_1 is associated with systole. The electrical activity of the heart is measured throughout diastole and systole by electrocardiography.

The second heart sound (S_2) results from closure of the semilunar valves (aortic and pulmonic) and correlates with the beginning of diastole. S_2 ("dubb") is also usually heard as one sound but may be heard as two sounds. If S_2 is heard as two sounds, the first component represents aortic valve closure (A_2) and the second component represents pulmonic valve closure (P_2).

NECK VESSELS

The internal jugular veins lie deep and medial to the sternocleidomastoid muscle. The external jugular veins lie lateral to the sternocleidomastoid muscle and above the clavicle. The jugular veins return blood to the heart from the head and neck by way of the superior vena cava.

The level of the jugular venous pressure reflects right atrial (central venous) pressure and right ventricular diastolic filling pressure. Right-sided heart failure raises pressure and volume, thus raising jugular venous pressure. *Decreased jugular venous pressure* occurs with reduced left ventricular output or blood volume. The right internal jugular vein is most directly connected to the right atrium and provides the best assessment of pressure changes. Components of the jugular venous pulse follow

- a wave—reflects rise in atrial pressure that occurs with atrial contraction.
- x descent—reflects right atrial relaxation and descent of the atrial floor during ventricular systole.
- v wave—reflects right atrial filling, increased volume, and increased atrial pressure.
- y descent—reflects right atrial emptying into the right ventricle and decreased atrial pressure.

Nursing Assessment
COLLECTING SUBJECTIVE DATA
Focus Questions

Chest pain—Onset? Location? Radiation? Quality? Rating on scale of 1 to 10 (10 being the worst)? Duration? How often? What brings it on? What relieves it? Does activity make it worse? Are there any other associated symptoms, such as nausea, vomiting, sweating? Irregular heartbeat, palpitations? Does your heart pound or beat too fast? Does your heart skip or jump? Difficulty breathing or shortness of breath? Dizziness? Lightheadedness? Swelling in feet ankles or legs? Heart burn—Onset? How often?

Relief? History of heart defect? Murmur? Rheumatic fever? Heart surgery? Cardiac balloon interventions? Last electrocardiogram and results? Cholesterol levels? Medications for heart disease? Usual blood pressure? Family history of hypertension, myocardial infarction, coronary heart disease, elevated cholesterol levels, or diabetes mellitus? Smoking? Packs per day? Over how many years? Twenty-four-hour dietary recall? Alcohol consumption each day? Form of exercise? How often? Over the last 5 years? Over the last 10 years? Ability to care for self? Any activities limited due to chest pain, shortness of breath, or fatigue? Effects of heart disease on sexual activities? Number of pillows used to sleep on at night? Daily stressors? Forms of relaxation? Fears regarding heart disease?

Risk Factors

Risk for coronary heart disease related to hypertension, increased low-density lipoprotein cholesterol and decreased high-density lipoprotein (HDL) cholesterol, diabetes mellitus, minimal exercise, cigarette smoking, diet high in saturated fat and trans fatty acids, postmenopausal without estrogen replacement (in females), family history, and upper body obesity.

COLLECTING OBJECTIVE DATA

Equipment Needed

- Stethoscope with bell and diaphragm
- Alcohol swab to clean ear and end pieces of stethoscope
- Watch with a second hand
- Small pillow
- Penlight or movable examination light
- Centimeter rulers (two)

Physical Assessment

See Figure 17-2 on page 346 for a diagram of the heart chambers, valves, and circulation. Additional data gathered during assessment of the blood pressure, skin, nails, head, thorax and lungs, and peripheral pulses all play a part in the complete cardiovascular assessment. Provide the client with as much modesty as possible. Explain that the client will need to move to different positions to facilitate auscultation of heart sounds. Tell the client you will be listening to the heart in several areas and that this does not necessarily mean that anything is wrong. *Note: If a client has large breasts, ask her to pull the breast upward and to the side when you are auscultating for heart sounds.*

NECK VESSELS

ASSESSMENT PROCEDURE	NORMAL FINDINGS	ABNORMAL FINDINGS
Inspection		
Observe the jugular venous pulse. Inspect the jugular venous pulse on client's right side in supine position with the torso elevated 30 to 45 degrees. Ask the client to turn the head slightly to left. Shine a tangential light source on neck to view pulsations. Inspect the suprasternal notch and area around clavicles for pulsations of the internal jugular veins.	The jugular venous pulse is not normally visible with the client sitting upright. This position fully distends the vein, and pulsations may or may not be discernible. It is normal for the jugular veins to be visible when the client is supine.	Fully distended jugular veins with the client's torso elevated more than 45 degrees indicate increased central venous pressure that may be the result of right ventricular failure, pulmonary hypertension, pulmonary emboli, or cardiac tamponade.
Evaluate jugular venous pressure by watching for distention of the jugular vein. To evaluate jugular vein distention, position the client supine with head of the bed elevated 30, 45, 60, and 90 degrees. Observe for distention, observe for protrusion, or bulging.	The jugular vein should not be distended, bulging, or protruding at 45 degrees or greater.	Distention, bulging, or protrusion at 45, 60, or 90 degrees may indicate right-sided heart failure. Clients with obstructive pulmonary disease may have elevated venous pressure only during expiration. An inspiratory increase in venous pressure, called Kussmaul sign, may occur in clients with severe constrictive pericarditis.

Continued on following page

NECK VESSELS (Continued)

ASSESSMENT PROCEDURE	NORMAL FINDINGS	ABNORMAL FINDINGS
Auscultation		
Auscultate the carotid arteries. Auscultate the carotid arteries if the client is middle-aged or older or if you suspect cardiovascular disease. Place the bell of the stethoscope over the carotid artery and ask the client to hold his or her breath for a moment so breath sounds do not conceal any vascular sounds (Fig. 17-4). *Note: Always auscultate the carotid arteries before palpating because palpation may increase or slow the heart rate, changing the strength of the carotid impulse heard.* 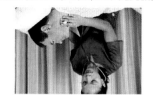 **FIGURE 17-4** Auscultating the carotid arteries.	No blowing or swishing or other sounds are heard.	A *bruit*, a blowing or swishing sound caused by turbulent blood flow through a narrowed vessel, is indicative of occlusive arterial disease. However, if the artery is more than two thirds occluded, a bruit may not be heard. Pulse inequality may indicate arterial constriction or occlusion in one carotid. Weak pulses may indicate *hypovolemia*, shock, or decreased cardiac output. A bounding, firm pulse may indicate *hypervolemia* or increased cardiac output. Variations in strength from beat to beat or with respiration are abnormal and may indicate a variety of problems. A delayed upstroke may indicate *aortic stenosis*.
	Pulses are equally strong; a 2+ or normal with no variation in strength from beat to beat. Contour is normally smooth and rapid on the upstroke and slower and less abrupt on the downstroke. The strength of the pulse is evaluated on a scale from 0 to 4 as follows. **Pulse Amplitude Scale** 0 = absent 1+ = weak 2+ = normal 3+ = increased 4+ = bounding	

ASSESSMENT PROCEDURE	NORMAL FINDINGS	ABNORMAL FINDINGS

Palpation

Palpate the carotid arteries. Palpate each carotid artery alternately by placing the pads of the index and middle fingers medial to the sternocleidomastoid muscle on the neck (Fig. 17-5). Note amplitude and contour of the pulse, elasticity of the artery, and any thrills.

Note: Palpate the carotid arteries individually because bilateral palpation could result in reduced cerebral blood flow.

Arteries are elastic and no thrills are noted.

Loss of elasticity may indicate *arteriosclerosis*. Thrills may indicate a narrowing of the artery.

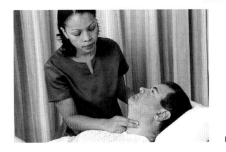

FIGURE 17-5 Palpating the carotid arteries.

HEART AND GREAT VESSELS

Inspection

Inspect chest to identify landmarks that aid in assessment of the heart (Fig. 17-6). Check for visibility of point of maximum impulse (PMI) and any abnormal pulsations.

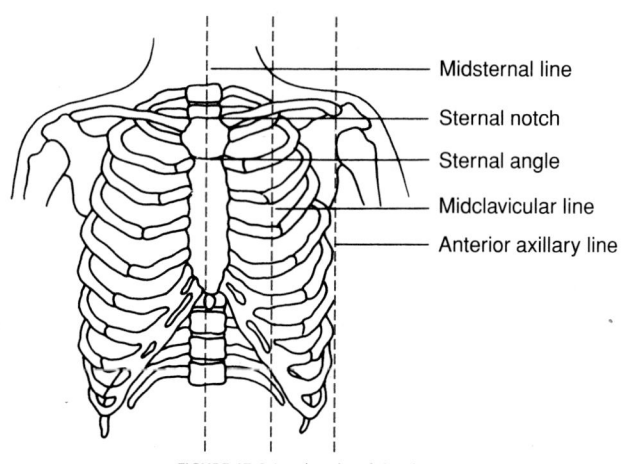

FIGURE 17-6 Landmarks of the chest.

ASSESSMENT PROCEDURE	NORMAL FINDINGS	ABNORMAL FINDINGS
Inspect the following: • Intercostal space (ICS): Locate by finding the sternal angle, which is felt as a ridge in the sternum approximately 5.08 cm (2 in) below the sternal notch (see Fig. 17-6). The adjacent rib is the second rib with the second ICS directly below it. Count from the second ICS to identify other ICSs. The fifth ICS is at the junction of the sternum and the xiphoid process. • Midsternal line (MSL): Imaginary line extending down the chest through the middle of the sternum. It divides the anterior chest in half (see Fig. 17-6). • Midclavicular line (MCL): Imaginary line extending from the middle of the clavicle down the chest, dividing the left or right anterior chest into two parts (see Fig. 17-6). • Anterior axillary line (AAL): Imaginary line extending along the lateral wall of the anterior chest and even with the anterior axillary fold (see Fig. 17-6).	• Small apical impulse ($\leq$2.5 cm) at or medial to left midclavicular line at fourth or fifth ICS. May not be visible in client with large chest.	• Impulses lateral to midclavicular line; pulsations (heaves or lifts) other than the apical pulsation are considered abnormal, and may be seen with an enlarged left ventricle due to work overload; apical impulse on right side of chest. Bulging and/or prominent pulsations (>3 cm) at the PMI. • Prominent impulse at right sternal border in pulmonic or aortic area.

Continued on following page

HEART AND GREAT VESSELS (Continued)

Palpation

The client should be lying down. Palpate using the fingertips and palmar surfaces of fingers in an organized fashion, beginning in the aortic area and moving down the chest toward the tricuspid area (Fig. 17-7).

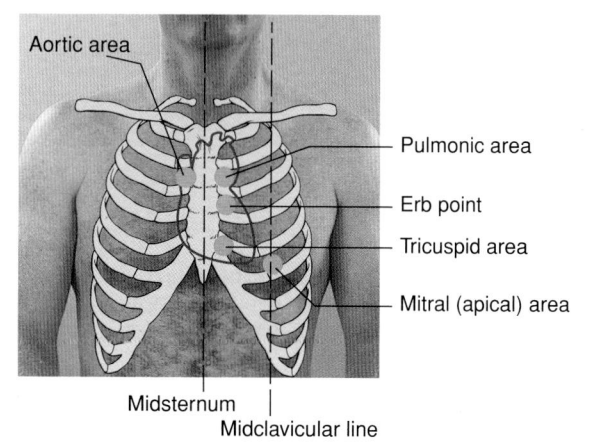

Aortic area

Pulmonic area

Erb point

Tricuspid area

Mitral (apical) area

Midsternum

Midclavicular line

FIGURE 17-7 Areas to auscultate and palpate on the chest.

ASSESSMENT PROCEDURE	NORMAL FINDINGS	ABNORMAL FINDINGS
Palpate the following: • Aortic area: Palpate second ICS at right sternal border (see Fig. 17-7). • Pulmonic area: Palpate second ICS at left sternal border (see Fig. 17-7). • Erb point: Palpate third ICS at left sternal border (see Fig. 17-7). • Tricuspid area: Palpate fifth ICS at lower left sternal border (see Fig. 17-7).	• No vibrations or pulsations are palpated in aortic, pulmonic, or tricuspid area.	• Thrill, which feels similar to a purring cat, or pulsation in any of these areas except the mitral area is usually associated with a grade 4 or higher murmur.
• Mitral (apical) area: Palpate fifth ICS at the left MCL. This is also called the PMI (Fig. 17-8). *Note: If this pulsation cannot be palpated, have the client assume a left lateral position. This displaces the heart toward the left chest wall and relocates the apical impulse farther to the left.*	PMI is felt as a pulsation and is approximately the size of a nickel. May not palpate in large chest.	No pulsation. If area of pulsation is the size of a quarter or larger, displaced, more forceful, or of longer duration, suspect cardiac enlargement.

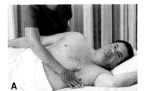 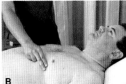

FIGURE 17-8 Locate the apical impulse with the palmar surface (**A**), and then palpate the apical pulse with the fingerpad (**B**).

Continued on following page

HEART AND GREAT VESSELS (Continued)

Percussion

Percussion may be done to define cardiac borders by identifying areas of dullness, but it is generally unreliable. Size of heart can be more accurately determined by chest x-ray.

Auscultation

Auscultate in an orderly, systematic fashion beginning with the aortic area. Move across and then down the chest. Focus on one sound at a time. Auscultate each area with the stethoscope diaphragm applied firmly to the chest. Repeat the sequence using the stethoscope bell applied lightly to the chest. Auscultate with the client in the supine position. Then listen specifically over the apex with the bell while client is in the left lateral position. Assist client to a sitting position, and auscultate the pericardium with the diaphragm. Then have the client lean forward and exhale while you listen over the aortic area with the diaphragm.

ASSESSMENT PROCEDURE	NORMAL FINDINGS	ABNORMAL FINDINGS
Auscultate to identify the **first heart sound** (S_1), or "lub," and the **second heart sound** (S_2), or "dub" (Fig. 17-9).	S_1 follows the long diastolic pause and precedes the short systolic pause and corresponds to each carotid pulsation. S_2 follows the short systolic phase and precedes the long diastolic phase (Fig. 17-10).	

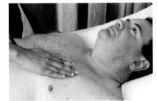

FIGURE 17-9 Auscultating S_1.

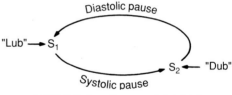

FIGURE 17-10 Normal heart sound: "lub dub."

Auscultate for **rate and rhythm**.	*Rate:* 60–100 beats per minute *Rhythm:* regular	Bradycardia (heart rate <60) tachycardia (heart rate >100) may result in decreased cardiac output; irregular rhythms (e.g., premature beats of atrial or ventricular premature contractions, atrial flutter and atrial fibrillation with varying block) need to be referred.

Continued on following page

HEART AND GREAT VESSELS (Continued)

ASSESSMENT PROCEDURE	NORMAL FINDINGS	ABNORMAL FINDINGS
If irregular rhythm is detected, **auscultate for pulse rate deficit** by comparing the radial pulse with the apical pulse for a full minute.	Radial and apical pulse should be identical.	A pulse deficit (difference between radial and apical pulses) may indicate atrial fibrillation, atrial flutter, premature ventricular contractions, and varying degrees of heart block.
Auscultate and focus on each sound and pause individually.	Crisp, distinct sound heard in each area but loudest at mitral and tricuspid areas.	
Auscultate S_1: Heard best with diaphragm	May become softer with inspiration. Split S_1 is normal in children, young adults, and pregnant women.	Split sound heard equally during inspiration and expiration.
Auscultate S_2: Heard best with diaphragm	Crisp, distinct sound heard loudest at the aortic and pulmonic areas. Split S_2 may be normal in adults if heard only during inspiration.	Split sound in middle-aged and older adults.
Auscultate systolic pause space: Heard between S_1 and S_2 (see Fig. 17-9).	Silent pause—should hear distinct end of S_1 and beginning of S_2, with nothing in between.	*Murmur:* Swishing sound heard at beginning, middle, or end of systolic pause (note intensity, pitch, and quality—Table 17-1, p. 363).
		Click: Sharp, high-pitched snapping sound heard immediately after S_1 or in the middle of the systolic pause.

ASSESSMENT PROCEDURE	NORMAL FINDINGS	ABNORMAL FINDINGS
• Auscultate diastolic pause space: Heard between S_2 and the next S_1 (see Fig. 17-9, p. 359).	• Silent pause—should hear distinct end of S_2 and distinct beginning of next S_1.	• *Murmur:* Swishing sound heard at beginning, middle, or end of diastolic pause (note intensity, pitch, and quality—Table 17-1). *Snap:* High-pitched snapping sound heard after S_2 during the diastolic pause in the mitral or tricuspid area.
• Auscultate S_3 with bell of stethoscope: Low, faint sound occurring at the beginning of the diastolic pause (Fig. 17-11).	• S_3 auscultated in children and young adults but disappears upon standing or sitting up; heard in people with a high cardiac output, and in women in the third trimester of pregnancy.	• S_3 auscultated in adults or that continues with standing or sitting in children and young adults; also called ventricular gallop (has rhythm of the word "Kentucky"); may be heard with ischemic heart disease, myocardial failure, volume overload of the ventricle from valvular disease; may be the earliest sign of heart failure.

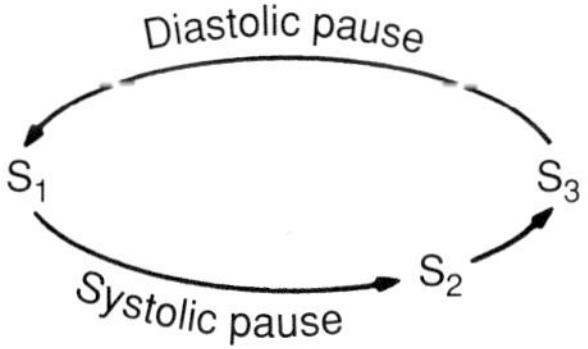

FIGURE 17-11 S_3 heart sound.

Continued on following page

HEART AND GREAT VESSELS (Continued)

ASSESSMENT PROCEDURE	NORMAL FINDINGS	ABNORMAL FINDINGS
• Auscultate S_4: Soft, low-pitched sound heard best with client in supine or left lateral position with stethoscope bell (Fig. 17-12).	• Auscultated in trained athletes and some older clients, especially after exercise.	• Auscultated in adults; also called atrial gallop (has rhythm of the word "Tennessee") and is associated with coronary artery disease, hypertension, aortic and pulmonic stenosis, and acute myocardial infarction.

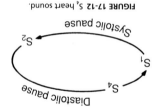

S_1

S_2

Systolic pause

Diastolic pause

S_4

FIGURE 17-12 S_4 heart sound.

TABLE 17-1 **Classification for Intensity, Pitch, and Quality of Murmurs**

Intensity
Grade 1—Very faint, heard only after the listener has "tuned in"; may not be heard in all positions
Grade 2—Quiet, but heard immediately upon placing stethoscope on the chest
Grade 3—Moderately loud
Grade 4—Loud with palpable thrill
Grade 5—Very loud, may be heard with stethoscope partly off the chest. Associated with thrills
Grade 6—May be heard with stethoscope entirely off the chest

Pitch
High, medium, or low

Quality
Blowing, rumbling, harsh, or musical

Adapted from: Bickley, L.S., & Szilagyi, P.G. (2012). *Bates' guide to physical examination and history taking* (11th ed.). Philadelphia: Lippincott Williams & Wilkins.

 PEDIATRIC VARIATIONS

Focus Questions

In addition to the focus questions for adults, inquire about the following: Mother's use of therapeutic drugs or drug abuse during pregnancy? Poor weight gain? Signs of delayed development (e.g., slowed social development, language development, or motor skills)? Difficulty in feeding (breast, bottle, acceptance of new foods)? Inability to tolerate physical activity or play with peers? Squatting behavior? Excessive irritability or crying? Circumoral cyanosis or central cyanosis?

PHYSICAL ASSESSMENT

ASSESSMENT PROCEDURE	NORMAL FINDINGS AND VARIATIONS
Inspect chest wall in semi-Fowler position from an angle for PMI.	PMI easily visible because heart is larger in proportion to chest size (Fig. 17-13). Heart lies more horizontally up to age of 5 to 6 years. Thus, the PMI may be lateral to the MCL.

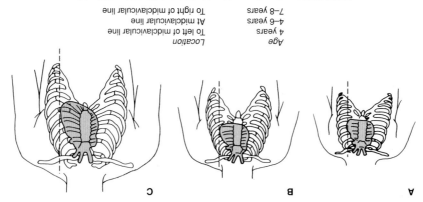

Age	Location
4 years	To left of midclavicular line
4–6 years	At midclavicular line
7–8 years	To right of midclavicular line

FIGURE 17-13 Location of apex of heart in (A) infant, (B) child, and (C) adult.

ASSESSMENT PROCEDURE	NORMAL FINDINGS AND VARIATIONS
Palpate peripheral pulse points in relation to apical pulse and to each other: Femoral, radial, brachial, and carotid. Palpate femoral and brachial pulses at the same time.	Symmetrical and equal rate, strength, and rhythm.
Percuss heart size. *Note: This is rarely done owing to inaccuracy of the method.*	Percussion area is slightly larger because of horizontal position and overlying thymus gland.
Auscultate S₁ and S₂ at: Pulmonic area (Erb point).	S_1 is louder than S_2, or S_2 is louder than S_1. Splitting of S_2 is heard best at Erb point (25–33% of all children). This is a frequent site of *innocent murmurs* (grade 3 or lower), which are common throughout childhood. They are of short duration with no transmission to other areas, are low pitched, musical, or of groaning quality that is variable in intensity in relation to position, respiration, activity, fever, and anemia with no other associated signs of heart disease. Other murmurs may indicate pathology.
Tricuspid area	S_1 louder, preceding S_2
Mitral area	S_1 loudest
Auscultate for sinus arrhythmia	Varies with respiration; very common and disappears with age. Heart rate may increase with inhaling and decrease with exhaling. If a child holds his/her breath, rhythm will become regular.
Auscultate for pulse rate	• See Table 17-2 for normal pediatric pulse rates.

TABLE 17-2 Average Heart Rate of Infants and Children at Rest

Age	Average Rate (beats per minute)	±2 Standard Deviations
Birth	140	90–190
First 6 months	130	80–180
6–12 months	115	75–155
1–2 years	110	70–150
2–6 years	103	68–138
6–10 years	95	65–125
10–14 years	85	55–115

Adapted from: Bickley, L.S., & Szilagyi, P.G. (2012). *Bates' Guide to physical examination and history taking* (11th ed.). Philadelphia: Lippincott Williams & Wilkins.

GERIATRIC VARIATIONS

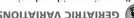

- Be cautious with palpating carotid arteries in older clients because atherosclerosis may have caused obstruction and compression may easily block circulation.
- Thickening of heart walls.
- Decreased elasticity of heart and arteries; reduced pumping ability of heart.

- Decreased cardiac output and cardiac reserve.
- Apical impulse may be difficult to palpate due to increased anteroposterior chest diameter.
- Location of heart sounds and PMI may be varied owing to kyphosis or scoliosis.
- Early and soft systolic murmurs are common.
- Atrial fibrillations often occur.
- Reduced maximum heart rate.

CULTURAL VARIATIONS

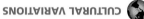

- African Americans have higher HDL levels, but higher lifestyle risk factors for congenital heart disease (CHD) than white Americans.
- African Americans have higher rates of hypertension, stroke, and CHD than white Americans. Hypertension in US black women has a higher incidence, earlier onset, and higher mortality than in white women.

POSSIBLE COLLABORATIVE PROBLEMS—RISK OF

Decreased cardiac output	Congenital heart disease
Congestive heart failure	Endocarditis
Myocardial ischemia	Angina
Cardiogenic shock	Dysrhythmia

Teaching Tips for Selected Nursing Diagnoses

Nursing Diagnosis: *Fear related to perceived increased risk of heart disease and family history of heart disease*

Explain what you are doing when auscultating so the client won't become alarmed by the amount of time you are taking. Explain that vigorous exercise (20 to 30 minutes three times a week) may decrease serum triglycerides and cholesterol, and therefore may prevent heart disease by increasing the working capabilities of the body and heart capillaries. Advise client to have a complete physical examination before starting a new fitness program.

Nursing Diagnosis: *Ineffective Therapeutic Regimen Management related to knowledge deficit: Taking pulse in order to assess heart rate before taking cardiac medications*

Teach client correct method for taking pulse. Instruct on heart rate necessary for taking prescribed medication.

Nursing Diagnosis: *Ineffective Sexuality Patterns related to fear of injury postmyocardial infarction*

Instruct client to discuss limitations on sexual activities as recommended by physician. (Usually, a client can safely engage in sexual intercourse by the time he or she is permitted to walk up a flight of stairs.)

Nursing Diagnosis: *Deficient knowledge related to optimal diet for preventing coronary heart disease*

Teach client the following dietary and lifestyle guidelines (American Heart Association, 2012a).

- Choose nutrient-rich foods high in vitamins, minerals, and fiber but low in calories.
- Eat lean meat without skin and cook without added saturated and trans fat.
- Choose fat free, 1% fat and low fat dairy products.
- Eat less than 300 mg cholesterol per day.
- Cut back on beverages and foods with added sugars.
- Try to eat less than 2,300 mg salt per day. Eat foods with little or no salt.
- If you drink, limit alcohol to one drink per day for women and two drinks per day for men.
- Eat only as many calories as you burn each day.

• Follow the AHA guidelines when you dine out and watch proportions.

Nursing Diagnosis: Ineffective Cardiopulmonary Tissue Perfusion related to excessive activity and congestive heart failure

Teach the client to follow physician's activity recommendations. Teach the client to cluster low-energy tasks (walk to bathroom, brush teeth, gather clothes, return to chair before putting on clothes). Teach the client to space higher energy tasks with adequate rest periods. Teach the client to take radial pulse and follow the physician's recommendations for maximum pulse rate with activity.

Nursing Diagnosis: Readiness for Enhanced activity planning related to stated interest in following physician's recommended exercise plan

Teach the client to seek physician's recommendation regarding an exercise plan and describe the following guidelines for healthy individuals (American Heart Association, 2008). Healthy adults age 18 to 65 years need moderate physical activity for a minimum of 30 minutes on 5 days per week or vigorous intensity aerobic activity for a minimum of 20 minutes on 3 days per week. Combinations of moderate and vigorous-intensity activity can be performed to meet this recommendation. In addition every adult should perform activities that maintain or increase muscular strength and endurance a minimum of 2 days each week (American Heart Association, 2007).

 Nursing Diagnosis: Fear related to unknown outcome of cardiac defect

Explain to the parents and the child in simple, comprehensive terms information regarding the new diagnosis. Explain all procedures to family and child prior to the event. Encourage family to spend time alone with child to provide comfort and support to the child. Bring items from home for the child while hospitalized for the comfort of the child (special toy, blanket, etc.). Use play therapy to encourage the child to ask questions and to assist the child in understanding what is happening at the time.

CHAPTER 18

Assessing Peripheral Vascular System

Structure and Function Overview.

The peripheral vascular system, composed of arteries, capillaries, and veins, carries blood to and from the heart and contributes to regulating blood pressure and to exchange oxygen, nutrients, and waste materials between the blood and tissue in the capillary network. The lymphatic system filters and returns tissue fluid back to the venous circulation.

Arteries carry blood from the heart to the capillaries. Artery walls are thicker and stronger than veins and contain elastic fibers to accommodate stretching as blood surges through the vessels. Each heartbeat forces a surge of blood through the arterial vessels under high pressure, which is the arterial pulse. These pulses that can be palpated include the brachial pulse, radial pulse, ulnar pulse, femoral pulse, popliteal pulse, dorsalis pedal pulse, posterior tibial pulse, and dorsalis pedal pulse (see Fig. 18-1).

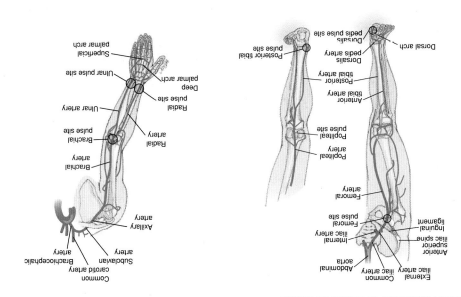

FIGURE 18-1 Major arteries of the arms and legs.

Assessment of the carotid pulse is discussed in Chapter 17: Assessing Heart and Neck Vessels.

CAPILLARY BED AND FLUID EXCHANGE

Capillaries, very small blood vessels, form the connecting network between the arterial and venous circulation, known as *arterioles* and *venules.* It allows balance between the vascular and interstitial spaces. The arterial vessels transport oxygen, water, and nutrients to microscopic capillaries (Fig. 18-2). Hydrostatic pressure is the mechanism by which interstitial fluid diffuses out of the capillaries into the tissue space to release oxygen, water, and nutrients and pick up waste products. Fluid re-enters the capillaries by osmotic pressure and is transported away from the tissues and interstitial spaces by venous circulation. *Lymphatic capillaries* function to remove excess fluid left behind in the interstitial spaces to maintain balance of interstitial fluid and prevent edema.

VEINS

Veins, blood vessels that carry deoxygenated, nutrient-depleted, waste-laden blood from the tissues back to the heart, contain 70% of the body's blood volume. The veins of the arms, upper trunk, head, and neck carry blood to the superior vena cava, where it passes into the right atrium. Blood from the lower trunk and legs drains upward into the inferior vena cava. This is a low-pressure system with no force to propel blood forward. The upward flow of blood back to the heart is a result of one-way valves in the veins, skeletal muscle contraction, and the pressure gradient in the chest and abdomen that occurs with breathing. Problems with any of these mechanisms can impede venous return resulting in venous stasis and edema in the lower extremities. Venous walls are thinner with a larger diameter than arteries. There are two *deep veins* in the leg: the *femoral vein* and *popliteal vein.* The *superficial veins* are the *great and small saphenous veins. Perforator veins* connect the superficial veins with the deep veins (Fig. 18-3). Assessment of the jugular vein is discussed in Chapter 17: Assessing Heart and Neck Vessels.

LYMPHATIC SYSTEM

The *lymphatic system,* a complex vascular system composed of *lymphatic capillaries, lymphatic vessels, and lymph nodes,* drains excess fluid and plasma proteins from tissues returning them back to the venous system to prevent edema. Fluids and proteins are absorbed into the *lymphatic vessels* by *lymphatic capillaries,*

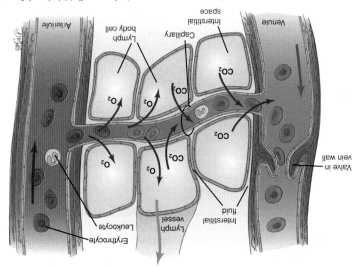

FIGURE 18-2 Normal capillary circulation ensures removal of excess fluid (edema) from the interstitial spaces as well as delivery of oxygen and nutrients and removal of carbon dioxide.

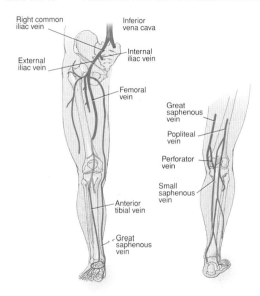

FIGURE 18-3 Major veins of the legs.

which form larger vessels that pass through *lymph nodes,* where microorganisms, foreign materials, dead cells, and abnormal cells are trapped and destroyed. After the lymph is filtered, it travels to either the *right lymphatic duct,* which drains the upper right side of the body or the *thoracic duct,* which drains the rest of the body back into the venous system through *subclavian veins* (Fig. 18-4).

This filtering defends the body against microorganisms and absorbs fats (lipids) from the small intestine into the bloodstream. The *superficial lymph nodes* assessed in this chapter include the *epitrochlear nodes* and the *superficial inguinal nodes.* The *epitrochlear nodes* drain the lower arm and hand. Lymph from the remainder of the arm and hand drains to the axillary lymph nodes. The *superficial inguinal nodes* drain the legs, external genitalia, and lower abdomen and buttocks (Fig. 18-5).

Nursing Assessment

COLLECTING SUBJECTIVE DATA

Focus Questions

Any changes in skin color, texture, or temperature? Pain in calves, feet, buttocks, or legs? What aggravates the pain?

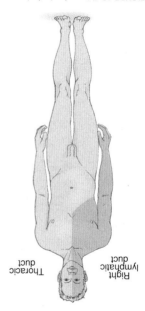

FIGURE 18-4 Lymphatic drainage.

Right lymphatic duct

Thoracic duct

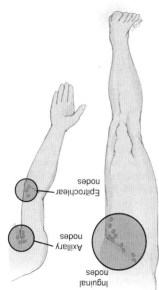

FIGURE 18-5 Superficial lymph nodes of the arms and legs.

Axillary nodes

Epitrochlear nodes

Inguinal nodes

Walking? Sitting for long periods? Standing for long periods? Does it awaken you? What relieves the pain? Elevating legs? Rest? Lying down? Is there associated coldness, cyanosis, edema, varicosities, paresthesia, or tingling in legs or feet? Any leg veins that are ropelike, bulging, or contorted? Any sores on legs? Location? Size? Appearance? Length of time? If client is male: Any changes in sexual activity? History of heart or blood vessel surgery? Family history of diabetes, hypertension, coronary artery disease, or elevated cholesterol or triglyceride levels? Is client taking any drugs that may mimic arterial insufficiency? Self-care activities: Does client have well-fitting shoes? Does client wear constricting garments or hosiery? In what type of chair does client usually sit? Does client cross legs frequently? What amount and type of exercise does the client do? Does client smoke? Amount and for how long?

Risk Factors

Risk for arterial peripheral vascular disease related to tobacco smoking, age greater than 50 years (if client has a history of diabetes or other risk factors then age *less than* 50 years is a risk factor), family history of hypertension, coronary or peripheral vascular disease.

Risk for venous peripheral vascular disease include pregnancy, prolonged standing, limited physical activity/poor physical fitness, congenital or acquired vein wall weakness, female gender, increasing age, genetics (e.g., African American), obesity, lack of dietary fiber, use of constricting corsets/clothes.

COLLECTING OBJECTIVE DATA

Equipment Needed

- Stethoscope
- Sphygmomanometer
- Doppler
- Tape measure (paper)
- Cotton (to detect light touch)
- Paper clip (tip used to detect sharp sensation—safer than pin tip)
- Tuning fork (to detect vibratory sensation)

Physical Assessment

After explaining what assessments you will be making, provide privacy while the patient changes into an examination gown. See Figures 18-1 and 18-3 for diagrams of major arteries and veins.

INSPECTION, PALPATION, AND AUSCULTATION OF CIRCULATION TO ARMS AND NECK

Inspection, palpation, and auscultation are performed together to assess blood pressure and circulation to the upper extremities while the client is in a sitting, then standing position. The Allen test is used to detect arterial insufficiency of hand.

ASSESSMENT PROCEDURE	NORMAL FINDINGS	ABNORMAL FINDINGS
Palpate **brachial artery,** and then auscultate **arterial blood pressure** alternately in both arms with client sitting.	May be difference of 5–10 mm Hg between each arm	More than 10 mm Hg difference between each arm
Palpate **brachial artery,** and then auscultate **arterial blood pressure** alternately in both arms with client standing.	*Systolic pressure:* <120 mm Hg *Diastolic pressure:* <80 mm Hg[a] (see Table 6-2, p. 125) *Systolic pressure:* Difference between arms of 15 mm Hg or less *Diastolic pressure:* Difference between arms of 5 mm Hg or less	*Systolic pressure:* ≥120 mm Hg[a] *Diastolic pressure:* ≥80 mm Hg[a] (see Table 6-2, p. 125) *Systolic pressure:* Difference between arms of more than 15 mm Hg *Diastolic pressure:* Difference between arms of more than 5 mm Hg
Inspect and palpate **upper extremities** for the following: • **Color**	• Pink; pink or red tones visible under dark pigmentation	• Pallor, cyanosis, rubor; rapid color changes—pallor, cyanosis, and redness seen with Raynaud disease
• **Edema**	• No edema bilaterally	• Swelling on one side may be the result of impaired lymph drainage such as with lymph-edema. Pitting edema may also be noted.

[a]Values may vary with individuals.

ASSESSMENT PROCEDURE	NORMAL FINDINGS	ABNORMAL FINDINGS
• Temperature	• Warm	• Cold; cool extremities seen with arterial insufficiency and Raynaud disease
• **Sensation:** Scatter stimuli over trunk and upper extremities with client's eyes closed • Mobility • **Radial pulses** (Fig. 18-6)	• Client can identify light and deep touch; nontender. • Mobile • Bilateral pulses strong and equal (Box 18-1 on page 388)	• Paresthesia, tenderness, pain; numbness seen in Raynaud disease • Paralysis • Bilateral/unilateral pulses weak, asymmetrical, or absent may indicate partial or complete obstruction; increased radial pulse may indicate hyperkinesis.

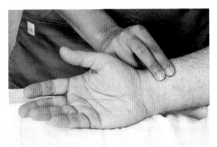

FIGURE 18-6 Palpating the radial pulse.

Continued on following page

INSPECTION, PALPATION, AND AUSCULTATION OF CIRCULATION TO ARMS AND NECK (Continued)

ASSESSMENT PROCEDURE	NORMAL FINDINGS	ABNORMAL FINDINGS
• **Ulnar pulses** (Fig. 18-7)	• Bilateral pulses strong and equal	• Bilateral/unilateral pulses weak, asymmetrical, or absent

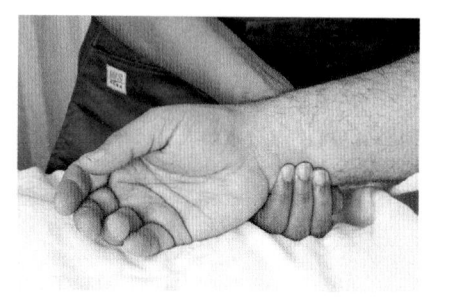

FIGURE 18-7 Palpating the ulnar pulse.

ASSESSMENT PROCEDURE	NORMAL FINDINGS	ABNORMAL FINDINGS
If client has weak radial and/or ulnar pulses, perform the **Allen test** to further assess circulation (Fig. 18-8).	Full palm of hand becomes pink with release of ulnar or radial artery.	Only half of palm of hand becomes pink with release of ulnar or radial artery; other half of palm remains whitish. Pallor persists with occlusion of ulnar artery.

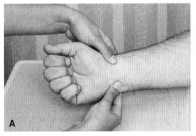 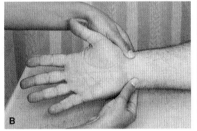 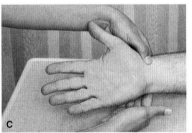

FIGURE 18-8 Allen test. **A:** Have the client rest the hand palm side up on the examination table and then make a fist. Use your thumbs to occlude the radial and ulnar arteries. **B:** Continue pressure to keep both arteries occluded and have the client release the fist. Note that the palm remains pale. **C:** Release the pressure on the ulnar artery and watch for color to return to the hand. To assess radial patency, repeat the procedure as before, but as the last step, release pressure on the radial artery.

Continued on following page

INSPECTION, PALPATION, AND AUSCULTATION OF CIRCULATION TO ARMS AND NECK (Continued)

ASSESSMENT PROCEDURE	NORMAL FINDINGS	ABNORMAL FINDINGS
Palpate for **epitrochlear lymph nodes** (Fig. 18-9). If able to feel nodes, evaluate for size, tenderness, and consistency. Repeat on opposite arm.	Usually epitrochlear lymph nodes are not palpable.	Enlarged epitrochlear nodes may indicate an infection in the hand or forearm. Generalized lymphadenopathy or a lesion may also cause enlarged nodes just above the elbow.

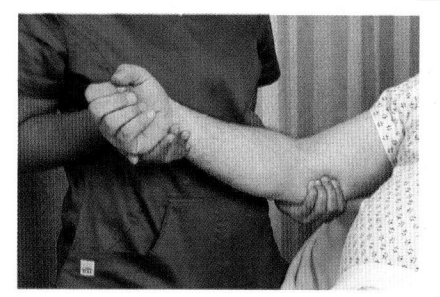

FIGURE 18-9 Palpating the epitrochlear lymph nodes by flexing the client's left elbow about 90 degrees. Use your left hand to palpate behind the elbow in the groove between the biceps and triceps muscles just above the elbow. Repeat on right elbow.

INSPECTION AND PALPATION OF JUGULAR VENOUS PRESSURE AND CIRCULATION OF LOWER EXTREMITIES

Inspection and palpation are performed together to assess circulation of the lower extremities with the client in a supine position. Finally, special maneuvers are performed to detect venous and arterial insufficiencies of the legs.

ASSESSMENT PROCEDURE	NORMAL FINDINGS	ABNORMAL FINDINGS
Inspect and palpate **legs** for the following:		
• **Color**	• Pink; pink or red tones visible under dark pigmentation	• Pallor, cyanosis, rubor; pallor on elevation and rubor on dependency suggest arterial insufficiency; rusty or brownish pigmentation around ankles indicates venous insufficiency (see Table 18-1 on page 388).
• **Temperature**	• Warm	• Cold; coolness in one leg suggests arterial insufficiency; increased warmth in leg may be due to thrombophlebitis; bilateral coolness in feet and legs suggests cold room, recent cigarette smoking, or anxiety
• **Sensation:** Scatter stimuli with client's eyes closed.	• Client can identify light and deep touch; nontender.	• Paresthesia, tenderness, pain
• **Mobility**	• Mobile	• Paralysis

Continued on following page

INSPECTION AND PALPATION OF JUGULAR VENOUS PRESSURE AND CIRCULATION OF LOWER EXTREMITIES (Continued)

ASSESSMENT PROCEDURE	NORMAL FINDINGS	ABNORMAL FINDINGS
• **Superficial veins**	• Slight venous distention with standing that collapses with elevation	• Severe venous distention and bulging are seen with varicose veins due to incompetent valves, vein wall weakness, or venous obstruction; superficial vein thrombophlebitis is characterized by redness, thickening, and tenderness along the vein.
• **Condition of skin**	• Intact	• Lesions
• Edema	• Not present	• Present
• **Femoral pulse** (Fig. 18-10)	• Bilateral pulses strong and equal	• Bilateral/unilateral pulses weak, asymmetrical, or absent in arterial occlusion

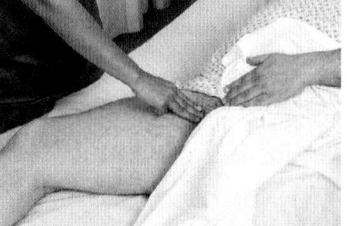

FIGURE 18-10 Palpating the femoral pulses.

ASSESSMENT PROCEDURE	NORMAL FINDINGS	ABNORMAL FINDINGS
• **Inguinal lymph nodes.** Because there are two chains of nodes, palpate for the horizontal chain on the anterior thigh just under the inguinal ligament and the vertical chain close to the great saphenous vein.	Usually inguinal lymph nodes are not palpable.	Enlarged inguinal nodes may indicate an infection in the leg, external genitalia, lower abdomen, or buttock.
• **Popliteal pulse:** Have client bend knees or, if on table, roll onto stomach and flex leg 90 degrees. Press deeply to feel (Fig. 18-11).	• Bilateral pulses strong and equal, but it is not unusual for popliteal pulse to be difficult or impossible to detect.	• Bilateral/unilateral pulses weak, asymmetrical, or absent may indicate occluded artery.

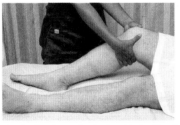 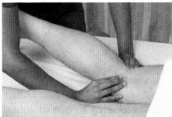

FIGURE 18-11 Palpating the popliteal pulse with the client (**left**) supine and (**right**) prone. If you cannot detect a pulse, try palpating with the client in a prone position. Partially raise the leg and place your fingers deep in the bend of the knee. Repeat palpation in opposite leg and note amplitude bilaterally.

Continued on following page

INSPECTION AND PALPATION OF JUGULAR VENOUS PRESSURE AND CIRCULATION OF LOWER EXTREMITIES (Continued)

ASSESSMENT PROCEDURE	NORMAL FINDINGS	ABNORMAL FINDINGS
• **Dorsalis pedis pulse:** Have client dorsiflex or extend foot (Fig. 18-12).	• Bilateral pulses strong and equal (congenitally absent in 5–10% of population)	• Bilateral/unilateral pulses weak, asymmetrical, or absent may indicate impaired arterial circulation.
• **Posterior tibial pulse** (located on medial malleolus of ankle; Fig. 18-13).	• Bilateral pulses strong and equal	• Bilateral/unilateral pulses weak or absent may indicate arterial occlusion.

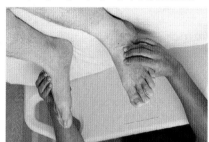

FIGURE 18-12 Palpating the dorsalis pedis pulse.

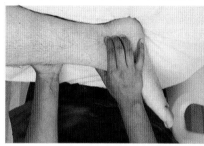

FIGURE 18-13 Palpating the posterior tibial pulse.

ASSESSMENT PROCEDURE	NORMAL FINDINGS	ABNORMAL FINDINGS
• Check for **arterial insufficiency** (Fig. 18-14) if leg pulses are decreased. Have client lie down on back while you support client's legs 30.4 cm (12 in) above heart level. Have client flap feet up and down at ankles for 60 seconds, then sit up and dangle legs.	• Feet pink to slight pale color with this maneuver; pink color returns to tips of toes in 10 seconds; veins on top of feet fill in 15 seconds.	• Extensive pallor with this maneuver in arterial insufficiency; toes and feet exhibit rubor (dusky red); venous return to feet is delayed 45 seconds or more in arterial insufficiency. (Refer to Tables 18-1 and 18-2 on pages 388 and 389 for comparisons and characteristics of venous and arterial insufficiency.)

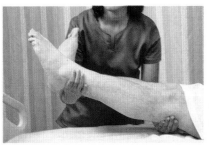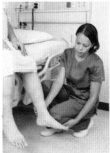

FIGURE 18-14 Testing for arterial insufficiency by (**left**) elevating the legs and then (**right**) having the client dangle the legs.

Continued on following page

INSPECTION AND PALPATION OF JUGULAR VENOUS PRESSURE AND CIRCULATION OF LOWER EXTREMITIES (Continued)

ASSESSMENT PROCEDURE	NORMAL FINDINGS	ABNORMAL FINDINGS
• Check for **competency of valves** (Fig. 18-15) (manual compression test) if client has varicose veins—compress dilated veins with one hand while using the other hand to feel pulsations 15.2–20.3 cm (6–8 in) above the first hand. Repeat in other leg.	• No pulsation palpated	• Pulsation felt with incompetent valves
Compare **venous and arterial insufficiency** of lower extremities (see Table 18-1 and Table 18-2).		*Note: See Tables 18-1 and 18-2 for comparison and characteristics of venous and arterial insufficiencies and differentiation of arterial and venous ulcers.*
Auscultation of Arteries		
If **arterial insufficiency** is found in legs, auscultate over the following areas.		
• **Aorta**	• NO sound	• Bruits
• **Renal arteries**	• NO sound	• Bruits
• **Iliac arteries**	• NO sound	• Bruits
• **Femoral arteries** (Fig. 18-16)	• NO sound	• Bruits

ASSESSMENT PROCEDURE	NORMAL FINDINGS	ABNORMAL FINDINGS

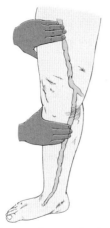

FIGURE 18-15 Performing manual compression to assess competence of venous valves in clients with varicose veins.

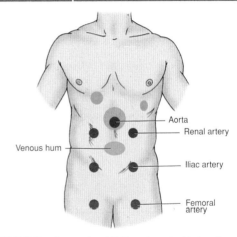

FIGURE 18-16 Vascular sounds and friction rubs can best be heard over these areas.

BOX 18-1   ASSESSING PULSE STRENGTH

Palpation of the pulses in the peripheral vascular examination is typically to assess amplitude or strength. Pulse amplitude is graded on a 0 to 3– scale, with 3+ being the strongest. Elasticity of the artery wall may also be noted during the peripheral vascular examination, by palpating for a resilient (bouncy) quality rather than a more rigid arterial tone, whereas pulse rate and rhythm are best assessed during examination of the heart and neck vessels.

PULSE AMPLITUDE

Pulse amplitude is typically graded as 0 to 3+:

Rating	Description
0	Absent
1+	Weak, diminished (easy to obliterate)
2+	Normal (obliterate with moderate pressure)
3+	Bounding (unable to obliterate or requires firm pressure)

TABLE 18-1   Comparison of Arterial and Venous Insufficiency

	Arterial Insufficiency	Venous Insufficiency
Pulse	Decreased or absent	Present
Color	Pale on elevation, dusky rubor on dependency	Pink to cyanotic, brown pigment at ankles
Temperature	Cool, cold	Warm
Edema	None	Present
Skin	Shiny skin, thick nails, absence of hair, ulcers on toes, gangrene may develop	Ulcers on ankles; discolored, scaly
Sensation	Leg pain aggravated by exercise and relieved with rest; pressure or cramps in buttocks or calves during walking, paresthesias	Leg pain aggravated by prolonged standing or sitting, relieved by elevation of legs, lying down, or walking; also relieved with use of support hose

TABLE 18-2 **Characteristics of Arterial and Venous Insufficiency**

Characteristic	Arterial	Venous
Pain	Intermittent claudication to sharp, unrelenting, constant	Aching, cramping
Pulses	Diminished or absent	Present, but may be difficult to palpate through edema
Skin characteristics	Dependent rubor—elevation pallor of foot, dry, shiny skin, cool-to-cold temperature, loss of hair over toes and dorsum of foot, nails thickened and ridged	Pigmentation in gaiter area (area of medial and lateral malleolus), skin thickened and tough, may be reddish blue, frequently associated dermatitis
Ulcer Characteristics		
Location	Tip of toes, toe webs, heel or other pressure areas if confined to bed	Medial malleolus; infrequently lateral malleolus or anterior tibial area
Pain	Very painful	Minimal pain if superficial or may be very painful
Depth of ulcer	Deep, often involving joint space	Superficial
Shape	Circular	Irregular border
Ulcer base	Pale to black and dry gangrene	Granulation tissue—beefy red to yellow fibrinous in chronic long-term ulcer
Leg edema	Minimal unless extremity kept in dependent position constantly to relieve pain	Moderate to severe

Used with permission from Smeltzer, S.C., Bare, B.G., Hinkle, J.L., & Cheever, K.H. (2012). *Brunner & Suddarth's textbook of medical-surgical nursing*. Philadelphia: Wolters Kluwer Health/Lippincott Williams & Wilkins.

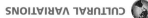

GERIATRIC VARIATIONS

- Hair loss of lower extremities occurs with aging and may not be an absolute sign of arterial insufficiency.
- Inspect for rigid, tortuous veins and arteries (decreased venous return and competency) because varicosities are common in older adults.
- Prominent, bulging veins are common. Varicosities are considered a problem only if ulcerations, signs of thrombophlebitis, or cords are present. Cords are nontender, palpable veins having a rubber tubing consistency (Fig. 18-17).
- Blood pressure increases as elasticity decreases in arteries with proportionately greater increase in systolic pressure resulting in a widening of pulse pressure.

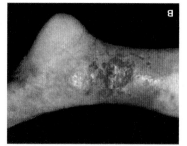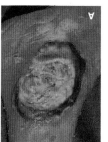

FIGURE 18-17 A: Characteristic ulcer of arterial insufficiency. (© 1994 Michael English, M.D.) **B:** Characteristic ulcer of venous insufficiency. (Courtesy of Dermik Laboratories, Inc.)

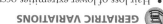

CULTURAL VARIATIONS

There are ethnic variations in rates of peripheral artery disease. South Asians have lower rates and African Americans in the United States have higher rates than non-Hispanic whites, even accounting for the differences in risk factors, which remains unexplained ("Ethnicity and peripheral artery disease," 2009).

POSSIBLE COLLABORATIVE PROBLEMS—RISK OF

- Hypertension
- Thrombophlebitis
- Arterial insufficiency
- Peripheral neuropathy
- Thrombosis/emboli

- Venous insufficiency
- Edema
- Gangrene
- Vasospasms
- Claudication
- Stasis ulcers

Teaching Tips for Selected Nursing Diagnoses and Collaborative Problems

Nursing Diagnosis: Impaired Skin Integrity related to arterial insufficiency

Instruct client on importance of exercise and diet (eat foods high in protein, vitamins A and C, and zinc to promote healing, unless contraindicated by other therapies) to aid healing of leg ulcers. Explain importance of keeping area clean and dry.

Nursing Diagnosis: Impaired Skin Integrity related to venous insufficiency

Instruct client on importance of rest, avoidance of restrictive clothing, elevation of extremities to reduce edema, and proper diet to aid healing of leg ulcers.

Nursing Diagnosis: Ineffective Peripheral Tissue Perfusion related to venous insufficiency

Teach client how to assess condition of extremities (color, temperature, sensation, movement, swelling). Teach client how to use assessment to determine activity level. Teach methods for accomplishing activities of daily living with restricted activity level.

Nursing Diagnosis: Risk for Ineffective Peripheral Tissue Perfusion related to increasing peripheral vascular disease

Teach client how to assess condition of extremities (color, temperature, sensation, movement, swelling).

Teach client how to modify activities of daily living in order to prevent injury and complications as recommended by "Peripheral Vascular Disease" (2013).

- Do not smoke.
- Eat nutritious, low-fat foods; avoid foods high in cholesterol.

- Maintain a healthy weight.
- Engage in moderately strenuous physical activity for at least 30 minutes a day. At least walk briskly for 20 to 30 minutes daily.
- Control high blood pressure.
- Lower high cholesterol (especially LDL cholesterol or the "bad cholesterol") and high triglyceride levels, and raise HDL or "the good cholesterol." If exercise fails to lower your cholesterol, certain medications (statin drugs) can be taken to decrease the bad cholesterol.
- If you have diabetes, control your blood sugar level and take scrupulous care of your feet. Ask your doctor what your HbA1c is, a measure of how well your blood sugar is controlled; it should be less than 7. If it is greater than 8, it is not controlled, and your risk of blood vessel complications (eyes, heart, brain, kidneys, legs) escalates.

Possible Collaborative Problem: Risk for Hypertension

Explain the effects of diet (low fat and low cholesterol), reduction of stress, vigorous exercise, not smoking, and decreased use of alcohol on promotion of adequate circulation. Blood pressure checks should be done on a regular basis. Blood pressures of 120 to 139/80 to 89 mm Hg are considered prehypertensive and require lifestyle modification (Seventh Report of the Joint National Committee on Prevention, Detection, and Treatment of High Blood Pressure, 2003). Refer any client with a reading ≥140/90 mm Hg for treatment.

CHAPTER 19

Assessing Abdomen

Structure and Function Overview

The abdomen is bordered superiorly by the costal margins, inferiorly by the symphysis pubis and inguinal canals, and laterally by the flanks. It is important to understand the anatomic divisions known as the abdominal quadrants, the abdominal wall muscles, the internal anatomy of the abdominal cavity, and the abdominal vasculature in order to perform an adequate assessment of the abdomen.

ABDOMINAL QUADRANTS

The abdomen is divided into four quadrants for purposes of physical examination. These are termed the right upper quadrant (RUQ), right lower quadrant (RLQ), left lower quadrant (LLQ), and left upper quadrant (LUQ) (Fig. 19-1). Note which organs are located within each quadrant (Box 19-1).

ABDOMINAL WALL MUSCLES

The abdominal contents are enclosed externally by the abdominal wall musculature, which includes three layers of muscle extending from the back, around the flanks, and to the front. The outermost layer is the external abdominal oblique; the middle layer is the internal abdominal oblique; and the innermost layer is the transverse abdominis (Fig. 19-2).

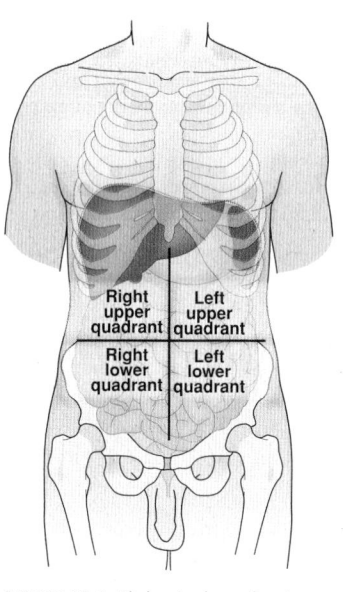

FIGURE 19-1 Abdominal quadrants.

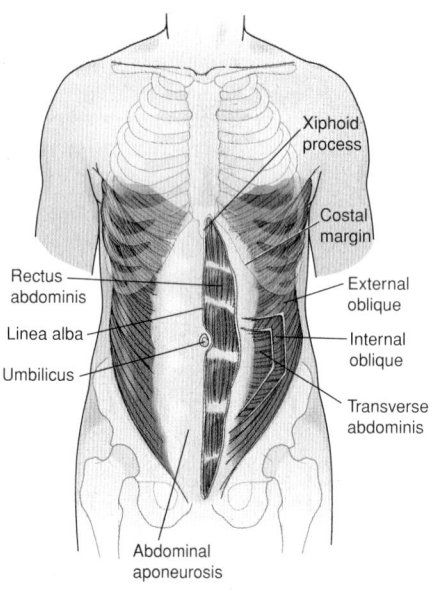

FIGURE 19-2 Abdominal wall muscles.

BOX 19-1 LOCATING ABDOMINAL STRUCTURES BY QUADRANTS

RUQ
   Ascending and transverse colon
   Duodenum
   Gallbladder
   Hepatic flexure of colon
   Liver
   Pancreas (head)
   Pylorus (the small bowel—or ileum—traverses all quadrants)
   Right adrenal gland
   Right kidney (upper pole)
   Right ureter
RLQ
   Appendix
   Ascending colon
   Cecum
   Right kidney (lower pole)
   Right ovary and tube
   Right ureter
   Right spermatic cord

LUQ
   Left adrenal gland
   Left kidney (upper pole)
   Left ureter
   Pancreas (body and tail)
   Spleen
   Splenic flexure of colon
   Stomach
   Transverse ascending colon
LLQ
   Left kidney (lower pole)
   Left ovary and tube
   Left ureter
   Left spermatic cord
   Sigmoid colon
MIDLINE
   Bladder
   Uterus
   Prostate gland

INTERNAL ABDOMINAL STRUCTURES

A thin, shiny, serous membrane lines the abdominal cavity and provides a protective covering (parietal peritoneum) for most of the internal abdominal organs (visceral peritoneum). Within the abdominal cavity are structures of several different body systems—gastrointestinal (GI), reproductive (female), lymphatic, and urinary. These structures are typically referred to as the abdominal viscera and can be divided into two types—solid viscera and hollow viscera. Solid viscera are those organs that maintain their shape consistently—the liver, pancreas, spleen, adrenal glands, kidneys, ovaries, and uterus. The hollow viscera consist of structures that change shape depending on their contents. These include the stomach, gallbladder, small intestine, colon, and bladder.

Solid Viscera

The liver is the largest solid organ in the body. It is located below the diaphragm in the RUQ of the abdomen (Fig. 19-3). The pancreas, located mostly behind the stomach, deep in the upper abdomen, is normally not palpable (see Figs. 19-3 and 19-4). The spleen is approximately 7 cm wide and is located above the left kidney, just below the diaphragm at the level of the ninth, tenth, and eleventh ribs (see Fig. 19-3). This soft, flat structure

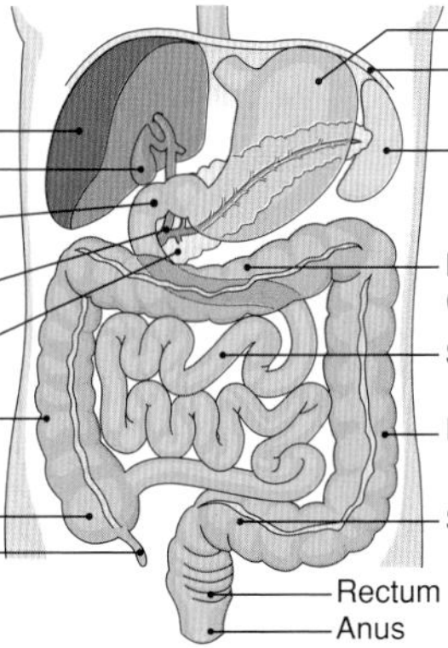

FIGURE 19-3 Abdominal viscera.

is normally not palpable. The kidneys are located high and deep under the diaphragm (see Fig. 19-4).

The pregnant uterus may be palpated above the level of the symphysis pubis in the midline (see Fig. 19-4). The ovaries are located in the RLQ and LLQ and are normally palpated only during a bimanual examination of the internal genitalia.

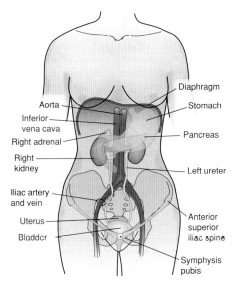

FIGURE 19-4 Abdominal and vascular structures (aorta and iliac artery and vein).

Hollow Viscera

The stomach is a distensible, flask-like organ located in the LUQ, just below the diaphragm and in between the liver and the spleen. The stomach is not usually palpable (see Fig. 19-3).

The gallbladder, a muscular sac approximately 10 cm long, is not normally palpated because it is difficult to distinguish between the gallbladder and the liver (see Fig. 19-3).

The small intestine is actually the longest portion of the digestive tract (approximately 7 m long). The small intestine, which lies coiled in all four quadrants of the abdomen, is not normally palpated (see Fig. 19-3).

The colon, or large intestine, has a wider diameter than the small intestine (approximately 6 cm) and is approximately 1.4 m long. The colon is composed of three major sections: Ascending, transverse, and descending.

The sigmoid colon is often felt as a firm structure on palpation, whereas the cecum and ascending colon may feel softer. The transverse and descending colon may also be felt on palpation (see Fig. 19-3).

The urinary bladder is a distensible muscular sac located behind the pubic bone in the midline of the abdomen. A bladder filled with urine may be palpated in the abdomen above the symphysis pubis (see Fig. 19-4).

VASCULAR STRUCTURES

The abdominal organs are supplied with arterial blood by the abdominal aorta and its major branches. Pulsations of the aorta are frequently visible and palpable midline in the upper abdomen (see Fig. 19-4).

COLLECTING SUBJECTIVE DATA

Focus Questions

Abdominal pain? Character? Onset? Location? Duration? Severity? Relieving and aggravating factors? Associated factors? (See Abnormal Findings 19-1.) Indigestion? Nausea? Vomiting? Precipitating/relieving factors? Change in appetite? Associated weight loss? Change in bowel elimination? Describe. Constipation? Diarrhea? Associated symptoms? Any past GI disorders (ulcers, gastroesophageal reflux, inflammatory or obstructive bowel, pancreatitis, gallbladder or liver disease, diverticulosis, appendicitis, history of viral hepatitis)? Family history of colon, stomach, pancreatic, liver, kidney, or bladder cancer? Use of medications—aspirin, ibuprofen, anti-inflammatory drugs, steroids? Chronic use of antacids or histamine-2 blockers? GI diagnostic tests? Surgeries? Health practices:

Usual diet? Exercise? Use of alcohol? Use of caffeine, typical dietary and fluid intake (24-hour recall), stressors? Effects of GI problems on activities of life style? Current life stressors?

Risk Factors

Risk for hepatitis B virus (HBV) exposure related to contact in population of high HBV endemicity, sexual contact with carriers, intravenous drug abusers, heterosexuals who have had more than one sex partner in past 6 months, sexually active homosexual or bisexual males, people with hemophilia, people undergoing hemodialysis, international travelers in high-risk HBV areas, health-care workers, long-term prison inmates.

Risk for gallbladder cancer related to female gender after menopause, increased parity, obesity, chronic inflammation or other diseases of the gallbladder or biliary system, and chronic infections of Helicobacter pylori or Salmonella.

Risk for colon cancer related to age greater than 50 years, family history of colorectal cancer, history of endometrial, breast, or ovarian cancer, history of inflammatory bowel disease, polyps, or colorectal cancer, diet low in fiber and high in fat, African American, sedentary lifestyle, heavy alcohol intake, and past radiation treatments for other cancers.

COLLECTING OBJECTIVE DATA

Equipment Needed

- Stethoscope (warm the diaphragm and bell)
- Centimeter ruler
- Marking pen
- Small pillow

Physical Assessment

Review Figures 19-1 to 19-4 for a diagram of landmarks of the abdomen.

Assessment of the abdomen differs from other assessments in that inspection and auscultation precedes percussion and palpation. This sequence allows accurate assessment of bowel sounds and delays more uncomfortable maneuvers until last. The client is placed in the supine position, with small pillows under the head and knees. The abdomen is exposed from the breasts to the symphysis pubis.

Examiner should warm hands and have short fingernails. Stand at the client's right side and carry out assessment systematically, beginning with the LUQ and progressing clockwise through the four abdominal quadrants (see Fig. 19-1). The client's bladder should be empty.

INSPECTION		
ASSESSMENT PROCEDURE	**NORMAL FINDINGS**	**ABNORMAL FINDINGS**
Inspect the **skin** for the following: • Color	• Normally paler, with white striae	• Dark bluish striae seen in Cushing syndrome, redness seen in inflammation, pale and taut with ascites, purple flank color (Grey Turner's sign) seen with bleeding within the abdominal wall

Continued on following page

INSPECTION (Continued)

ASSESSMENT PROCEDURE	NORMAL FINDINGS	ABNORMAL FINDINGS
• Venous pattern	• Fine veins observable	• Engorged, prominent veins seen with cirrhosis of the liver, inferior vena cava obstruction, portal hypertension, or ascites
• Integrity	• No rashes or lesions	• Rashes, lesions
Perform the following special maneuver for **prominent abdominal veins:** • Compress a section of vein with two fingers next to each other, remove one finger, and observe for filling; repeat procedure, removing other finger.	• Blood fills from upper to lower abdomen	• Blood fills from lower to upper abdomen (obstructed inferior vena cava)
Inspect the **umbilicus** for the following:		
• Position	• Sunken, centrally located	• Deviated from midline with mass, hernia, enlarged organs, or fluid; everted with abdominal distention or umbilical hernia
• Color	• Pinkish	• Inflamed, crusted; bluish color (Cullen sign) seen in intra-abdominal hemorrhage

ASSESSMENT PROCEDURE	NORMAL FINDINGS	ABNORMAL FINDINGS
Observe the **abdomen** for the following (Fig. 19-5): • Contour	• Rounded or flat	• Generalized distention seen with air or fluid accumulation; distention below umbilicus due to full bladder, uterine enlargement, ovarian tumor or cyst; distention above the umbilicus seen with pancreatic mass or gastric dilation. Major causes of abdominal distention may be referred to as "6 Fs": Fat, feces, fetus, fibroids, flatulence, and fluid.
• Symmetry	• Symmetrical	• Asymmetrical with organ enlargement, large masses, hernia, diastasis recti, or bowel obstruction

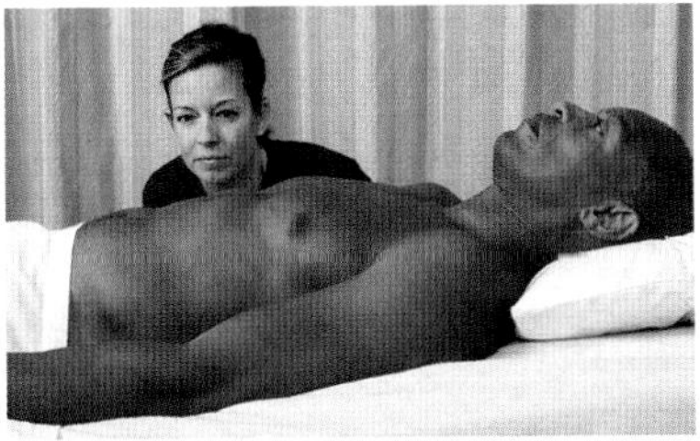

FIGURE 19-5 View abdominal contour from the client's side.

Continued on following page

INSPECTION (Continued)

ASSESSMENT PROCEDURE	NORMAL FINDINGS	ABNORMAL FINDINGS
Surface motion	• No movement or slight peristalsis visualized over aorta	• Diminished abdominal movement with peritoneal irritation; bounding peristalsis; bounding pulsations with abdominal aortic aneurysm (AAA); peristaltic, ripple waves seen with intestinal obstruction.
Observe color of stools	Brown to dark brown	Black, tarry (melena), bright red
Observe color of emesis	Varies	Bloody (hematemesis), coffee grounds (old blood)

AUSCULTATION

Note: Using the diaphragm of a warm stethoscope, apply light pressure to auscultate for bowel sounds for up to 5 minutes in each quadrant. Use the bell to auscultate for vascular sounds.

Auscultate for **bowel sounds**	A series of intermittent, soft clicks and gurgles are heard at a rate of 5–30 per minute. Postoperatively, bowel sounds may resume gradually with the small intestine functioning normally in first few hours post-op; stomach emptying takes 24–48 hours to recover; and the colon requires 3–5 days to recover propulsive activity.	Absent bowel sounds with peritonitis or paralytic ileus; hypoactive in abdominal surgery, late bowel obstruction, or pneumonia. Hyperactive sounds heard in diarrhea, gastroenteritis, or early bowel obstruction; high-pitched tinkling and rushes (borborygmus) heard in bowel obstruction

ASSESSMENT PROCEDURE	**NORMAL FINDINGS**	**ABNORMAL FINDINGS**
Auscultate for **vascular sounds** (Fig. 19-6). *Caution: If bruits are heard, do not palpate abdomen as part of the assessment. (Bruits may be indicative of a narrowed vessel or aneurysm.)*	No bruits, no venous hums, no friction rubs	Bruits heard over aorta, renal arteries, or iliac arteries; venous hum auscultated over epigastric or umbilical area may indicate increased collateral circulation between portal and systemic venous systems as with cirrhosis of the liver.

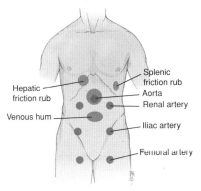

Hepatic friction rub

Venous hum

Splenic friction rub

Aorta

Renal artery

Iliac artery

Femoral artery

FIGURE 19-6 Vascular sounds and friction rubs can best be heard over these areas.

Continued on following page

PERCUSSION

ASSESSMENT PROCEDURE	NORMAL FINDINGS	ABNORMAL FINDINGS

Note: Percussion notes will vary from dull to tympanic, with tympany dominating over the hollow organs. The hollow organs include the stomach, intestines, bladder, aorta, and gallbladder. Dull percussion notes will be heard over the liver, spleen, pancreas, kidneys, and uterus. Percuss from areas of tympany to dullness to locate borders of these solid organs.

Percuss abdomen in **all four quadrants** for percussion tones (notes); see Figure 19-7.	Generalized tympany over bowels	Increases dullness over enlarged organs; hyperresonance over gaseous, distended abdomen

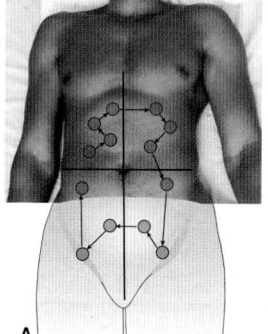

B
Abdominal percussion Technique

A
Abdominal percussion pattern

FIGURE 19-7 Abdominal percussion sequences may proceed clockwise or up and down over the abdomen.

ASSESSMENT PROCEDURE	NORMAL FINDINGS	ABNORMAL FINDINGS
Percuss the **liver** for span as follows: • Percuss starting below umbilicus at client's right midclavicular line (MCL), and percuss upward until you hear dullness; mark this point. Percuss downward from lung resonance in the right MCL to dullness and mark this point.	Liver span is 6–12 cm (2.5–5 in) in the right MCL (Fig. 19-8). The lower border of liver dullness is located at the costal margin to 1–2 cm below. On deep inspiration, the lower border of liver dullness may descend from 1–4 cm below the costal margin. *Note: Liver span is greater in men.*	• Liver span is greater than 12 cm in the right MCL with enlarged liver as seen in tumors, cirrhosis, abscess, and vascular engorgement. A liver in a lower position may be caused by emphysema, and a liver in a higher position may be caused by a mass, ascites, or paralyzed diaphragm.

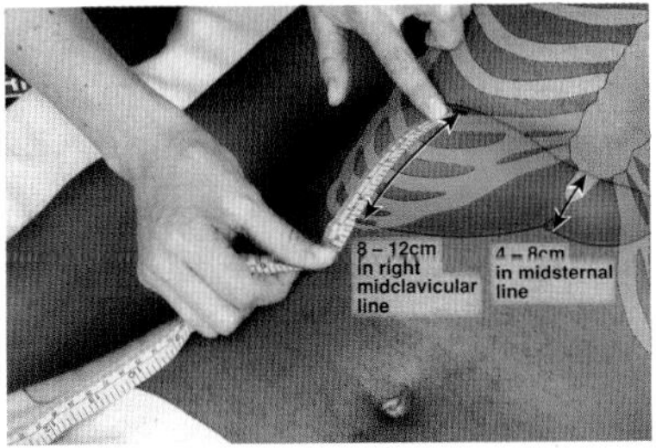

FIGURE 19-8 Normal liver span.

Continued on following page

PERCUSSION (Continued)

ASSESSMENT PROCEDURE	NORMAL FINDINGS	ABNORMAL FINDINGS
• Repeat in midsternal line.	• Liver span is 4–8 cm in midsternal line.	• Liver span is greater than 8 cm in right midsternal line.
Percuss the **spleen** (Fig. 19-9) as follows: • Percuss for dullness by percussing downward in left midaxillary line, beginning with lung resonance until you hear splenic dullness. *Note: Location fluctuates with respiration.*	• Small area of dullness at sixth to tenth ribs.	• Dullness extends above sixth rib or covers larger area. Enlarged spleen is seen with portal hypertension, mononucleosis, or trauma.

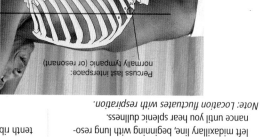

Percuss last interspace: normally tympanic (or resonant)

Anterior axillary line

Midaxillary line

Dull tone over spleen (9th–11th ribs)

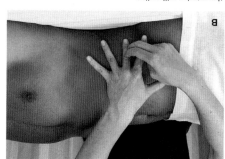

B

FIGURE 19-9 Last left interspace at the anterior axillary line.

ASSESSMENT PROCEDURE	NORMAL FINDINGS	ABNORMAL FINDINGS
• Splenic percussion sign: Ask client to inhale deeply and hold breath; percuss lowest interspaces at left anterior axillary line.	• Percussion note remains tympanic on inhalation.	• Percussion note becomes dull on inhalation.

PALPATION

Note: Light palpation precedes deep palpation to detect tenderness and superficial masses. Deep palpation is used to detect masses and size of organs.

Watch the client's facial expressions and body posture carefully to help assess pain. Examine tender areas last. Never use deep palpation over tender organs in client with polycystic kidneys, after renal transplant, or after hearing an abnormal bruit. Use deep palpation with caution.

Lightly palpate all **four quadrants** for the following: *Note: Do not palpate a pulsating midline mass as it may be a dissecting aneurysm that can rupture from the pressure of palpation. Also avoid deep palpation over tender organs as in the case of polycystic kidneys, Wilms' tumor, transplantation, or suspected splenic trauma.*		

Continued on following page

PALPATION (Continued)

ASSESSMENT PROCEDURE	NORMAL FINDINGS	ABNORMAL FINDINGS
• Tenderness	• Nontender	• Tender, painful with infection, inflammation, pressure from gaseous distention, tumors, or enlarged organs
• Consistency	• Soft, nontender	• Rigid, board-like
• Masses	• No masses	• Superficial masses (A superficial mass becomes more prominent against examiner's hand when client lifts head from examination table, whereas a deep abdominal mass does not.)
Deeply palpate all four quadrants for the following:		
• Tenderness	• Mild tenderness over midline at xiphoid, cecum, and sigmoid colon	• Tenderness, severe pain seen with tumor, cyst, abscess, enlarged organ, aneurysm, or adhesions
• Guarding	• Voluntary guarding	• Involuntary guarding is seen with peritoneal irritation; right-sided guarding is seen with acute cholecystitis.
• Masses	• No masses; aorta; feces in colon	• Masses

ASSESSMENT PROCEDURE	NORMAL FINDINGS	ABNORMAL FINDINGS
Palpate deeply for **liver border** at right costal margin (Assessment Guide 19-1, page 416) for the following: • Tenderness • Consistency	• Nontender • Smooth, firm sharp edge, no masses	• Tenderness seen in trauma or diseased liver • Hard, firm liver may indicate cancer; nodularity may occur with tumors, metastatic cancer, late cirrhosis, or syphilis.
Palpate deeply for **splenic border,** using bimanual technique (see Assessment Guide 19-1). Check for the following: • Size	• Not normally palpable	• Enlarged and palpable with trauma, mononucleosis, blood disorders, and malignancies *Caution: To avoid traumatizing and possibly rupturing the organ, be gentle when palpating an enlarged spleen.*
• Tenderness	• Nontender	• Tender
Palpate deeply for the **kidneys** by using bimanual technique (Assessment Guide 19-2, page 417). Assess for the following: • Size	• Not normally palpable	• Enlarged and palpable owing to cyst, tumor, or hydronephrosis

Continued on following page

PALPATION (Continued)		
ASSESSMENT PROCEDURE	**NORMAL FINDINGS**	**ABNORMAL FINDINGS**
• Tenderness • Masses	• Nontender • No masses	• Tender • Masses
Special maneuvers for **ascites**: • Measure abdominal girth at same point every day.	• No increase in abdominal girth	• Increase in abdominal girth
• Fluid wave test: Place palmar surfaces of fingers and hand firmly on one side of abdomen. Tap with other hand on opposite abdominal wall side. Have assistant put lateral side of lower arm firmly on center of abdomen (Fig. 19-10).	• No fluid wave transmitted	• Fluid wave palpated with ascites

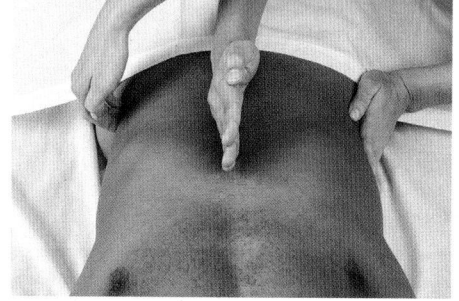

FIGURE 19-10 Performing fluid wave test.

ASSESSMENT PROCEDURE	NORMAL FINDINGS	ABNORMAL FINDINGS
• Shifting dullness: Place client in supine position and percuss from midline to flank, noting level of dullness. Then assist client to side position and percuss again for level of dullness (Fig. 19-11).	• Level of dullness does not change	• Level of dullness is higher when client turns on side

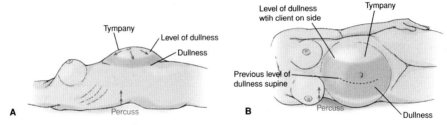

FIGURE 19-11 Percussing for level of dullness with (**A**) client supine and (**B**) client lying on side.

Continued on following page

PALPATION (Continued)

ASSESSMENT PROCEDURE	NORMAL FINDINGS	ABNORMAL FINDINGS
Special tests for **appendicitis**: • Rebound tenderness: Palpate deeply in one of client's four abdominal quadrants, and quickly withdraw palpating hand. Do this at the end of the abdominal examination (Fig. 19-12). *Note: Test for rebound tenderness at the end of the examination because a positive response produces pain and muscle spasm that can interfere with the remaining examination.*	• No pain present	• Pain is present in peritoneal irritation (as in appendicitis); because of danger of rupture do not repeat if pain is present.

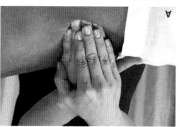

A

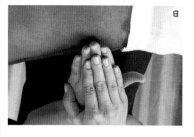

B

FIGURE 19-12 Assessing for rebound tenderness. **A:** Palpating deeply. **B:** Releasing pressure rapidly.

ASSESSMENT PROCEDURE	NORMAL FINDINGS	ABNORMAL FINDINGS
• Psoas sign: Ask client to lie supine and raise right leg. Place pressure on client's thigh.	• No abdominal pain present	• Right lower abdominal pain present with irritation of the iliopsoas muscle due to appendicitis
• Obturator sign: Ask client to flex right leg at hip and knee. Then rotate leg internally and externally.	• No abdominal pain present	• Lower abdominal pain present with irritation of the obturator muscle due to appendicitis
Special test for **acute cholecystitis** (Murphy's sign):		
• Place thumb below right costal margin and ask patient to inhale deeply.	• Client has no increase in pain	• Client has sharp increase in pain with cholecystitis
Testing for **asterixis** (classic sign of hepatic coma):		
• Dorsiflex client's wrist with fingers extended.	• No tremor noted	• Persistent, involuntary flapping tremor

ABNORMAL FINDINGS **19-1** **Mechanisms and Sources of Abdominal Pain**

TYPES OF PAIN

Abdominal pain may be formally described as visceral, parietal, or referred.

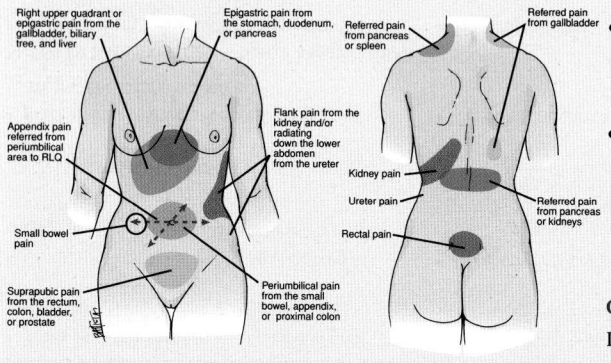

Right upper quadrant or epigastric pain from the gallbladder, biliary tree, and liver

Epigastric pain from the stomach, duodenum, or pancreas

Appendix pain referred from periumbilical area to RLQ

Flank pain from the kidney and/or radiating down the lower abdomen from the ureter

Small bowel pain

Suprapubic pain from the rectum, colon, bladder, or prostate

Periumbilical pain from the small bowel, appendix, or proximal colon

Referred pain from pancreas or spleen

Referred pain from gallbladder

Kidney pain

Ureter pain

Rectal pain

Referred pain from pancreas or kidneys

• *Visceral pain* occurs when hollow abdominal organs, such as the intestines, become distended or contract forcefully or

when the capsules of solid organs such as the liver and spleen are stretched. Poorly defined or localized and intermittently timed, this type of pain is often characterized as dull, aching, burning, cramping, or colicky.

• *Parietal pain* occurs when the parietal peritoneum becomes inflamed, as in appendicitis or peritonitis. This type of pain tends to localize more to the source and is characterized as a more severe and steady pain.

• *Referred pain* occurs at distant sites that are innervated at approximately the same levels as the disrupted abdominal organ. This type of pain travels, or refers, from the primary site and becomes highly localized at the distant site. The accompanying illustrations show common clinical patterns and referents of pain.

CHARACTER OF ABDOMINAL PAIN AND IMPLICATIONS

Dull, aching
  Appendicitis
  Acute hepatitis
  Biliary colic

ABNORMAL FINDINGS 19-1 Mechanisms and Sources of Abdominal Pain (Continued)

Cholecystitis
Cystitis
Dyspepsia
Glomerulonephritis
Incarcerated or strangulated hernia
Irritable bowel syndrome
Hepatocellular cancer
Pancreatitis
Pancreatic cancer
Perforated gastric or duodenal ulcer
Peritonitis
Peptic ulcer disease
Prostatitis
Burning, gnawing
  Dyspepsia
  Peptic ulcer disease
  Cramping ("crampy")
  Acute mechanical obstruction
  Appendicitis

Colitis
Diverticulitis
Gastroesophageal reflux disease (GERD)
Pressure
  Benign prostatic hypertrophy
  Prostate cancer
  Prostatitis
  Urinary retention
Colicky
  Colon cancer
Sharp, knife-like
  Splenic abscess
  Splenic rupture
  Renal colic
  Renal tumor
  Ureteral colic
  Vascular liver tumor
Variable
  Stomach cancer

ASSESSMENT GUIDE 19-1   Liver and Spleen Palpation

Liver Palpation

1. Stand at client's right side and place your left hand under client's back at the eleventh and twelfth ribs.
2. Place right hand parallel to right costal margin.
3. Ask client to breathe deeply, and press upward with your right fingers with each inhalation.

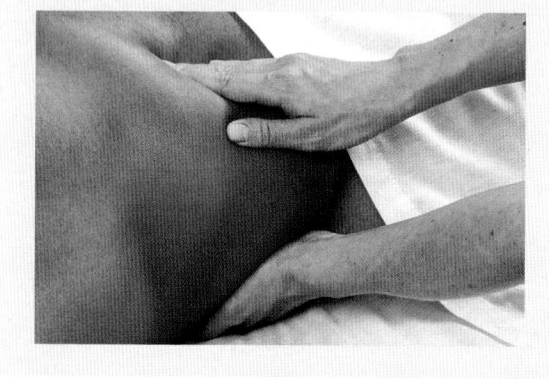

Spleen Palpation

1. Stand at client's right side; reach across client to place your left hand under client's posterior lower ribs, and push-up.
2. Place your right hand below rib margin.
3. Ask client to breathe deeply.
4. Press hands together to palpate spleen on inhalation.

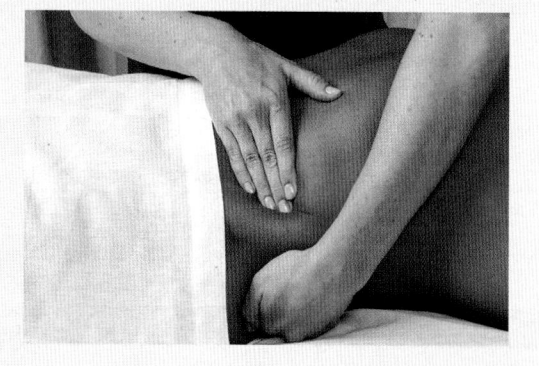

ASSESSMENT GUIDE 19-2 Kidney Palpation

1. Place one of your hands behind lower edge of rib cage and above iliac crest.
2. Place the other hand over corresponding anterior surface.
3. Instruct client to breathe deeply.
4. Lift up lower hand and push in with upper hand as client exhales.
5. Repeat on other side.

Note: The kidneys are rarely palpable.

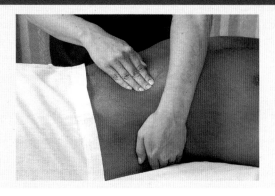

 PEDIATRIC VARIATIONS

Questions to ask the parents when collecting *subjective data* include the following.

- Types of food, fluids, and formula?
- Bowel patterns?
- Frequent spitting up?
- Ability to feed self?
- Milk intake?
- Food intolerances?
- History of eating disorders?
- History of pica?

When collecting *objective data* note the following.

ASSESSMENT PROCEDURE	NORMAL FINDINGS
INSPECTION	
Inspect **contour and size of abdomen.**	Prominent/cylindrical (protuberant) when erect, flat when supine. Superficial veins may be present in infants. An umbilical hernia is commonly seen in the infant and toddler, especially when the infant or toddler strains or cries. As the muscles in the abdomen grow and strengthen, this benign hernia will commonly resolve on its own. In adolescents, if piercing of the umbilicus is present, assess for signs of infection.
Inspect **abdominal movement** in children younger than 8 years.	Rises with inspiration in synchrony with chest; may have visible pulsations in epigastric region
PALPATION	
Palpate **liver border.**	Normal, shortened liver span on percussion. May not extend below costal margin. *Infants and young children:* Liver may be felt 1–3 cm below costal margin; may descend with inspiration.
Palpate **splenic border** (may have child roll on right side).	*Infants and young children:* Spleen may be felt 1–3 cm below costal margin.
Palpate for **abdominal tenderness.**	Extremely difficult to assess in young children, who may confuse pressure of palpation with pain. Distraction is important.
Palpate **kidney borders.**	Difficult to locate except in newborns.

GERIATRIC VARIATIONS

- Decline in appetite and at risk for nutritional imbalance
- Dilated superficial capillaries visible
- Abdomen is softer and organs more easily palpated owing to a decrease in tone of abdominal musculature
- Decreased production of saliva, decreased peristalsis, decreased enzymes, weaker gastric acid
- Gastric mucosa and parietal cell degeneration result in a loss of intrinsic factor, which decreases absorption of vitamin B_{12}
- Bowel sounds 5–30 sounds per minute
- Shortened liver span on percussion due to a decrease in liver size after the age of 50 years
- Liver border is more easily palpated
- Decreased nerve sensation to lower bowel contributes to constipation
- The U.S. Preventive Services Task Force (2005) recommends one-time screening for AAA for men between 65 and 75 years of age who have smoked at least 100 cigarettes in their lifetime.

POSSIBLE COLLABORATIVE PROBLEMS—RISK OF

- Bowel strangulation
- Intestinal obstruction
- Peritonitis
- Ascites
- Paralytic ileus
- Malabsorption syndrome
- Metabolic acidosis/alkalosis
- Diverticulitis
- Pancreatitis
- GI bleeding
- Hepatic failure
- Stromal changes
- Gastric ulcer
- Evisceration
- Gallbladder disease (stones and cancer)

Teaching Tips for Selected Nursing Diagnoses

Nursing Diagnosis: *Imbalanced Nutrition: More or less than body requirements*

Discuss essential components of a well-balanced diet in relation to client's level of physical development and energy expenditure and limiting alcohol consumption to no more than two drinks daily for men and one drink daily for women. Advise client to eat a varied diet, maintain a desirable weight, eliminate tobacco use, and be physically active. Physical activity is associated with a reduced risk of colon cancer (Healthy People 2010).

Nursing Diagnosis: Readiness for Enhanced Nutrition of Child

Teach parents nutritional needs of the child at various ages.

Infant: Exclusive breast-feeding is the ideal nutrition for the first 6 months. Gradually introduce iron-enriched solid food at 6 months to complement breast-feeding. When possible, continue breast-feeding for at least 1 year. Do not give cow's milk before 12 months of age. Introduce finger foods by 1 year. The American Academy of Pediatrics (Abrams, 2011) doubled the recommended intake of vitamin D in foods or as supplements for infants to 400 IU per day for infants less than 1 year of age and 600 IU for older children. Breast-fed infants should get oral iron supplements. Fluoride supplements are required only if the water supply is severely deficient in fluoride.

Toddlers: Food fads are common. Accept this as long as child gets balanced diet over period of days versus every day.

(basal metabolic rate). Teach client how to keep a daily food diary in order to assess intake.

Discuss with client the following.

- Decreasing calories
- Increasing carbohydrates (whole grains and vegetables)
- Decreasing saturated fats
- Decreasing refined sugars
- Decreasing intake of cholesterol to 300 mg/day and salt to 5 g/day

Provide information on support groups such as Weight Watchers, TOPS (Take Off Pounds Sensibly).

Nursing Diagnosis: Risk for Constipation

Discuss bowel habits that are "normal" for client. Caution against overuse of laxatives. Discourage overuse of mineral oil as a laxative because it decreases absorption of vitamins A, D, E, and K. Explain the effects of nutrients, bulk, fluids, and exercise on elimination. The American Cancer Society (*Cancer facts and figures,* 2009) recommends maintaining a healthy weight, engaging in 30 minutes of moderate to vigorous activity per day, eating five or more servings of vegetables and fruits each day, eating whole grains rather than processed (refined grains), limiting processed and red meats,

Nursing Diagnosis: *Deficit Fluid Volume related to vomiting or diarrhea*

Teach parents to give child small amounts of clear liquids (approximately 1 oz every hour for 8 hours) until symptoms subside. May recommend Pedialyte for fluid and electrolyte replacement.

 Nursing Diagnosis: *Risk for Aspiration related to improper feeding and small size of stomach in newborns*

Explain size of infant's stomach to parents (holds 60 mL), and demonstrate proper burping technique to use after every ½ oz feeding.

CHAPTER 20

Assessing Musculoskeletal System

Structure and Function Overview

The body's bones, muscles, and joints compose the musculoskeletal system. Two hundred and six bones make up the axial skeleton (head and trunk) and the appendicular skeleton (extremities, shoulders, and hips; Fig. 20-1). There are varying shapes including short bones (e.g., carpals), long bones (e.g., humerus, femur), flat bones (e.g., sternum, ribs), and irregular-shaped bones (e.g., vertebrae). **Bones**, composed of osseous tissue, provide structure, give protection, serve as levers, store calcium, and produce blood cells. There are two types: **Compact bone** (hard and dense) making up the bone shaft and outer layers; and **spongy bone** (numerous spaces) making up the bone ends and centers. Bone tissue is formed by **osteoblasts** and broken down by cells referred to as **osteoclasts**. The **periosteum** covers the bones and contains osteoblasts and blood vessels.

The body consists of three types of muscles: Skeletal, smooth, and cardiac. The musculoskeletal system is made up of 650 skeletal (voluntary) muscles, which are under conscious control (Fig. 20-2). Skeletal muscles attach to bones by way of strong, fibrous

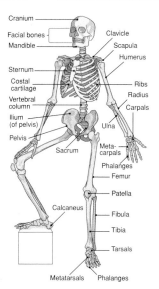

FIGURE 20-1 Major bones of the skeleton. The axial skeleton is shown in yellow and the appendicular in blue.

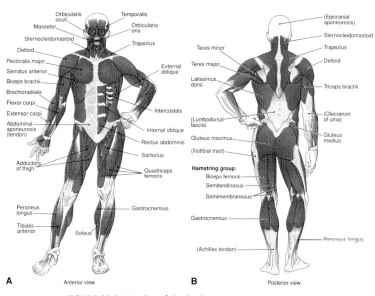

FIGURE 20-2 Muscles of the body. **A:** Anterior. **B:** Posterior.

cords called **tendons** and assist with posture, produce body heat, and allow the body to move.

The joint (or articulation) is the place where two or more bones meet and provide a variety of range of motion (ROM) for the body parts. There are three types of joints. **Fibrous joints** (e.g., sutures between skull bones) are joined by fibrous connective tissue and are immovable. **Cartilaginous joints** (e.g., joints between vertebrae) are joined by cartilage. Synovial joints (e.g., shoulders, wrists, knees, hips, ankles; Fig. 20-3) contain a space between the bones that is filled with synovial fluid, a lubricant that promotes a sliding movement of the bones. Bones in synovial joints are joined by ligaments, which are strong, dense bands of fibrous connective tissue. A fibrous capsule made of connective tissue and connected to the periosteum of the bone encloses synovial joints. Some synovial joints contain **bursae** (small sacs filled with synovial fluid) that cushion the joint.

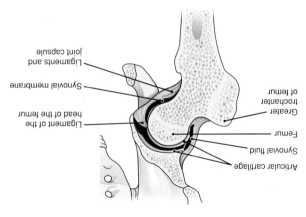

FIGURE 20-3 Components of synovial joints (right hip joint).

Ligaments and joint capsule

Synovial membrane

Ligament of the head of the femur

Greater trochanter of femur

Femur

Synovial fluid

Articular cartilage

Nursing Assessment

COLLECTING SUBJECTIVE DATA

Focus Questions

Pain in joints, muscles, or bones? At rest? With exercise? Changes in size or shape of an extremity? Changes in ability to carry out activities of daily living, sports, work? Stiffness? Time of day? Relation to weight bearing and exercise? Decreased, altered, or absent sensations? Redness or swelling of joints? History of past problems with bones, joints, muscles, fractures? Treatment?

Orthopedic surgery? Last tetanus and polio immunizations? History of osteoporosis or osteomyelitis? Family history of rheumatoid arthritis, gout, osteoporosis, muscular dystrophy? Age of menopause, if applicable? Occupational and recreational history? Self-care: Exercise, weight lifting, weight reduction, diet, use of tobacco or alcohol? Last bone density screening?

Risk Factors

Risk for osteoporosis related to lack of exercise, low calcium intake, excessive caffeine or alcohol consumption, smoking, use of steroids, low estrogen levels in women or postmenopausal women not on estrogen replacement therapy. Risk for sports injury related to lack of wearing protective gear, poor physical fitness, lack of warm-up exercises, and overuse of joints.

COLLECTING OBJECTIVE DATA

Equipment Needed

- Tape measure
- Goniometer (measures angles of joints)
- Marking pen

Physical Assessment

See Figures 20-1 and 20-2 for diagrams of the bones and muscles of the body.

Inspection and palpation are performed while client is standing, sitting, and supine. ROM can be measured by degrees, using approximation or a goniometer. (Normal trunk ROM is given as an example—see Fig. 20-5, p. 428.) In assessing muscle weakness or swelling, size is compared bilaterally by measuring circumference with a tape measure. Joints should not be forced into painful positions. Muscle strength can be estimated using a muscle strength scale (Table 20-1).

TABLE 20-1 **Scale for Muscle Strength**

Rating	Explanation	Strength Classification
5	Active motion against full resistance	Normal
4	Active motion against some resistance	Slight weakness
3	Active motion against gravity	Average weakness
2	Passive ROM (gravity removed and assisted by examiner)	Poor ROM
1	Slight flicker of contraction	Severe weakness
0	No muscular contraction	Paralysis

Inspection: Observe for ROM, swelling, deformity, atrophy, condition of surrounding tissues, and pain.

Palpation: Palpate for heat, strength, tone, edema, crepitus, and nodules. (*Note: Dominant side is normally stronger in muscle strength and tone.*)

INSPECTION OF STANCE AND GAIT

Observe stance and gait as client enters and walks around the room.

ASSESSMENT PROCEDURE	NORMAL FINDINGS	ABNORMAL FINDINGS
Inspect the **stance** for the following:		
Base of support	Weight evenly distributed	Uneven base, with unequal weight bearing, wide-based
Weight-bearing stability	Able to stand on right/left heels, toes	Weakness or inability to use either extremity
Posture	Erect	Stooped
Inspect the **gait** for the following:		
Position of feet	Toes point straight ahead	Toes point in or out
Posture	Erect	Stooped
Stride	Equal on both sides	Wide-based, propels forward, shuffling, or limping
Arm swing	Swing in opposition	No swing

INSPECTION OF THE SPINE, SHOULDER, AND POSTERIOR ILIAC CREST

With client standing, observe in the erect position and as the client bends forward to touch toes. Stabilize client at the waist, and evaluate ROM of the upper trunk.

ASSESSMENT PROCEDURE	NORMAL FINDINGS	ABNORMAL FINDINGS
Inspect the **spine** for the following: • Curves 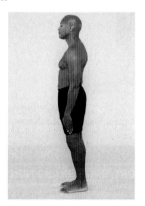 **FIGURE 20-4** Normal spinal curves.	• Cervical concave; thoracic convex; lumbar concave (Fig. 20-4) • Spinal processes in alignment	• Kyphosis, scoliosis, lordosis (see Abnormal Findings 20-1, page 445); a flattened lumbar curve is seen with herniated lumbar disk or ankylosing spondylitis; lateral curvature of spine is seen with scoliosis; and exaggerated lumbar curve (lordosis) is seen with pregnancy or obesity.

Continued on following page

INSPECTION OF THE SPINE, SHOULDER, AND POSTERIOR ILIAC CREST (Continued)

ASSESSMENT PROCEDURE	NORMAL FINDINGS	ABNORMAL FINDINGS
• Posture • ROM—flexion, lateral bending, rotation, extension (Fig. 20-5)	• Erect • Full ROM	• Stooped • Limited ROM with pain or crepitation

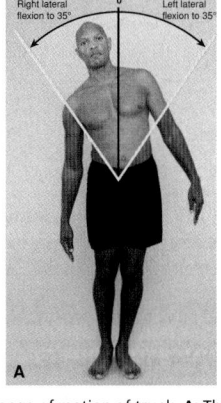 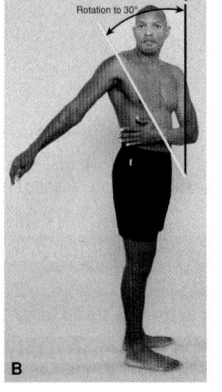 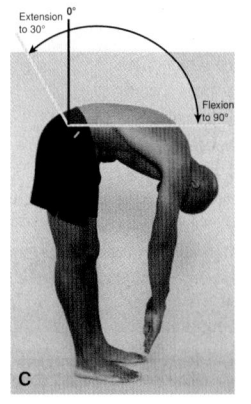

FIGURE 20-5 Range of motion of trunk. **A:** Thoracic and lumbar spines: Lateral bending. **B:** Thoracic and lumbar spines: Rotation. **C:** Thoracic and lumbar spines: Flexion.

PALPATION OF THE SPINE, SHOULDER, AND POSTERIOR ILIAC CREST

With client in standing or sitting position, palpate the paravertebral muscles, using both moderate pressure and gentle sweeping motions. Ask client to shrug shoulders against resistance.

ASSESSMENT PROCEDURE	NORMAL FINDINGS	ABNORMAL FINDINGS
Palpate the **paravertebrals** for the following:		
• Muscle strength and tone	• Equally strong	• Weak, spasm
• Temperature	• Warm	• Hot and swollen
• Sensation	• Nontender	• Tender, painful
Palpate the **shoulder** (trapezius muscle) for the following:		
• Muscle strength and tone	• Able to shrug shoulders against resistance (3–5)	• Weakness with shrugging of shoulders; pain (0–2)
• Sensation	• Nontender	• Tender, painful with shoulder strains, sprains, arthritis, bursitis, and degenerative joint disease
Palpate the shoulder, scapula, and posterior hip for the following:		
• Bony prominences	• Smooth and nontender, no swelling	• Bony enlargement and tenderness, swelling, pain

Continued on following page

PALPATION OF THE SPINE, SHOULDER, AND POSTERIOR ILIAC CREST (Continued)

ASSESSMENT PROCEDURE	NORMAL FINDINGS	ABNORMAL FINDINGS
• Muscle size, strength, and tone	• Equal in size bilaterally, equally strong (3–5)	• Muscle atrophy, weakness, flabbiness, or
• Temperature	• Warm to cool	• Hot • swelling (0–2)

INSPECTION OF THE HEAD, THORAX, AND NECK

With client in sitting position facing you, inspect body parts. Ask client to open and close mouth to assess temporomandibular joint (TMJ) function.

ASSESSMENT PROCEDURE	NORMAL FINDINGS	ABNORMAL FINDINGS
Observe the **head** for the following:		
• Facial structure and muscle development	• Symmetrical structure and development of muscles	• Asymmetrical structure and development of muscles
• TMJ function	• Can open mouth 5.08 cm (2 in)	• Limited ROM; audible crepitation, click; trismus (muscle spasms), pain, tenderness, and swelling seen with TMJ syndrome.
Observe the **thorax** for posture.	Erect, slight kyphosis	Stooped; abnormal spinal curves
Observe the **neck** for ROM: Flexion, extension, rotation, lateral bending (Fig. 20-6).	Full ROM; no pain	Limited ROM with crepitation or pain; nuchal rigidity; neck pain with radiation to back, shoulder, or arms seen with cervical disk degeneration. Neck pain with weakness or loss of sensation in legs is seen with cervical spine compression.

ASSESSMENT PROCEDURE	NORMAL FINDINGS	ABNORMAL FINDINGS
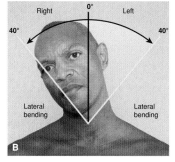		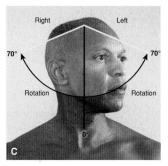

FIGURE 20-6 Normal range of motion of cervical spine. **A:** Flexion–hyperextension. **B:** Lateral bending. **C:** Rotation.

Continued on following page

PALPATION OF THE HEAD, THORAX, AND NECK

While inspecting the TMJ, palpate it bilaterally anterior to the ear as client opens mouth and clenches teeth. Ask client to turn head laterally against resistance.

ASSESSMENT PROCEDURE	NORMAL FINDINGS	ABNORMAL FINDINGS
Palpate the TMJ for the following (Fig. 20-7):		
• Joint function	• Smooth movement bilaterally on opening, with no clicks or pain	• Palpable click, pain
• Joint contour	• Symmetrical	• Asymmetrical
• Temperature	• Warm	• Hot and swollen

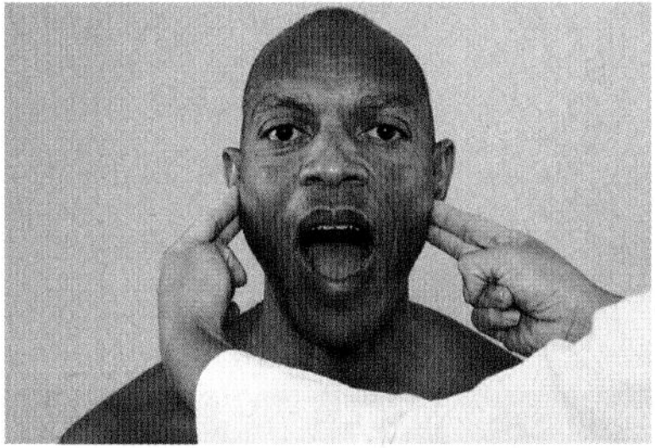

FIGURE 20-7 Palpating the temporomandibular joint.

Palpate the **neck** (sternocleidomastoid) for muscle strength and tone.	Can turn head laterally against resistance without pain (3–5).	Weakness or pain when turning head against resistance (0–2).

INSPECTION OF THE UPPER EXTREMITIES

Position client in the sitting position facing you, with the upper extremities exposed. Inspect each joint and determine ROM. Both active and passive ROM may be assessed. It is easier for the client to carry out ROM if you demonstrate movements first.

ASSESSMENT PROCEDURE	NORMAL FINDINGS	ABNORMAL FINDINGS
Observe the **shoulder, elbow, wrist, hand, and fingers** for bone structure, bony prominences, muscle mass, joint structure, and symmetry.	Bilaterally symmetrical	Bony deformity, muscle atrophy, swelling, deviation, contractures, nodes, tophi. Swelling of wrists, tenderness, and nodules are seen in rheumatoid arthritis; nontender, round, enlarged, swollen cysts may be ganglion of the wrists.
Observe the **shoulder, elbow, wrist, and fingers** for ROM. See Table 20-2 on page 444, and Figures 20-8 to 20-11 for normal ROM.	Full ROM	Limited ROM with crepitation or pain. Catches of pain with ROM in shoulder are seen with rotator cuff tendinitis; chronic pain and limited ROM seen with calcified tendinitis; pain-limited abduction of shoulder seen with rotator cuff tear; redness and heat of elbows with bursitis; ulnar deviation of wrists and fingers with limited ROM seen in rheumatoid arthritis; inability to extend ring finger seen in Dupuytren contracture; painful extension of finger with tenosynovitis.

Continued on following page

INSPECTION OF THE UPPER EXTREMITIES (Continued)

ASSESSMENT PROCEDURE	NORMAL FINDINGS	ABNORMAL FINDINGS

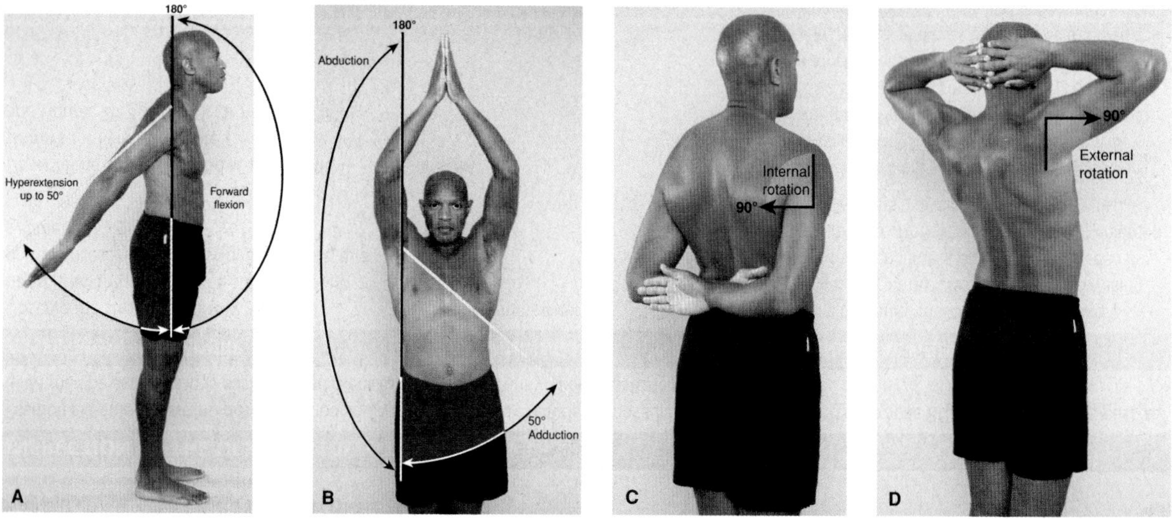

FIGURE 20-8 Normal range of motion of the shoulder. **A:** Flexion–extension. **B:** Adduction–abduction. **C:** Internal rotation. **D:** External rotation.

ASSESSMENT PROCEDURE	**NORMAL FINDINGS**	**ABNORMAL FINDINGS**

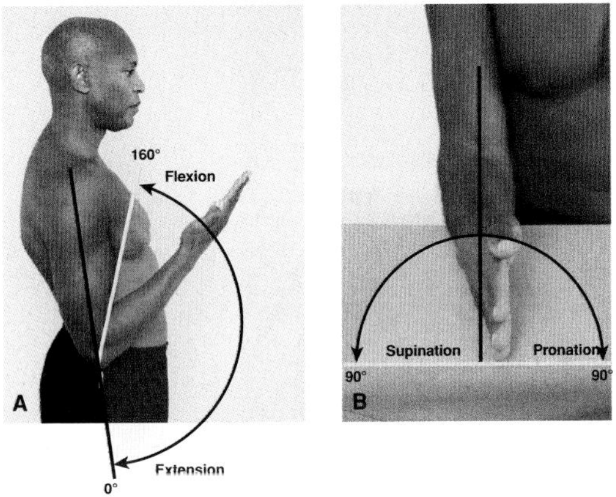

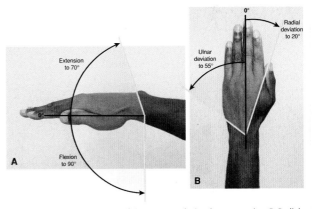

FIGURE 20-9 Normal range of motion of the elbow. **A:** Flexion–extension. **B:** Pronation–supination.

FIGURE 20-10 Range of motion of the wrists. **A:** Flexion–hyperextension. **B:** Radial–ulnar deviation.

Continued on following page

INSPECTION OF THE UPPER EXTREMITIES (Continued)

ASSESSMENT PROCEDURE	NORMAL FINDINGS	ABNORMAL FINDINGS

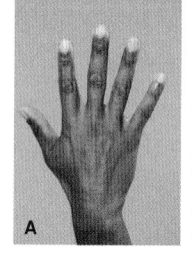
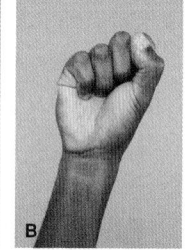
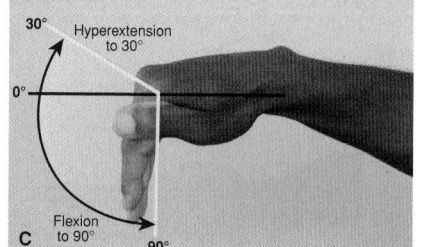

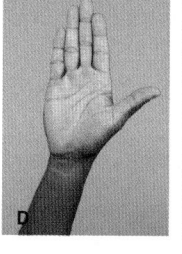
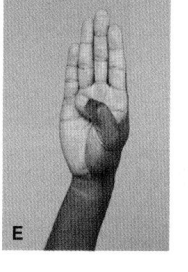

FIGURE 20-11 Normal range of motion of the fingers. **A:** Abduction. **B:** Adduction. **C:** Flexion–hyperextension. **D:** Thumb away from fingers. **E:** Thumb touching base of small finger.

PALPATION OF THE UPPER EXTREMITIES

As the musculoskeletal structure of the upper extremity is going through active or passive ROM, palpate bones, muscles, tendons, and joints. Assess muscle strength and tone.

ASSESSMENT PROCEDURE	NORMAL FINDINGS	ABNORMAL FINDINGS
Palpate the **arm** (biceps, triceps) for muscle strength and tone.	Can flex and extend arm against resistance (3–5)	Weakness paralysis (0–2)
Palpate the **hand** for the following: • Muscle strength, tone • Sensation	• Grip is firm and equal. • Nontender (3–5)	• Weakness, paralysis • Tenderness, pain (0–2)
Palpate the **elbow, wrist, hand, and fingers** for the following: • Bony landmarks • Muscle size • Joint structure • Strength • Temperature • Sensation	• Nontender, smooth • Regular and equal bilaterally • Symmetrical and equal • Equally strong (3–5) • Warm • Nontender	• Bony enlargement • Muscle atrophy • Loss of joint structure; joint bogginess; nodules, swelling • Unilateral or bilateral weakness (0–2) • Hot • Tender, painful, swollen joints seen in acute rheumatoid arthritis (see Abnormal Findings 20-2, page 446).

Continued on following page

PALPATION OF THE UPPER EXTREMITIES (Continued)

ASSESSMENT PROCEDURE	NORMAL FINDINGS	ABNORMAL FINDINGS
Ask client to close eyes for 20–30 seconds with arms extended in front of body with palms up.	Arms remain up with no drifting.	• Chronic swelling and thickening of joints, and limited ROM seen in chronic rheumatoid arthritis (see Abnormal Findings 20-2, page 446). • Hard, painless nodules known as Heberden nodes over distal interphalangeal joints seen in osteoarthritis (see Abnormal Findings 20-2). • Bouchard's nodes seen over proximal interphalangeal joints (see Abnormal Findings 20-2). • Arm tends to drift downward and pronate.

INSPECTION OF THE LOWER EXTREMITIES

Position the client in standing or supine position to inspect the hips, and in sitting position with legs hanging freely to inspect the knees, ankles, feet, and toes. If the client is unable to sit or stand, assessments may be made in the supine position. Both active and passive ROM may be assessed.

ASSESSMENT PROCEDURE	NORMAL FINDINGS	ABNORMAL FINDINGS
Observe the hip, knee, ankle, foot, and toes for the following: • Muscle mass • Bone structure and bony landmarks	• Bilaterally symmetrical and equal • Symmetrical and equal	• Bony deformity • Muscle atrophy

ASSESSMENT PROCEDURE	NORMAL FINDINGS	ABNORMAL FINDINGS
• Joint structure	• Feet maintain straight position	• Swelling, deviation, or contractures; bunion, hammer toe • Deviation of great toe seen in hallux valgus
• Leg length	• Bilateral leg lengths within 2.5 cm (1 in) of each other	• Unequal lengths
Observe the **hip, knee, ankle, and toes** for ROM. See Table 20-3 on page 444, and Figures 20-12 to 20-14, pp. 440–442 for normal ROM.	Full ROM	Limited ROM with crepitation or pain in joint and muscle disease. Hip pain, decreased ROM, crepitus in hip inflammation, and degenerative joint disease; tenderness and warmth with boggy consistency in synovitis; turned-in knees (genu valgum), knees turned out (genu varum); fluid bulge in knee joint effusion; pain or clicking in torn meniscus. Hyperextension at the metatarsophalangeal joint with flexion at the proximal interphalangeal joint (hammer toe) commonly occurs with the second toe (see Abnormal Findings 20-2, p. 446).

Continued on following page

INSPECTION OF THE LOWER EXTREMITIES (Continued)

ASSESSMENT PROCEDURE	NORMAL FINDINGS	ABNORMAL FINDINGS

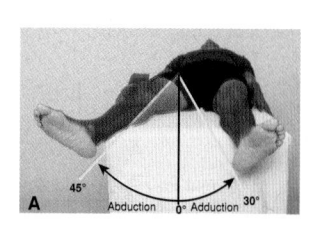 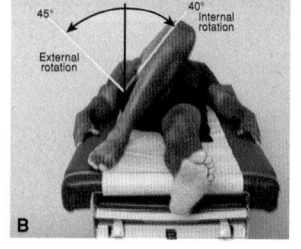 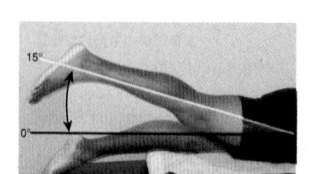

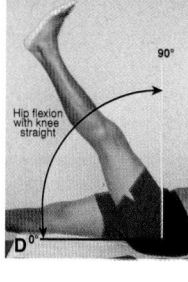 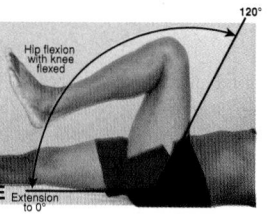 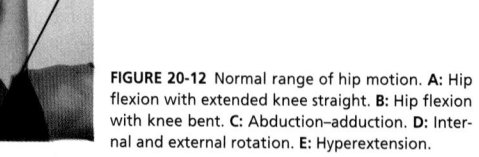

FIGURE 20-12 Normal range of hip motion. **A:** Hip flexion with extended knee straight. **B:** Hip flexion with knee bent. **C:** Abduction–adduction. **D:** Internal and external rotation. **E:** Hyperextension.

ASSESSMENT PROCEDURE	NORMAL FINDINGS	ABNORMAL FINDINGS
		Hallux valgus is an abnormality in which the great toe is deviated laterally and may overlap the second toe. An enlarged, painful, inflamed bursa (bunion) may form on the medial side (see Abnormal Findings 20-2, p. 446).

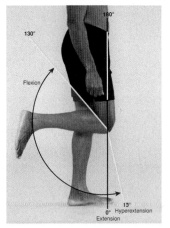

FIGURE 20-13 Normal range of motion of knee.

Continued on following page

INSPECTION OF THE LOWER EXTREMITIES (Continued)		
ASSESSMENT PROCEDURE	**NORMAL FINDINGS**	**ABNORMAL FINDINGS**
	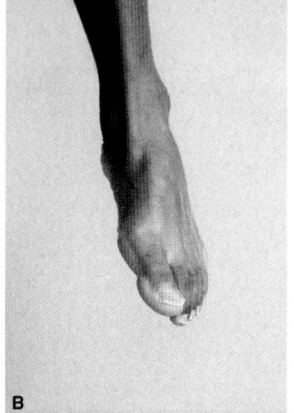	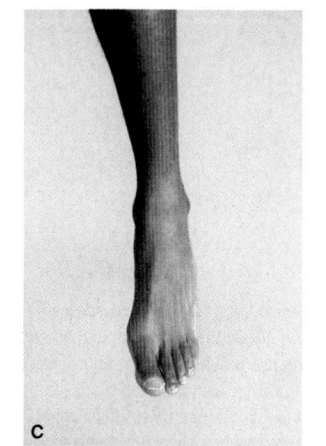
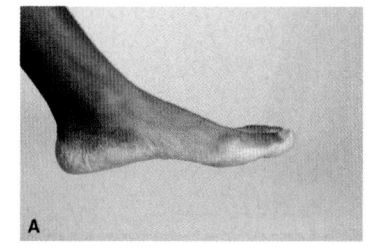		

FIGURE 20-14 Normal range of motion of the feet and ankles. **A:** Dorsiflexion–plantar flexion. **B:** Eversion–inversion. **C:** Abduction–adduction.

PALPATION OF THE LOWER EXTREMITIES

As the musculoskeletal structure of the lower extremity is going through active or passive ROM, palpate bones, bony landmarks, muscles, and joints. Assess muscle strength and tone.

ASSESSMENT PROCEDURE	NORMAL FINDINGS	ABNORMAL FINDINGS
Palpate the **hip** (quadriceps, gastrocnemius) for the following: • Bony landmarks • Muscle size and strength • Joint structure • Temperature • Sensation	• Bilaterally symmetrical and equal • Smooth, regular, strong (3–5) • Bilaterally symmetrical; strong • Warm • Nontender	• Bony enlargement • Muscle atrophy and weakness (0–2) • Loss of joint structure; joint bogginess • Hot and swollen • Tenderness, pain

TABLE 20-2 Normal Range of Motion for Joints of the Upper Extremities

Shoulder	Elbow	Wrist	Fingers
Flexion	Flexion	Flexion	Flexion
Extension	Extension	Hyperextension	Hyperextension
Abduction	Supination	Deviation	Abduction
Adduction	Pronation	Radial	Adduction
Rotation (internal and external)		Ulnar	Thumb away from fingers
			Thumb to base of small finger

TABLE 20-3 Normal Range of Motion for Joints of the Lower Extremities

Hip	Knee	Ankle	Toes
Rotation (internal and external)	Flexion	Dorsiflexion	Flexion
Flexion	Extension	Plantar flexion	Extension
Extension		Inversion	
Abduction		Eversion	
Adduction			

ABNORMAL FINDINGS | **20-1** | **Abnormal Spinal Curves**

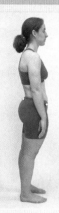

Lordosis (Photo from Oatis, C.A. (2004). *Kinesiology: The mechanics and pathomechanics of human movement*. Baltimore: Lippincott Williams & Wilkins.)

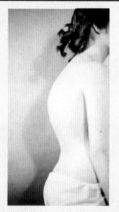

Kyphosis (Photo courtesy of Martin Herman, MD)

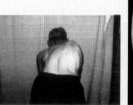

Scoliosis (*left* Berg D & Worzala K. (2006). *Atlas of adult physical diagnosis*. Philadelphia: Lippincott Williams & Wilkins; *right* Used with permission from SIU/Biomedical Communications/Custom Medical Stock Photography.)

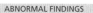

ABNORMAL FINDINGS

| ABNORMAL FINDINGS | 20-2 | **Abnormal Upper and Lower Extremity Findings** |

Acute rheumatoid arthritis

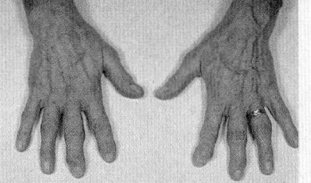

(© 1991 National Medical Slide Bank/CMSP.)

Chronic rheumatoid arthritis

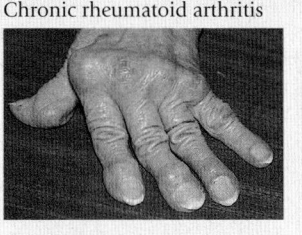

(© 1995 Science Photo Library.)

Heberden nodes

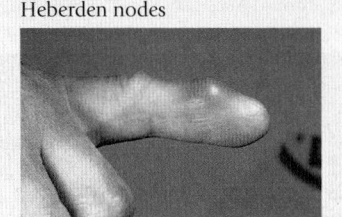

(© 1991 National Medical Slide Bank/CMSP.)

Bouchard's nodes

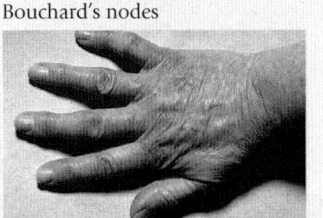

(© 1991 National Medical Slide Bank/CMSP.)

Hammer toe

Hallux valgus

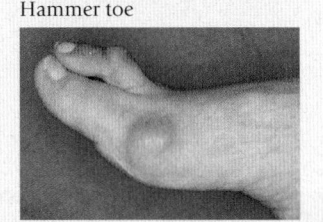

PEDIATRIC VARIATIONS

Questions to ask the parents when collecting *subjective data* include the following.
- Birth injuries?
- Alignment of hips?
- Trauma?
- Participation in sports or outdoor activities?
- Frequent pain in joints?
- Any previous injury or fracture?
- Any recent surgery?
- Any concerns from parent or client regarding mobility, strength, or movement of any joints, arms, legs?

When collecting *objective data* note the following.

ASSESSMENT PROCEDURE	NORMAL FINDINGS
Infant: Inspect lower extremities. 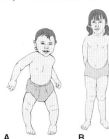 **FIGURE 20-15 A:** Genu varum (bow legs). **B:** Genu valgum (knock knees).	A distinct bowlegged growth pattern persists and begins to disappear at 18 months. At the age of 2 years, a knock-kneed pattern is common (Fig. 20-15), persisting until the age of 6–10 years, when legs straighten. A greater ROM in joints is present in infants. Legs are wide set until the child begins walking; weight is borne on the inside of the feet.

Continued on following page

ASSESSMENT PROCEDURE	NORMAL FINDINGS
Perform Ortolani maneuver to test for congenital hip dysplasia. With the infant supine, flex the knees while holding your thumbs on midthigh and your fingers over the greater trochanters; abduct the legs, moving the knees outward and down toward the table (Fig. 20-16A).	Positive Ortolani sign: A click heard along with feeling the head of the femur slip in or out of the hip.
Perform Barlow maneuver. With the infant supine, flex the knees while holding your thumbs on midthigh and your fingers over the greater trochanters; adduct legs until thumbs touch (Fig. 20-16B).	Positive Barlow sign: A feeling of the head of the femur slipping out of the hip socket (acetabulum).

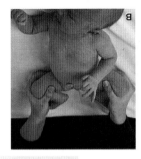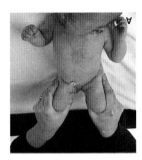

FIGURE 20-16 **A:** Ortolani maneuver. **B:** Barlow maneuver.

ASSESSMENT PROCEDURE	NORMAL FINDINGS
Greater than the age of 2 years: Inspect gait.	Wide-based gait common until the age of 2 years
Measure distance between knees with ankles together.	Less than 5.1 cm (2 in)
3–7 years of age: Measure distance between ankles with knees together. Longitudinal arch of foot is often obscured by adipose until the age of 3 years, and infant appears flat-footed.	Less than 7.6 cm (3 in)
4–13 years of age: See also Appendix 5 for developmental milestones.	
Inspect **curvature of spine** (Fig. 20-17): • Stand behind erect child and note asymmetry of shoulders and hips.	• Shoulders symmetrical, parallel with hips
• Have child bend forward at waist until back is parallel to floor; observe from side, looking for asymmetry or prominence of rib cage.	• Shoulders, scapulae, iliac crests symmetrical

Continued on following page

ASSESSMENT PROCEDURE	NORMAL FINDINGS

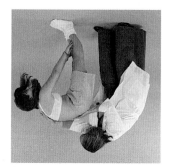

FIGURE 20-17 Assessing spinal curvature for scoliosis.

A preparticipation sports evaluation should be performed on all children and adolescents before participating in sports. Perform careful evaluation of the musculoskeletal system. This examination will assess mobility/motion of joints, strength of muscles, symmetry of hands, arms, legs, and shoulders, and motion of the spine and hips. Each state school program has its own form to be completed for the student athlete.

GERIATRIC VARIATIONS

- Decrease in total bone mass due to decreased activity level, change in hormones, and bone resorption; this results in weaker, softer bones.
- Slower gait with wide-based stance and smaller arm swing
- Accentuated dorsal spinal curve (kyphosis)
- Loss of muscle bulk and tone
- Decreased ROM of spine, neck, extremities
- Decrease in height (1.2 cm of height lost every 20 years)
- Shoulder width decreases; chest and pelvis widths increase.
- May have bowlegged appearance due to decreased muscle control

CULTURAL VARIATIONS

- Some variation in muscle size and mass and in bone length and density are seen in different racial/ethnic groups. Overfield (1995), Rush et al. (2007), and Ward et al. (2007) noted that the peroneus tertius in foot or palmaris longus muscles in wrist may be absent in some groups; the number of vertebrae may differ (black women may have 23, Eskimo and Native American men, 25). A large gluteal prominence in some blacks may be mistaken as lordosis, and the ulna and radius may have unequal lengths (e.g., Swedes and Chinese). Bone density (and osteoporosis) varies with men having denser bones, blacks denser than whites, and most East Asians (except Polynesian women) less dense than Caucasians (Overfield, 1995).
- In growth and development, Caucasian American youth tends to mature faster than European youth, but those of African and Asian American origins mature faster than Caucasians (Berk, 2012).

POSSIBLE COLLABORATIVE PROBLEMS—RISK OF

Bone fractures	Osteoporosis	Osteoarthritis
Sprains	Dislocation of joints	Rheumatoid arthritis
Contractures of joints	Compartment syndrome	

Teaching Tips for Selected Nursing Diagnoses

Nursing Diagnosis: *Readiness for Enhanced Mobility related to (specify)*

Teach client the importance of maintaining an ideal weight. Explain the importance of doing weight-bearing and muscle-toning exercises at least three times per week. Encourage client to wear seat belts in vehicles, to wear low well-fitted shoes, and to use walking aids (e.g., cane) as needed to prevent injury.

Nursing Diagnosis: *Chronic Pain (muscles and joints) related to (specify)*

Discuss independent pain management measures the client may find useful (e.g., massage, relaxation, distraction). Weight loss may also reduce discomfort if obesity is straining the bones, muscles, and joints. Explain use and side effects of pain medications.

Nursing Diagnosis: *Risk for injury related to excessive exercise/ improper body mechanics*

Caution the client against the dangerous effects of excessive exercise. Teach proper body mechanics and correct posture.

 Nursing Diagnosis: *Risk for injury (child) related to parent's knowledge deficit of correlating musculoskeletal development and home safety*

Caution parents on home safety precautions (e.g., gates at stairways, removal of objects that may cause unnecessary falls, avoiding leaving child near water alone) based on child's level of musculoskeletal development. Develop home safety checklist with parents. Teach normal milestones of musculoskeletal development, and advise parent to encourage these skills as appropriate.

 Nursing Diagnosis: *Risk for injury related to decalcification of bones secondary to sedentary lifestyle and postmenopausal state*

Discuss importance of calcium supplements in diet for postmenopausal women. Explain effects of exercise on decreasing bone decalcification.

 Nursing Diagnosis: *Risk for injury related to unstable gait secondary to aging process*

Explain the correct use of aids (e.g., crutches, canes, walkers) and other prostheses. Use referrals as necessary. Instruct client on measures to prevent falls (e.g., adequate lighting, avoidance of loose board ends and scatter rugs on floor). Discourage use of sleeping pills and suggest alternate methods of promoting sleep (e.g., watching TV, reading, warm bath, music, warm milk).

Nursing Diagnosis: *Impaired Physical Mobility related to decreased activity secondary to aging process*

Instruct client on the hazards of immobility and methods to prevent complications (e.g., turning, coughing, deep breathing, repositioning, ROM, adequate diet, plentiful fluid intake, and diversional activities). Encourage mild exercise to loosen joint stiffness.

Nursing Diagnosis: *Ineffective Self-health Management (specify) related to decreased mobility and/or weakness*

Assess safe level of activity with the client, and teach methods to increase activity gradually to that level. Explore alternate self-help methods of maintaining self-care (e.g., feeding aids, wheelchairs, crutches, hygienic aids). Assist the client with identifying and utilizing services and groups to assist with activities of daily living (e.g., Meals on Wheels). Support and teach family caregivers.

CHAPTER 21

Assessing Neurologic System

Structure and Function Overview

The very complex neurologic system is responsible for coordinating and regulating all body functions. It consists of two structural components: the central nervous system (CNS) and the peripheral nervous system.

The CNS encompasses the brain and spinal cord, which are covered by three layers of protective meninges. The subarachnoid space surrounding the brain and spinal cord is filled with cerebrospinal fluid, which cushions the brain and spinal cord, nourishes the CNS, and removes waste materials. Electrical activity of the CNS is governed by neurons located in the sensory and motor neural pathways. The CNS contains upper motor neurons that influence lower motor neurons located mostly in the peripheral nervous system.

Located in the cranial cavity, the brain has four major divisions: the cerebrum, the diencephalon, the brainstem, and the cerebellum (Fig. 21-1).

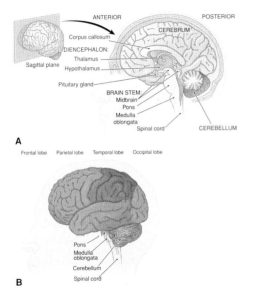

FIGURE 21-1 A: Structures of the brain (sagittal section). **B:** Lobes of the brain.

The cerebrum is divided into the right and left cerebral hemispheres, joined by the corpus callosum—a bundle of nerve fibers responsible for communication between the hemispheres. Each hemisphere sends and receives impulses from the opposite sides of the body and consists of four lobes (frontal, parietal, temporal, and occipital) which mediate higher-level functions (Table 21-1). Damage to a lobe impairs its specific function.

The diencephalon lies beneath the cerebral hemispheres and consists of the thalamus and hypothalamus. Most sensory impulses travel through the thalamus, which is responsible for screening and directing impulses to specific areas in the cerebral cortex. The hypothalamus (a part of the autonomic nervous system, which in turn is a part of the peripheral nervous system) is responsible for regulating many body functions including water balance, appetite, vital signs (temperature, blood pressure, pulse, and respiratory rate), sleep cycles, pain perception, and emotional status.

Located between the cerebral cortex and the spinal cord, the brainstem consists of the midbrain, pons, and medulla oblongata. The midbrain serves as a relay center for ear and eye reflexes and relays impulses between the higher cerebral centers and the lower pons, medulla, cerebellum, and spinal cord. The pons

TABLE 21-1 Lobes of the Cerebral Hemispheres and Their Function

Lobe	Function
Frontal	Directs voluntary, skeletal actions (left side of lobe controls right side of body and right side of lobe controls left side of body). Also influences communication (talking and writing), emotions, intellect, reasoning ability, judgment, and behavior. Contains Broca area, which is responsible for speech.
Parietal	Interprets tactile sensations, including touch, pain, temperature, shapes, and two-point discrimination.
Occipital	Influences the ability to read with understanding and is the primary visual receptor center.
Temporal	Receives and interprets impulses from the ear. Contains Wernicke area, which is responsible for interpreting auditory stimuli.

links the cerebellum to the cerebrum and the midbrain to the medulla. It is responsible for various reflex actions. The medulla oblongata contains the nuclei for cranial nerves and has centers that control and regulate respiratory function, heart rate and force, and blood pressure.

The cerebellum, located behind the brainstem and under the cerebrum, has two hemispheres and is responsible for coordination and smoothing of voluntary movements, maintenance of equilibrium, and maintenance of muscle tone.

The spinal cord (Fig. 21-2) is located in the vertebral canal and extends from the medulla oblongata to the first lumbar vertebra. The inner part of the cord has an H-shaped appearance and is made up of two pairs of columns (dorsal and ventral) consisting of gray matter. The outer part is made up of of white matter and surrounds the gray matter. The spinal cord conducts sensory impulses up ascending tracts to the brain, conducts motor impulses down descending tracts to neurons that stimulate glands and muscles throughout the body, and is responsible for simple reflex activity. The simplest stretch reflex involves one sensory neuron (afferent), one motor neuron (efferent), and one synapse, such as the knee jerk, elicited by tapping the patellar tendon. More complex reflexes involve three or more neurons.

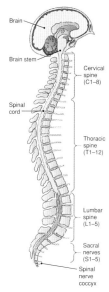

FIGURE 21-2 Spinal cord.

Neural Pathways

Sensory impulses travel to the brain by way of two ascending neural pathways (the spinothalamic tract and posterior columns) (Fig. 21-3). These impulses originate in the afferent fibers of the peripheral nerves and are carried through the posterior (dorsal) root into the spinal cord. Sensations of pain, temperature, and crude and light touch travel by way of the spinothalamic tract, whereas sensations of position, vibration, and fine touch travel by way of the posterior columns. Motor impulses are conducted to the muscles by two descending neural pathways: the pyramidal (corticospinal) tract and the extrapyramidal tract (Fig. 21-4). The motor neurons of the pyramidal tract originate in the motor cortex and travel down to the medulla where they cross over to the opposite side; then they travel down the spinal cord where they synapse with a lower motor neuron in the anterior horn of the spinal cord. These impulses are carried to muscles and produce voluntary movements that involve skill and purpose. The extrapyramidal tract motor neurons consist of those motor neurons that originate in the motor cortex, basal ganglia, brainstem, and spinal cord outside the pyramidal tract. They travel from the frontal lobe to the pons where they cross over to the opposite side and down the spinal cord where they connect with lower motor neurons that

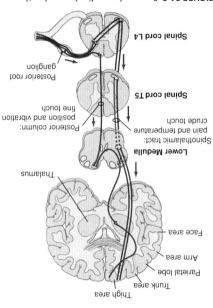

FIGURE 21-3 Sensory (ascending) neural pathways.

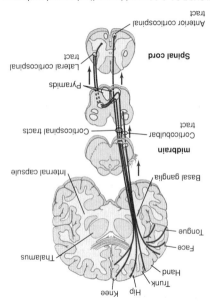

FIGURE 21-4 Motor (descending) neural pathways.

conduct impulses to the muscles. These neurons conduct impulses related to maintenance of muscle tone and body control.

PERIPHERAL NERVOUS SYSTEM

Carrying information to and from the CNS, the peripheral nervous system consists of 12 pairs of cranial nerves (Table 21-2) and 31 pairs of spinal nerves. Comprising 8 cervical, 12 thoracic, 5 lumbar, 5 sacral, and 1 coccygeal nerve, the 31 pairs of spinal nerves are named after the vertebrae below each one's exit point along the spinal cord (Fig. 21-2, p. 457). Each nerve is attached to the spinal cord by two nerve roots. The sensory (afferent) fiber enters through the dorsal (posterior) roots of the cord, whereas the motor (efferent) fiber exits through the ventral (anterior) roots of the cord. The sensory root of each spinal nerve innervates an area of the skin called a dermatome (Fig. 21-5). These nerves are categorized as two types of fibers: somatic and autonomic. Somatic fibers carry CNS impulses to voluntary skeletal muscles, whereas autonomic fibers carry CNS impulses to smooth, involuntary muscles (in the heart and glands). The somatic nervous system mediates conscious, or voluntary, activities, whereas the autonomic nervous system mediates unconscious, or involuntary, activities.

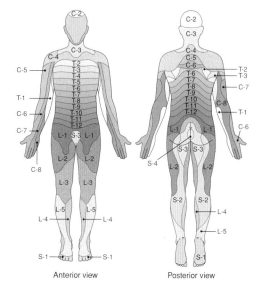

FIGURE 21-5 Anterior and posterior dermatomes (areas of the skin innervated by spinal nerves).

TABLE 21-2 Cranial Nerves: Type and Function

Cranial Nerve (Name)	Type of Impulse	Function
I (olfactory)	Sensory	Carries smell impulses from nasal mucous membrane to brain
II (optic)	Sensory	Carries visual impulses from eye to brain
III (oculomotor)	Motor	Contracts eye muscles to control eye movements (inferior lateral, medial, and superior), constricts pupils, and elevates eyelids
IV (trochlear)	Motor	Contracts one eye muscle to control inferomedial eye movement
V (trigeminal)	Sensory	Carries sensory impulses of pain, touch, and temperature from the face to the brain; Influences clenching and lateral jaw movements (biting, chewing)
VI (abducens)	Motor	Controls lateral eye movements
VII (facial)	Sensory	Contains sensory fibers for taste on anterior two thirds of tongue and stimulates secretions from salivary glands (submaxillary and sublingual) and tears from lacrimal glands; Supplies the facial muscles and affects facial expressions (smiling, frowning, closing eyes)
VIII (acoustic, vestibulocochlear)	Sensory	Contains sensory fibers for hearing and balance
IX (glossopharyngeal)	Sensory	Contains sensory fibers for taste on posterior third of tongue and sensory fibers of the pharynx that result in the "gag reflex" when stimulated; Provides secretory fibers to the parotid salivary glands; promotes swallowing movements
X (vagus)	Sensory	Carries sensations from the throat, larynx, heart, lungs, bronchi, gastrointestinal tract, and abdominal viscera; Promotes swallowing, talking, and production of digestive juices
XI (spinal accessory)	Motor	Innervates neck muscles (sternocleidomastoid and trapezius) that promote movement of the shoulders and head rotation. Also promotes some movement of the larynx
XII (hypoglossal)	Motors	Innervates tongue muscles that promote the movement of food and talking

Nursing Assessment

The neurologic assessment is performed last because several of its components may have been integrated into previous parts of the examination. For example, the eighth cranial nerve (CN VIII) may have been tested during the ear examination and therefore will not need to be tested again. A complete neurologic assessment consists of examining: (1) mental status (see Chapter 4), (2) cranial nerve function, (3) motor function (see Chapter 21), (4) cerebellar function, (5) sensory function, and (6) reflexes.

Perform the examinations in an order that moves from a level of higher cerebral integration (mental status) to a lower level (reflex activity).

COLLECTING SUBJECTIVE DATA

Focus Questions

Numbness? Paralysis? Tingling? Neuralgia? (Timing, duration, associated factors?) Seizures? Auras? Medications taken for seizures? Wear MedicAlert identification? Tremors? Headaches? (Frequency, duration, character, precipitating/relieving factors?) Loss of consciousness? Dizziness? Fainting? Loss of memory? Confusion? Visual loss, blurring, pain? Facial pain, weakness, twitching? Speech problems (aphasia—expressive/receptive)? Swallowing problems? Drooling? Neck weakness, spasms? Any muscle weakness or loss of bowel or urinary control? History of head injury? Meningitis? Encephalitis? Treatment? Family history of high blood pressure, stroke, Alzheimer disease, epilepsy, brain cancer, or Huntington chorea?

Self-care: Use of medications? Alcohol intake? Use of drugs such as marijuana, tranquilizers, barbiturates, or cocaine? Smoking? Use of seat belt, head gear for sports? Daily diet and exercise? Prolonged exposure to lead, insecticides, pollutants, or other chemicals?

Risk Factors

Risk for cerebrovascular accident (stroke) related to age more than 60 years, male sex (slightly higher risk), hypertension, smoking, chronic alcohol intake, history of cardiovascular disease, sleep apnea, high levels of fibrinogen, diabetes mellitus, drug abuse, oral contraceptives, high estrogen levels, postmenopausal women not taking estrogen replacement, obesity, African American, and newly industrialized environment.

COLLECTING OBJECTIVE DATA

Equipment Needed

General

• Gloves

Equipment needed for a cranial nerve examination includes the following.

• Cotton-tipped applicators
• Newsprint to read
• Ophthalmoscope
• Paper clip
• Penlight
• Snellen chart
• Sterile cotton ball
• Substances to smell or taste such as soap, coffee, vanilla, salt, sugar, lemon juice
• Tongue depressor
• Tuning fork

Equipment needed for a motor and cerebellar examination includes the following.

• Tape measure

Equipment needed for a sensory examination includes the following.

• Cotton ball
• Objects to feel such as a quarter or key
• Paper clip
• Test tubes containing hot and cold water
• Tuning fork (low-pitched)

Equipment needed for a reflex examination includes the following.

• Cotton-tipped applicator
• Reflex (percussion) hammer

Physical Assessment

Ask the client to remove all clothing and jewelry and to put on an examination gown. Have the client sit on the exam table, but explain that several different position changes are needed throughout the exam. Explain the length of the exam and allow rest periods as needed. You may perform over two different time periods to avoid client fatigue. Explain some requests (i.e., counting backward or hopping on one foot) may seem unusual but that these activities are parts of a total neurologic evaluation. Demonstrate what you want the client to do, especially during the cerebellar examination, when the client will need to perform several movements.

See Chapter 5 for an examination of mental status.

CRANIAL NERVES

Assess CN I through XII.

ASSESSMENT PROCEDURE	NORMAL FINDINGS	ABNORMAL FINDINGS
CN I—Olfactory: Hold scent (e.g., coffee, orange) under one nostril with the other occluded while client close eyes. Repeat with the other nostril (Fig. 21-6).	Identifies scent correctly with each nostril	Unable to identify correct odor
CN II—Optic: Assess **vision.** Assess visual fields. Perform funduscopic examination for direct visualization of optic nerve.	See Chapter 12, *Assessing Eyes*.	See Chapter 12, *Assessing Eyes*.

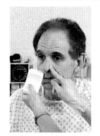

FIGURE 21-6 Testing cranial nerve I.

Continued on following page

CRANIAL NERVES (Continued)		
ASSESSMENT PROCEDURE	**NORMAL FINDINGS**	**ABNORMAL FINDINGS**
CN III—Oculomotor **CN IV—Trochlear** **CN VI—Abducens:** Assess **extraocular movements**. Assess PERRLA (pupils equal, round, and reactive to light and accommodation).	See Chapter 12, *Assessing Eyes*.	See Chapter 12, *Assessing Eyes*.
CN V—Trigeminal: Assess **sensory function** by: • Touching cornea lightly with wisp of cotton (Fig. 21-7)	• Eyelids blink bilaterally.	• Absent blink of eyelids with lesion of CN V (trigeminal) or lesions of the motor part of CN VII (facial)

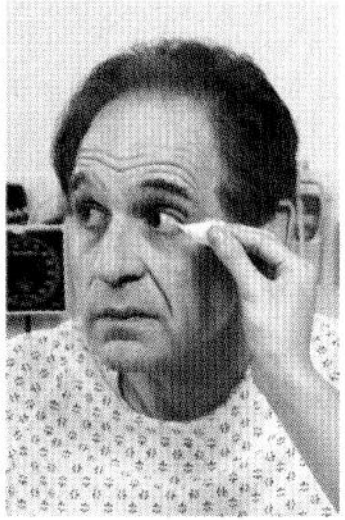

FIGURE 21-7 Testing corneal reflex with wisp of cotton.

ASSESSMENT PROCEDURE	NORMAL FINDINGS	ABNORMAL FINDINGS
• Testing client's ability to feel light touch, dull, and sharp facial sensations on both sides of face at the forehead, cheek, and chin areas (with client's eyes closed; Fig. 21-8)	• Identifies light touch, dull, and sharp sensations to forehead, cheeks, and chin	• Unable to identify or feel facial sensations with lesions of CN V, spinothalamic tract, or posterior columns
Assess **motor function** by palpating masseter and temporal muscles as client clenches teeth (Fig. 21-9).	Muscles contract bilaterally.	Asymmetrical or no muscle contractions; irregular facial movements; pain or bilateral muscle weakness is seen with peripheral or CNS dysfunction. Unilateral weakness is seen with lesion of CN V.

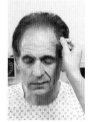

FIGURE 21-8 Testing sensory function of cranial nerve V: dull stimulus using a paper clip.

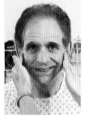
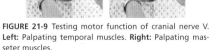

FIGURE 21-9 Testing motor function of cranial nerve V. **Left:** Palpating temporal muscles. **Right:** Palpating masseter muscles.

Continued on following page

CRANIAL NERVES (Continued)

ASSESSMENT PROCEDURE	NORMAL FINDINGS	ABNORMAL FINDINGS
CN VII—Facial: Assess **sensory function** by asking the client to identify sugar, salt on anterior two thirds of tongue, with eyes closed and tongue protruded.	Identifies taste correctly	Unable to taste or to identify taste correctly with impaired CN VII
Assess **motor function** by asking client to do the following:		
• Smile • Frown • Show teeth • Blow out cheeks • Raise eyebrows and tightly close eyes	• Smiles • Frowns • Shows teeth • Blows out cheeks • Raises eyebrows and closes eyes tightly as instructed; facial movements are symmetrical.	• Unable to perform facial movements as instructed, or movements asymmetrical on one side of face. Unable to do facial movements along with paralysis of the face of the face in Bell palsy; paralysis of lower part of face on opposite side is seen with central lesion affecting upper motor neurons from cerebrovascular accident.
CN VIII—Acoustic: Assess hearing	See Chapter 13, *Assessing Ears.*	See Chapter 13, *Assessing Ears.*
CN IX—Glossopharyngeal: Assess **taste and gag reflex.**	See CN VII and CN X for gag reflex.	See CN VII (taste) and CN IX (gag reflex).

ASSESSMENT PROCEDURE	NORMAL FINDINGS	ABNORMAL FINDINGS
Ask the client to identify lemon juice and salt on posterior one third of tongue with eyes closed.	• Identifies taste and gag reflex present	Unable to identify correct taste with lesion of CN IX
CN X—Vagus: Ask client to open mouth and say "ah."	Bilateral, symmetrical rise of soft palate and uvula	Unequal or absent rise of soft palate and uvula with lesions of CN X
Touch back of tongue or soft palate with tongue blade (Fig. 21-10).	Gag reflex present	Gag reflex absent with lesions of CN IX or X

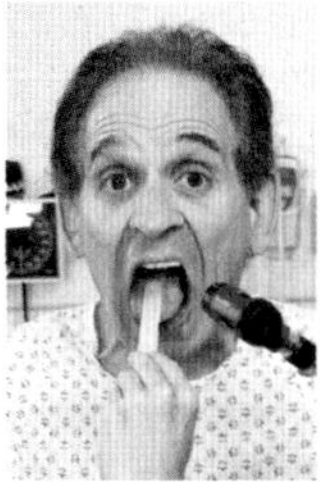

FIGURE 21-10 Testing cranial nerves IX and X: checking uvula rise and gag reflex.

Continued on following page

CRANIAL NERVES (Continued)

ASSESSMENT PROCEDURE	NORMAL FINDINGS	ABNORMAL FINDINGS
CN XI—Spinal Accessory: Palpate **strength of trapezius muscles** by asking the client to shrug shoulders against your hands (Fig. 21-11).	Symmetrical, strong contraction of trapezius muscles	Asymmetrical, weak, or absent contraction of trapezius muscles seen with paralysis or muscle weakness
Palpate **strength of sternocleidomastoid muscles** by asking the client to turn head against your hand (Fig. 21-12).	Strong contraction of sternocleidomastoid muscle on the opposite side of which the head is turned	Weak or absent contraction of sternocleido-mastoid muscle on the opposite side of which the head is turned is seen with peripheral nerve disease

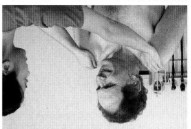

FIGURE 21-11 Testing cranial nerve XI: assessing strength of trapezius muscle.

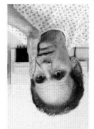

FIGURE 21-12 Testing cranial nerve XI: assessing strength of sternocleidomastoid muscle.

ASSESSMENT PROCEDURE	NORMAL FINDINGS	ABNORMAL FINDINGS
CN XII—Hypoglossal: Ask the client to protrude tongue and move it to each side against tongue blade.	Symmetrical tongue with smooth outward movement and bilateral strength	Asymmetrical tongue; deviation to one side seen with unilateral lesion; fasciculations and atrophy of tongue seen with peripheral nerve disease; unequal or no strength

MOTOR

For the Motor System, assess muscle size, tone, movement, voluntary movements, and strength. See Chapter 20, *Assessing Musculoskeletal System*.

CEREBELLAR SYSTEMS

For the Cerebellar System, ask the client to perform the following actions, after you demonstrate them, in order to assess coordination.

ASSESSMENT PROCEDURE	NORMAL FINDINGS	ABNORMAL FINDINGS
Close eyes, and hold arms overhead and straight out in front.	Holds arms over head and straight out steadily for 20 seconds	Downward drift; a flexion of one or both arms
With arms extended to the sides, touch each forefinger alternately to nose, first with eyes open and then with eyes closed (Fig. 21-13).	Smooth accurate movements while touching finger to nose	Uncoordinated jerky movements, inability to touch nose seen with cerebellar disease

Continued on following page

CEREBELLAR SYSTEMS (Continued)

ASSESSMENT PROCEDURE	NORMAL FINDINGS	ABNORMAL FINDINGS
Put the palms of both hands down on both legs, then turn the palms up, and then turn the palms down again. Ask client to increase speed (Fig. 21-14).	Rapidly turns palms up and down	Uncoordinated movements or tremors are seen with cerebellar disease
Button and unbutton coat/shirt.	Buttons and unbuttons clothes smoothly	Clumsy attempts to button and unbutton clothes
Run each heel down opposite shin one at a time (Fig. 21-15).	Runs each heel smoothly down each shin	Unable to place heel on shin and move it down shin with coordination with cerebellar disease

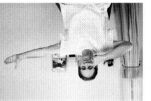

FIGURE 21-13 Testing coordination: finger-to-nose test.

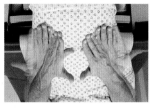

FIGURE 21-14 Testing rapid alternating movements: palms.

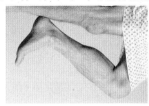

FIGURE 21-15 Performing heel-to-shin test.

ASSESSMENT PROCEDURE	NORMAL FINDINGS	ABNORMAL FINDINGS
Stand erect with feet together and arms at sides, first with eyes open and then with eyes closed. (Put your arms around client to prevent falls—Romberg test.)	Stands straight with minimal swaying	Sways, moves feet out to prevent fall with disease of posterior column, vestibular dysfunction, or cerebellar disorders
Walk naturally.	Steady gait with opposite arm swing	Unsteady gait, uncoordinated arm swing; uses wide foot stance; shuffles or drags feet; lifts feet high off ground; crosses feet when walking. Gait is affected by disorders of the motor, sensory, vestibular, and cerebellar systems.
Walk in a heel-to-toe fashion (tandem walk, Fig. 21-16).	Maintains balance with tandem walk	Unsteady tandem walk; unable to walk tandem style

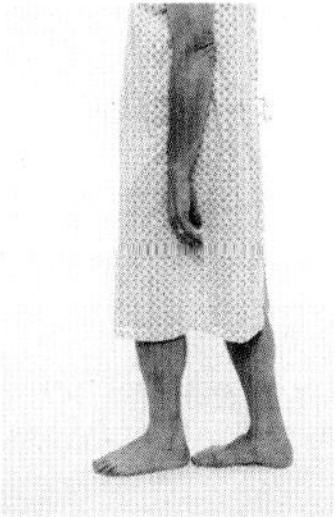

FIGURE 21-16 Testing balance: tandem walking.

Continued on following page

CEREBELLAR SYSTEMS (Continued)		
ASSESSMENT PROCEDURE	**NORMAL FINDINGS**	**ABNORMAL FINDINGS**
Stand on each foot (one at a time).	Stands on one foot at a time	Unable to stand on one foot at a time
Hop on each foot (one at a time) (Fig. 21-17).	Hops on each foot without losing balance	Inadequate strength or balance to hop on each foot with muscle weakness or disease of the cerebellum
Walk on heels, then toes.	Walks on heels, then toes	Unable to walk on heels or toes

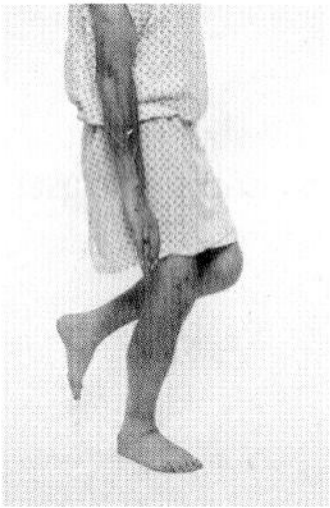

FIGURE 21-17 Hopping on one foot.

SENSORY SYSTEM

To test the client's ability to perceive various sensations over the extremities and abdomen, stimuli must be scattered to cover all dermatomes. The client is asked to close his or her eyes and identify the type of sensation perceived and the body area where it was felt. If a perceptual deficit is identified, the area is mapped out to determine the extent of impaired sensation.

ASSESSMENT PROCEDURE	NORMAL FINDINGS	ABNORMAL FINDINGS
Test for **primary sensations** with client's eyes closed by touching client with the following:		
• Piece of cotton	• Identifies area of light touch	• Unable to identify location or light touch sensation
• Alternately with sharp tip and dull tip of paper clip	• Identifies area touched and differentiates between sharp and dull sensations	• Unable to identify location or differentiate touch sensations
• Vibrating tuning fork on major distal bony prominences of wrist, sternum	• Identifies vibratory sensation	• Unable to identify vibratory sensation
Test for **cortical and discriminatory sensation** with client's eyes closed by asking the client to identify the following.		
• The number of points touching him or her while you touch the client with two points simultaneously (two-point discrimination; Fig. 21-18)	• Identifies two points on forearm at 40 mm apart; back at 40–70 mm apart; dorsal hands at 20–30 mm apart; fingertips at 2–5 mm apart	• Unable to identify two points at normal ranges with lesions of the sensory cortex
• The object (e.g., a coin) you place in the client's hand (stereognosis)	• Identifies correct object	• Unable to identify object with lesions of the sensory cortex

Continued on following page

SENSORY SYSTEM (Continued)

ASSESSMENT PROCEDURE	NORMAL FINDINGS	ABNORMAL FINDINGS
• A number you write on the client's palm with a tongue blade (graphesthesia)	• Identifies correct number	• Unable to identify number with lesions of the sensory cortex
• The direction you move a part of the client's body (e.g., move fingers or toes up or down with eyes closed; kinesthesia; Fig. 21-19)	• Identifies correct direction in which the body part is moved	• Unable to identify direction in which the body part is moved with lesions of the sensory cortex

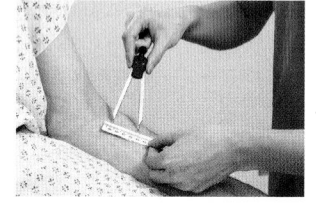

FIGURE 21-18 Two-point discrimination.

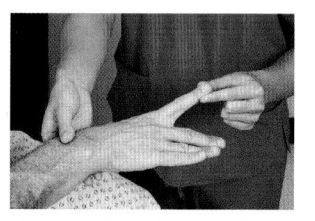

FIGURE 21-19 Testing position sense (kinesthesia).

REFLEXES

The reflex (or percussion) hammer is used to elicit deep tendon reflexes (see Assessment Guide 21-1, page 479). To elicit superficial reflexes, lightly stroke the skin with a moderately sharp instrument (e.g., key, tongue blade). Finally, certain maneuvers are performed to elicit any pathologic reflexes.

ASSESSMENT PROCEDURE	NORMAL FINDINGS	ABNORMAL FINDINGS
*Elicit **deep tendon reflexes** as follows:* • Biceps reflex: With reflex hammer, tap your thumb placed over biceps tendon with client's arm flexed (tests nerve roots C5, C6; Fig. 21-20). • Brachioradialis reflex: Tap brachioradialis tendon just above wrist on radial side with client's arm resting midway between supination and pronation (tests nerve roots C5, C6; Fig. 21-21).	• Biceps contract (1+, 2+, 3+ biceps reflex). • Elbow flexes with pronation of forearm (1+, 2+, 3+ brachioradialis reflex).	• Absent or hyperactive contraction of biceps (0, 4+ biceps reflex) • Absent or hyperactive flexion of elbow and forearm pronation (0+, 4+ brachioradialis reflex)

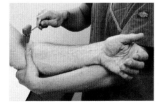

FIGURE 21-20 Eliciting biceps reflex.

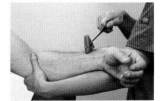

FIGURE 21-21 Eliciting brachioradialis reflex.

Continued on following page

REFLEXES (Continued)

ASSESSMENT PROCEDURE	NORMAL FINDINGS	ABNORMAL FINDINGS
• Triceps reflex: Tap triceps tendon (just above elbow) with client's arm abducted and forearm hanging freely (tests nerve roots C6, C7, C8; fig. 21-22).	• Elbow extends (1+, 2+, 3+ triceps reflex).	• Absent or hyperactive elbow extension (0, 4+ triceps reflex)
• Patellar reflex: Tap patellar tendon with client's knee flexed and thigh stabilized (tests nerve roots L2, L3; fig. 21-23).	• Extension of knee (1+, 2+, 3+ patellar reflex)	• Absent or hyperactive extension of knee (0, 4+ patellar reflex)
• Achilles reflex: Tap Achilles tendon with client's foot slightly dorsiflexed and stabilized (tests nerve roots S1, S2; fig. 21-24).	• Plantar flexion of foot (1+, 2+, 3+ Achilles reflex)	• Absent or hyperactive plantar flexion of foot (0, 4+ plantar flexion)

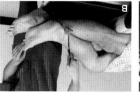
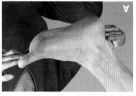
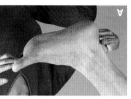
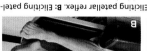

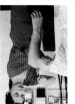

FIGURE 21-22 Eliciting triceps reflex.

FIGURE 21-23 A: Eliciting patellar reflex. **B:** Eliciting patellar reflex (supine position).

FIGURE 21-24 A: Eliciting Achilles reflex. **B:** Eliciting Achilles reflex (supine position).

ASSESSMENT PROCEDURE	NORMAL FINDINGS	ABNORMAL FINDINGS
Elicit **superficial reflexes** *as follows:* • Lightly stroke each side of abdomen above and below umbilicus (umbilicus reflexes; Fig. 21-25). • Stroke gluteal area. • Stroke inner upper thigh of males. *Assess for* **pathologic reflexes** *as follows:* • Plantar reflex: Use end of reflex hammer to stroke lateral aspect of sole from heel to ball of foot (Fig. 21-26).	• Bilateral upward and downward movements of umbilicus toward stroke; abdomen contracts. • Anal sphincter contracts. • Scrotum elevates on side stimulated. • Flexion of all toes (plantar response) seen in adults (Fig. 21-26)	• Absent or unilateral movement of umbilicus; no abdominal contraction • Absent contraction of gluteal reflex • No elevation of scrotum • Except in infancy, extension (dorsiflexion) of the big toe and fanning of all toes (positive plantar reflex; Babinski response) are seen with lesions of upper motor neurons. Unconscious states resulting from drug and alcohol intoxication or subsequent to an epileptic seizure may also cause it.

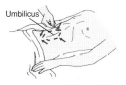

FIGURE 21-25 Umbilicus reflex.

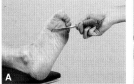 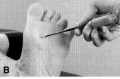

FIGURE 21-26 A: Eliciting plantar reflex. **B:** Normal plantar response.

Continued on following page

REFLEXES (Continued)

ASSESSMENT PROCEDURE	NORMAL FINDINGS	ABNORMAL FINDINGS
• Ankle clonus: Sharply dorsiflex foot with knee supported and partially flexed, and hold this way (Fig. 21-27).	• Foot stays dorsiflexed with no movement. 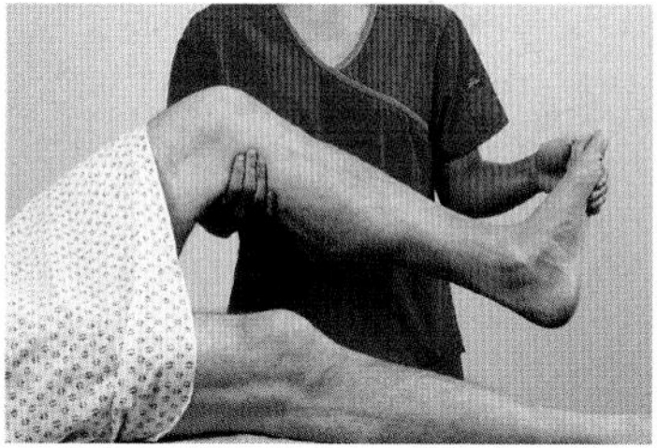 **FIGURE 21-27** Testing for ankle clonus.	• Foot oscillates between dorsiflexion and plantar flexion.
• Brudzinski sign: Ask the client to flex the neck; watch the hips and knees in reaction to the maneuver.	• Hips and knees remain relaxed and motionless.	• Flexion of the hips and knees is a positive Brudzinski sign and suggests meningeal inflammation
• Kernig sign: Flex the client's leg at both the hip and the knee, and then straighten the knee.	• No pain felt. Discomfort behind the knee during full extension occurs in many normal people.	• Pain and increased resistance to extending the knee are a positive Kernig sign. When Kernig sign is bilateral, the examiner suspects meningeal irritation.

ASSESSMENT GUIDE 21-1 Eliciting Deep Tendon Reflexes

Proceed as follows to elicit a deep tendon reflex.

1. Encourage the client to relax and position the client properly.
2. Hold the handle of the reflex hammer between your thumb and index finger so it swings freely.

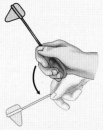

3. Palpate the tendon and use a rapid wrist movement to strike the tendon briskly. Observe the response.
4. Compare the response of one side with the other.
5. For arm reflexes, ask the client to clench his or her jaw or to squeeze one thigh with the opposite hand, and then immediately strike the tendon. For leg reflexes, ask the client to lock the fingers of both

hands and pull them against each other, and then immediately strike the tendon.

6. Rate and document reflexes using the following scale and figure.

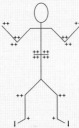

- Grade 4+: Hyperactive, very brisk, rhythmic oscillations (clonus); abnormal and indicative of disorder
- Grade 3+: More brisk or active than normal, but not indicative of a disorder
- Grade 2+: Normal, usual response
- Grade 1+: Decreased, less active than normal
- Grade 0: No response

PEDIATRIC VARIATIONS

Cranial Nerve Examination

The cranial nerves are difficult to assess in the newborn and young child. Assessment of cranial nerves may be performed in middle to later childhood and adolescence.

Motor and Cerebellar Examination

Cerebellar functioning may be assessed in older children and adolescents by performing the following: Romberg test, finger-to-nose, finger-to-finger, heel-to-shin and rapid alternating movements with hands and fingers.

Sensory Examination

Sensory nerve assessment may be assessed by asking the child to close his/her eyes and lightly touching the child in different places on the face, arm, hand, lower legs.

Reflex Examination

Assess deep tendon reflexes in all children with the reflex hammer. The first finger may be used to assess infants if desired. Average reflexes for children are 2+ to 3+. Newborns tend to have more brisk reflexes (3+).

INFANT REFLEXES (Birth to age 1 year; See Appendix 5 for developmental milestones for ages 1 to 3 years)	NORMAL VARIATIONS
Cough	No cough reflex until 1–2 days of age; after 1–2 days, cough should be strong and present even during sleep throughout infancy.
Rooting: Infant turns head toward side of face stroked.	Disappears at about age 3–12 months
Extension: When tongue is pressed or touched, infant forces tongue outward.	Disappears at about age 4 months

INFANT REFLEXES	NORMAL VARIATIONS
Grasp: Touch to palm of hand or soles of feet causes flexion of hands/toes.	Palmar grasp should disappear at about age 3 months
Plantar reflex: Stroking outer sole of foot from heel to toe causes big toe to rise (dorsiflexion) and other toes to fan out.	Disappears after 1 year
Moro: Sudden jarring or change in equilibrium causes sudden extension and abduction of extremities, with thumb forming "C" shape; crying.	Disappears at about age 3–4 months
Startle: Sudden noise caus es abduction of arms, clenched hands.	Disappears at about age 4 months
Crawling: Infant on abdomen will make crawling movements with arms and legs.	Disappears at about age 6 weeks
Dance: Infant held so soles of feet touching table will simulate walking movements.	Disappears at about age 3–4 weeks
Neck righting: In supine infant, if head is turned to one side, shoulder and trunk will turn to that side.	Disappears around age 10 months
Asymmetrical tonic neck: Infant's head quickly turns to one side, arm and leg on that side will extend, and opposite leg and arm will flex	Disappears at about age 3–4 months

GERIATRIC VARIATIONS

Cranial Nerve Examination

• Decreased ability to see, hear, taste, and smell

Motor and Cerebellar Examination

• Slowed coordination and voluntary movements
• Decreased fine motor coordination
• May see tremors of the hand or head, or repetitive movements of the lips, jaw, or tongue
• May have slower and less certain gait; tandem walking may be very difficult for older client
• Hopping on one foot is often impossible because of decreased flexibility and strength; it is best to avoid this test with the older client because of risk for injury

Sensory Examination

• Touch sensations may diminish normally with aging due to atrophy of peripheral nerve endings
• Decreased light touch and pain perception
• Vibratory sensation at ankles often decreased after age 70 years

Reflex Examination

• Generalized decreased deep tendon reflexes and slowed reflexes
• Decrease in transmission of impulses along with a delay in reaction time

POSSIBLE COLLABORATIVE PROBLEMS—RISK OF

• Cranial nerve
  • Cranial nerve impairment
  • Corneal ulceration
  • Increased intraocular pressure
• Motor/cerebellar
  • Increased intracranial pressure
  • Meningitis
  • Paralysis
  • Spinal cord compression
  • Seizures
• Sensory
  • Peripheral nerve impairment
  • Neuropathies

Teaching Tips for Selected Nursing Diagnoses

Nursing Diagnosis: *Sensory/Perceptual Alterations (specify) related to injury or aging*

Explain to family the use and benefits of sensory therapy. Refer for hearing/visual aids as necessary. Teach client slowly and concisely. Speak clearly and demonstrate instructions from client's best side for hearing and seeing. Teach client how to prevent thermal injuries.

Nursing Diagnosis: *Risk for Injury related to seizure activity*

Teach appropriate precautions and care, including the following.
- Use of padded tongue blade, wallet, or cloth to maintain airway
- Protection of client from harm during seizures
- Positioning on side after seizure
- Significance of drug maintenance

Nursing Diagnosis: *Risk for Adult Failure to Thrive*

Teach the client and family or caregivers to assess behavior patterns that suggest anorexia, fatigue, dehydration, onset of incontinence (bowel or bladder), increase in chronic health problems such as pneumonia and urinary tract infections, cognitive decline, self-neglect, apathy, sadness. Teach the client and caregivers to seek appropriate referrals if pattern is detected.

Nursing Diagnosis: *Risk for Injury related to decreased tactile sensations*

Instruct on proper inspection and protective care of extremities. Caution client on dangers of exposure to extreme hot and cold temperatures, contact with sharp objects, and wearing tight-fitting shoes or garments.

CHAPTER 22

Assessing Male Genitalia and Rectum

Structure and Function Overview

EXTERNAL GENITALIA

The penis is the male reproductive organ (Fig. 22-1). The penile shaft is composed of three masses of vascular erectile tissue bound by fibrous tissue—two corpora cavernosa on the dorsal side and the corpus spongiosum on the ventral side, which forms the acorn-shaped glans. The urethra is located in the center of the corpus spongiosum and opening at the glans tip as the urethral meatus. The frenulum, a fold of foreskin, extends ventrally from

the urethral meatus. The scrotum, a thin-walled sac suspended below the pubic bone posterior to the penis, contains sweat and sebaceous glands and consists of skin folds (rugae) and the cremaster muscle. The scrotum protects the testes, epididymis, and vas deferens and maintains a temperature (less than 37 °C) required for sperm production.

INTERNAL GENITALIA

The internal genitalia consists of the testes, a pair of ovoid-shaped organs located in the scrotal sac that produce spermatozoa and

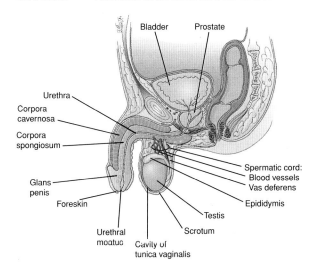

FIGURE 22-1 External and internal male genitalia.

Labels on figure:
- Bladder
- Prostate
- Urethra
- Corpora cavernosa
- Corpora spongiosum
- Glans penis
- Foreskin
- Urethral meatus
- Cavity of tunica vaginalis
- Spermatic cord: Blood vessels, Vas deferens
- Epididymis
- Testis
- Scrotum

testosterone (see Fig. 22-1). The testes are covered by the tunica vaginalis, a serous membrane that protects the testes. The testes are suspended by a spermatic cord that contains blood vessels, lymphatic vessels, nerves, and the vas deferens, which transports spermatozoa away from the testes. The left side of the spermatic cord is usually longer; thus the left testis hangs lower than the right testis. The epididymis, a comma-shaped, coiled tubular structure curves up over the upper and posterior surfaces of the testis. It is here that the spermatozoa mature. The vas deferens is a firm, muscular tube continuous with the lower portion of the epididymis, which travels up within the spermatic cord through the inguinal canal into the abdominal cavity. It joins with the duct of the seminal vesicle to form the ejaculatory duct, which empties into the urethra. The vas deferens transports sperm from the testes to the urethra for ejaculation. Along the way, secretions from the vas deferens, seminal vesicles, prostate gland, and Cowper's or bulbourethral glands mix with the sperm to form semen.

INGUINAL AREA

The inguinal (groin) area, located between the anterior superior iliac spine and the symphysis pubis, is a common area for hernias

(Fig. 22-2). Located within this area is the inguinal canal, a tube-like structure through which the vas deferens travels as it passes through the lower abdomen. The external inguinal ring can be palpated above and lateral to the symphysis pubis. The internal inguinal ring cannot be palpated. The femoral canal located posterior to the inguinal canal and medial to the femoral artery and vein is another area in which hernias may occur.

ANUS AND RECTUM

The **anal canal,** 2.5 to 4 cm long, begins at the anal sphincter and ends at the anorectal junction (Fig. 22-3). It is lined with somatic sensory nerves, making it susceptible to painful stimuli. The **anal opening** is hairless and overlies the external anal sphincter. Within the anus are the two sphincters that hold the anal canal closed except when passing gas and feces. The **external anal sphincter,** composed of skeletal muscle, is under voluntary control. The **internal sphincter,** composed of smooth muscle, is under involuntary control by the autonomic nervous system. Just above the internal sphincter is the **anorectal junction,** the dividing point of the anal canal and the rectum. The rectum is lined with mucosal folds (columns of Morgagni) that contain

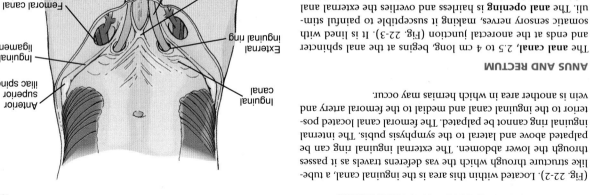

FIGURE 22-2 Inguinal area.

Anterior superior iliac spine

Inguinal ligament

Femoral canal with femoral artery & vein

External inguinal ring

Inguinal canal

Suspensory ligament of penis

Spermatic cord

Scrotum

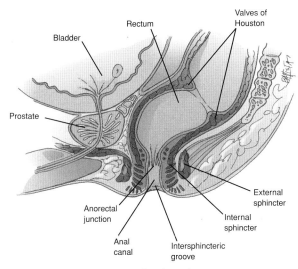

FIGURE 22-3 Anal and rectal structures.

arteries, veins, and visceral nerves. These tissues may engorge from chronic pressure and form hemorrhoids. The **rectum** (12 cm long) extends from the **sigmoid colon** to the anorectal junction. It enlarges above the anorectal junction and proceeds toward the hollow of the sacrum and coccyx, forming the rectal ampulla. The inside of the rectum contains three foldings (valves of Houston).

PROSTATE

The **prostate gland** (2.5 to 4 cm in diameter) surrounds the bladder neck and urethra and lies between these structures and the rectum. It has two lobes separated by a shallow groove (median sulcus). It secretes a milky substance that promotes sperm motility and neutralizes acidic vaginal secretions. This organ can be palpated through the anterior wall of the rectum. The **seminal vesicles,** located on the sides and above the prostate, produce the ejaculate that nourishes and protects sperm. The **Cowper or bulbourethral glands** are pea-sized glands located posterior to the prostate, which produce mucus.

Health Assessment

COLLECTING SUBJECTIVE DATA

Focus Questions

Pain in penis, scrotum, testes, or groin? Lesions in penis or genital area? Discharge from penis? Color? Odor? Lumps, masses, or swelling in scrotum, groin, or genital area? Heavy, draggy feeling in scrotum? Difficulty voiding—hesitancy, frequency, starting or maintaining stream? Change in color, odor, or amount of urine? Pain or burning when urinating? Incontinence or dribbling? Change in sexual activities? Difficulty with maintaining an erection? Problem with ejaculation? Trouble with fertility? Any bulges or pain when straining or lifting heavy objects? History of inguinal or genitalia surgery? History of STD? Self-care: Last testicular exam? Self-examination? Tested for HIV? Result? History of cancer in family? Number of sexual partners? Contraceptive form? Exposure to chemical or radiation? Fertility concerns? Comfort with communicating with sexual partner?

Usual bowel pattern? Changes? Diarrhea? Constipation? Color of stools? Mucus in stools? Pain? Itching? Bleeding after stools? History of rectal or anal surgery? Proctosigmoidoscopy? Family history of polyps, colon, rectal, or prostate cancer? Self-care: Use of laxatives? Engage in anal sex? Amount of roughage, fat, and water in diet? Last digital rectal examination by a physician or health-care provider?

Risk Factors

- Risk for colorectal cancer related to age greater than 40 years, history of rectal or colon polyps, inflammatory bowel disease, history of colorectal cancer, diet high in fat, protein, beef, and low in fiber.

- Risk for prostate cancer related to dietary fat intake, age greater than 60 years, African American or Hispanic origin, exposure to cadmium, dioxin, agent orange, high-risk occupations (e.g., tire and rubber manufacturers, farmers, mechanics, sheet metal workers), lack of circumcision, brother or father with prostate cancer, high testosterone levels may be a factor, excessive alcohol consumption, and lack of sleep or sleeping with light on.

- Risk for HIV/AIDS related to having unprotected sex (especially male-on-male anal intercourse), having multiple sexual partners, bisexual partners or partner who uses intravenous drug, having another STD, using intravenous drugs especially sharing needles, being an uncircumcised male, being the fetus of an HIV-positive mother (mother–infant transmission during pregnancy or delivery), exchanging blood or body fluids through blood transfusions or needle sticks, breastfeeding by HIV-infected mother, and having body piercings with nonsterilized instruments.

COLLECTING OBJECTIVE DATA

Equipment Needed

- Stool to sit on
- Gown
- Disposable nonlatex gloves
- Flashlight (for possible transillumination)
- Stethoscope (for possible auscultation)
- Drape
- Pillow
- Water-soluble lubricant for rectal examination

Physical Assessment

Review Figures 22-1 to 22-3 for anatomy of the external and internal genital structures, the inguinal area, and the anus and rectal area. Explain the purpose of the exam and procedure to put client at ease. Preserve the client's modesty and privacy. Teach client the importance of testicular self-examination (TSE) and explain how to perform the examination as you are performing it. Ask a third person to be present to protect the client and examiner from false allegations. Wear gloves for every step of this examination to ensure safety for the nurse and the client.

ASSESSMENT PROCEDURE	NORMAL FINDINGS	ABNORMAL FINDINGS
Observe for sexual maturity.	See norms on Table 22-1 on page 501.	• Under development or excessive development noted in relation to Table 22-1 on page 501.

Continued on following page

PENIS

ASSESSMENT PROCEDURE	NORMAL FINDINGS	ABNORMAL FINDINGS
Inspect the shaft of the penis with the client in a standing position. Ensure the client's privacy.		
Observe **penis** for the following:		
• Skin texture	• Wrinkled	• Nodules, growths, lesions (see Abnormal Findings 22-1, p. 504)
	• Hairless	• Swelling
		• Phimosis
		• Paraphimosis
Inspect the glans of the penis for the following:		
• Size, shape, and lesions	• Size varies; rounded, broad, or pointed; free of lesions	• Chancres (red, oval ulcerations from syphilis); pimple lesions in herpes; venereal warts (see Abnormal Findings 22-1)
• Urinary meatus	• Located at the tip of glans penis	• Displaced to ventral side (hypospadias) or dorsal side (epispadias) of penis
• Discharge	• No discharge	• Any drainage—yellow discharge is seen with gonorrhea; clear or white discharge is seen with urethritis.

ASSESSMENT PROCEDURE	NORMAL FINDINGS	ABNORMAL FINDINGS
Palpate **the penis.** With client standing, gently palpate the shaft and glans of penis between gloved thumb and fingers. If foreskin is present, retract from tip of penis, then replace.		
Palpate for the following:		
• Masses	• None	• Nodules, masses, or lesions anywhere on the shaft or glans may indicate STDs or cancer.
• Tenderness	• Slightly tender	• Very tender or painful; hardness along central shaft may indicate cancer; tenderness is seen with infection or inflammation.
• Discharge (see Fig. 22-4)	• None	• Clear or purulent from lesions or urinary meatus.
• Foreskin	• May not be present; should retract and return easily with clean, smooth skin underneath	• Unable to retract owing to phimosis or adherence to underlying tissue; any drainage or sores under skin; discoloration of foreskin seen with scarring or infection.

Continued on following page

PENIS (Continued)

ASSESSMENT PROCEDURE	NORMAL FINDINGS	ABNORMAL FINDINGS

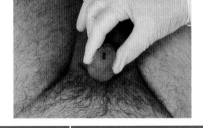

FIGURE 22-4 Palpating for urethral discharge (Photo by B. Proud).

SCROTUM AND TESTES

With client standing, inspect **scrotum** for the following:

- Size
- Color
- Texture

- Varies in size; left side of scrotal sac hangs slightly lower than right side.
- Pink or normal skin color
- Many skin folds

- Unilateral or bilateral enlargement due to presence of blood (hematocele), fluid (hydrocele), bowel (hernia), or tumor (cancer)
- Red, shiny, bruised
- Lesions, ulcers, taut skin

ASSESSMENT PROCEDURE	NORMAL FINDINGS	ABNORMAL FINDINGS
Palpate each **testis.** Grasp each testicle between thumb and fingers. Gently roll testicle so all surfaces are palpated (Fig. 22-5). Client may do self-examination with instructions and report findings (Box 22-1) on page 503.	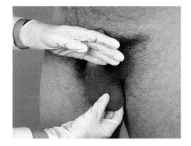 FIGURE 22-5 Palpating the scrotal contents (Photo by B. Proud).	
Palpate each testis for the following: • Location • Shape • Texture • Tenderness	• Each should be entirely in sac, left slightly lower than right. • Oval, symmetrical • Smooth, firm • Very tender	• One or both are absent or cannot be palpated at inguinal border (partially descended). • Enlarged, different sizes • Grainy or coarse; lumps or nodules • Pain; dull ache in lower abdomen or groin with feeling of heaviness

Continued on following page

SCROTUM AND TESTES (continued)

ASSESSMENT PROCEDURE	NORMAL FINDINGS	ABNORMAL FINDINGS
Transilluminate the scrotal contents if an abnormal mass or swelling is noted in the scrotum. Darken the room and shine a light from the back of the scrotum through the mass. Look for a red glow.	Scrotal contents do not transilluminate.	Swellings or masses that contain serous fluid—hydrocele, spermatocele—light up with a red glow. Swellings or masses that are solid or filled with blood—tumor, hernias, or varicocele—do not light up with a red glow.
Inspect and palpate for scrotal hernia. If you discovered a mass during inspection and palpation of the scrotum and you suspect it may be a hernia, ask the client to lie down; note whether the bulge disappears. If the bulge remains, auscultate it for bowel sounds. Finally, gently palpate the mass and try to push it upward into the abdomen.	If the bulge disappears, no scrotal hernia is present, but the mass may result from something else. Refer the client for further evaluation. A mass on or around the scrotum should be considered malignant until testing proves otherwise.	If the bulge disappears when the client lies down, a scrotal hernia is present. Bowel sounds auscultated over the mass indicate the presence of bowel and thus a scrotal hernia. If you cannot push the mass into the abdomen, suspect an *incarcerated hernia*. A hernia is *strangulated* when its blood supply is cut off. The client typically complains of extreme tenderness and nausea.

INGUINAL AREA

Have client stand so inguinal area is visible. Inspect **inguinal area.**	Smooth, symmetrical	Bulging on one or both sides that increase with straining indicates inguinal or femoral hernia.

ASSESSMENT PROCEDURE	NORMAL FINDINGS	ABNORMAL FINDINGS
Palpate **inguinal area.** Then have client strain down as you palpate inguinal area (Fig. 22-6). Use right hand for right side and left hand for left side.	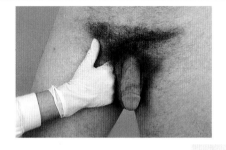 FIGURE 22-6 Palpating for an inguinal hernia (Photo by B. Proud).	
Palpate for the following: • Lymph nodes • Masses	• Nonpalpable • Smooth, no masses	• Palpable, tender • Bulge of soft tissue that increases with straining indicates hernia.
Palpate for femoral hernia. Palpate on the front of the thigh in the femoral canal area. Ask the client to bear down or cough. Feel for bulges. Repeat on the opposite thigh.	Bulges or masses are not normally palpated.	Bulge or mass palpated as client bears down or coughs.

Continued on following page

ANUS, RECTUM, AND PROSTATE

ASSESSMENT PROCEDURE	NORMAL FINDINGS	ABNORMAL FINDINGS

The most frequently used position for examining the anus, rectum, and prostate is the left lateral position, which allows adequate inspection and palpation of the anus, rectum, and prostate and promotes client comfort. Drape client's torso and legs. Ask client to lie on the left side, with the buttocks as close to the edge of the examining table as possible, and to bend the right knee. Support leg on pillow if needed and provide a pillow for head. Another method is to perform the male anus, rectum, and prostate exam while the client stands and bends over the examining table with his hips flexed (Fig. 22-7). Use the position best for the particular client and promotion of comfort. The rectum will be able to be examined only to a certain point with the examiner's finger. If an exam of the upper rectum and sigmoid colon is necessary, refer client for a sigmoidoscopy.

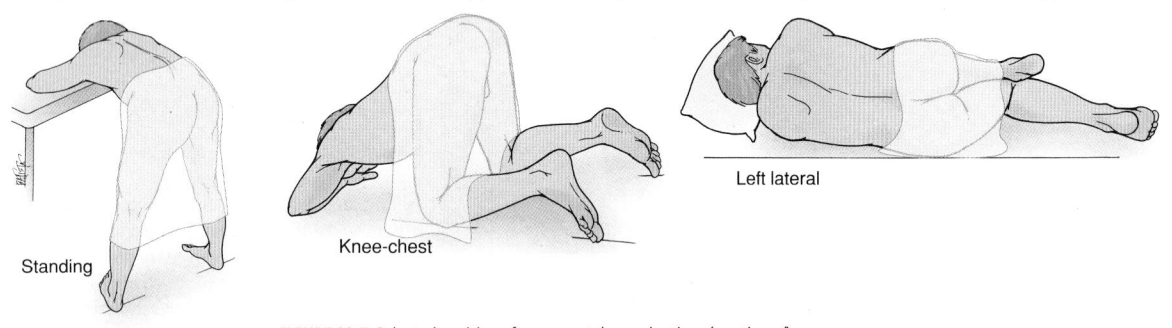

Standing   Knee-chest   Left lateral

FIGURE 22-7 Selected positions for anorectal examination. (*continued*)

ASSESSMENT PROCEDURE	NORMAL FINDINGS	ABNORMAL FINDINGS

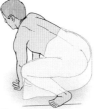
Squatting

FIGURE 22-7 (Continued)

Inspect **perianal area** (Fig. 22-8). Spread the client's buttocks and inspect the anal opening and the surrounding area for the following:
- Lumps
- Ulcers
- Lesions
- Rashes
- Redness
- Fissures
- Thickening of the epithelium

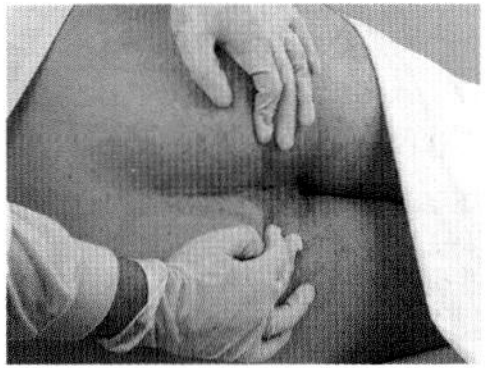

FIGURE 22-8 Inspecting the perianal area (Photo by B. Proud).

Anal opening is hairless, moist, and tightly closed. The surrounding perianal area is free of redness, lumps, ulcers, lesions, or rashes.

Lesions may indicate sexually transmitted diseases, cancer, or hemorrhoids. A thrombosed external hemorrhoid appears swollen. It is itchy, painful, and bleeds when the client passes stool. A previously thrombosed hemorrhoid appears as a skin tag that protrudes from the anus.

Continued on following page

ANUS, RECTUM, AND PROSTATE (Continued)

ASSESSMENT PROCEDURE	NORMAL FINDINGS	ABNORMAL FINDINGS
Inspect **sacrococcygeal area** for color, hair, and texture.	Smooth, free of hair, and redness	Red, swollen area covered by a small tuft of hair located in the lower sacrum suggests the presence of a pilonidal cyst.
Ask the client to perform Valsalva maneuver by straining or bearing down. Inspect the anal opening for any bulges or lesions.	No bulging or lesions appear.	Bulges of red mucous membrane may indicate a rectal prolapse. Hemorrhoids or an anal fissure may also be seen.
Palpate the anus. Explain to the client what you are going to do. Explain that the client may feel like his bowels will move. With one hand, gently separate buttocks so rectum is exposed. Lubricate gloved index finger and ask client to bear down. Then place the pad of your index finger on the anal opening (Fig. 22-9).	Sphincter relaxes.	Sphincter tightens, preventing further examination.

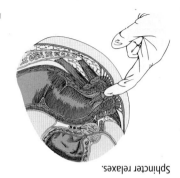

FIGURE 22-9 Palpating the anus.

ASSESSMENT PROCEDURE	NORMAL FINDINGS	ABNORMAL FINDINGS
Assess **sphincter tone.**	Can close sphincter around gloved finger	Poor tone may be a result of spinal cord injury, previous surgery, trauma, prolapsed rectum, or sexual abuse. Tightened sphincter may be the result of anxiety, scarring, or inflammation.
Palpate for **tenderness, nodules, and hardness.**	Normally smooth, nontender, without nodules or hardness	Tenderness indicates hemorrhoids, fistula, fissure; nodules indicate polyps, cancer; hardness scarring, cancer.
Palpate **rectum.** Insert finger farther into rectum. Turn finger clockwise, then counterclockwise. Note tenderness irregularities, nodules, and hardness.		
Palpate the **prostate gland.** On the anterior surface of the rectum, turn the hand fully counterclockwise so the pad of your index finger faces toward the client's umbilicus. Tell the client he may feel an urge to urinate but will not. Move the pad of your index finger over the prostate gland, trying to feel the sulcus between the lateral lobes (Fig. 22-10).	Prostate nontender and rubbery with two lateral lobes that are divided by a median sulcus. The lobes are normally smooth, 2.5 cm long, and heart-shaped.	A swollen, tender prostate may indicate acute prostatitis. An enlarged, smooth, firm, slightly elastic prostate that may not have a median sulcus suggests benign prostatic hypertrophy (BPH). A hard area on the prostate or hard, fixed, irregular nodules on the prostate suggest cancer (see Abnormal Findings 22-2).

Continued on following page

ANUS, RECTUM, AND PROSTATE (Continued)

ASSESSMENT PROCEDURE	NORMAL FINDINGS	ABNORMAL FINDINGS
Inspect the **stool.** Withdraw your gloved finger. Inspect any fecal matter on your glove. Assess the color, and test the feces for occult blood. Provide the client with a towel to wipe the anorectal area.	Stool is normally semisolid, brown, and free of blood.	Black stool seen in upper gastrointestinal bleeding, gray or tan stool results from the lack of bile pigment, yellow stool suggests steatorrhea (increased fat content). Blood in stool may indicate cancer of the rectum or colon. An endoscopic examination of the colon should be performed if blood is detected.

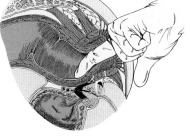

FIGURE 22-10 Palpating the prostate gland.

TABLE 22-1 Tanner Sexual Maturity Rating: Male Genitalia Development and Pubic Hair Growth

Developmental Stage	Genitalia	Pubic Hair
Stage 1	Prepubertal	Prepubertal: No pubic hair; fine vellus hair
Stage 2	Initial enlargement of scrotum and testes with rugation and reddening of the scrotum.	Sparse, long, straight, downy hair
Stage 3	Elongation of the penis; testes and scrotum further enlarge	Darker, coarser, curly; sparse over entire pubis

Continued on following page

TABLE 22-1 **Tanner Sexual Maturity Rating: Male Genitalia Development and Pubic Hair Growth** (Continued)

Developmental Stage		Genitalia	Pubic Hair
Stage 4		Increase in size and width of penis and the development of the glans; scrotum darkens	Dark, curly, and abundant in pubic area; no growth on thighs or up toward umbilicus
Stage 5		Adult configuration	Adult pattern (growth up toward umbilicus may not be seen); growth continues until mid 20s

Used with permission from Tanner, J.M. (1962). *Growth at adolescence* (2nd ed.). Oxford, UK: Blackwell Scientific Publications.

BOX 22-1 SELF ASSESSMENT: TESTICULAR SELF-EXAMINATION

Testicular self-examination (TSE) is to be performed once a month; it is neither difficult nor time-consuming. A convenient time is often after a warm bath or shower when the scrotum is more relaxed.

1. Stand in front of a mirror and check for scrotal swelling.
2. Use both hands to palpate the testis; the normal testicle is smooth and uniform in consistency.
3. With the index and middle fingers under the testis and the thumb on top, roll the testis gently in a horizontal plane between the thumb and fingers **(A)**.
4. Feel for any evidence of a small lump or abnormality.
5. Follow the same procedure and palpate upward along the testis **(B)**.
6. Locate the epididymis **(C)**, a cord-like structure on the top and back of the testicle that stores and transports sperm.
7. Repeat the examination for the other testis. It is normal to find that one testis is larger than the other.
8. If you find any evidence of a small, pea-like lump, consult your physician. It may be due to an infection or a tumor growth.

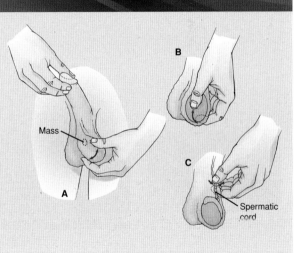

ABNORMAL FINDINGS 22-1 Abnormalities of the Penis

Syphilitic chancre

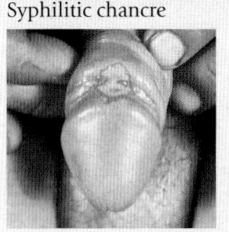

(Courtesy of UpJohn Co.)

Herpes progenitalis

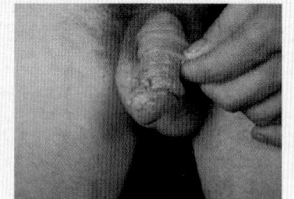

Genital warts

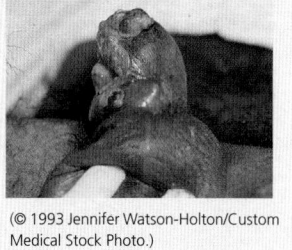

(Courtesy of Reed & Carnick Pharmaceuticals.)

Cancer of the Glans Penis

(© 1993 Jennifer Watson-Holton/Custom Medical Stock Photo.)

ABNORMAL FINDINGS **22-2** **Abnormalities of the Prostate Gland**

Acute prostatitis

Benign prostatic hypertrophy

Cancer of the Prostate

Swelling and inflammation characteristic of acute prostatitis.

Enlargement characteristic of benign prostatic hypertrophy.

Mass characteristic of prostate cancer.

PEDIATRIC VARIATIONS

Questions to ask the parents or the adolescent when collecting *subjective data* include the following.

- Development of secondary sexual characteristics?
- Previous education on sexual development and activities?
- Use of contraceptives? Type?

When collecting *objective data* note the following.

Inspection and palpation of external genitalia constitute the *total* genitourinary assessment until puberty. Assessment of the level of sexual development usually begins at approximately the age of 11 years. This determination involves assessment of secondary characteristics associated with sexual maturity. Refer to Table 22-1 for a summary of the timing of sexual development for boys.

 GERIATRIC VARIATIONS

- Pubic hair may be gray and sparse
- Penis becomes smaller and the testes hang lower in the scrotum
- Decrease in size and firmness of testicles
- Loss of tone in musculature of scrotum
- Slowed erections and less forceful ejaculations
- Enlargement of medial lobe of prostate

 CULTURAL VARIATIONS

Male genitalia are mutilated in pubertal rites in some cultures. Examples include circumcision or surgical incision along penile shaft and into its base for passage of urine and semen.

POSSIBLE COLLABORATIVE PROBLEMS—RISK OF

Bladder perforation	Obstruction of urethra	Renal calculi
Urinary tract infection	Hemorrhage	Hormonal imbalances
Genitalia ulcers or lesions	Renal failure	Hemorrhoids
	Sexually Transmitted Diseases	
	BPH	

Teaching Tips for Selected Nursing Diagnoses and Collaborative Problems

Nursing Diagnosis: Readiness for Enhanced Self-health Management: Urinary Elimination and Reproductive Pattern

Teach the client to drink eight glasses of fluid per day and to limit intake of alcohol, caffeine, and carbonated beverages.

Nursing Diagnosis: Readiness for Enhanced Self-health Management: Testicular Self-Examination

Instruct the client on proper method of TSE, performed once a month after a warm bath or shower. Instruct the client to roll each testicle gently between thumb and fingers of both hands, feeling for lumps or nodules (see Box 22-1). Have client demonstrate. Begin at puberty, because testicular cancer is one of the most common cancers in men between 15 and 34 years old.

Nursing Diagnosis: *Risk for Infection (STD) related to unprotected intercourse with multiple partners*

Teach early warning signs and symptoms. Discuss methods of prevention (limit to one uninfected partner and use of condoms) and modes of transmission. Routine screening for infection is recommended during pelvic exam (Healthy People, 2010).

Nursing Diagnosis: *Ineffective Health Maintenance related to a lack of knowledge of birth control methods*

Teach alternate forms of birth control, proper use of methods, and advantages and disadvantages of each.

Nursing Diagnosis: *Sexual Dysfunction: Impotence related to unknown etiology*

Explore possible etiologies and alternate forms of sexual satisfaction. Refer to urologist for information on penile implants, surgery, and other alternatives.

Nursing Diagnosis: *Sexual Dysfunction related to poor partner communication and deficient knowledge of psychological and physical health and sexual performance*

Teach effects and benefits of exercise. Explore communication with partner. Refer to counselor (psychiatric, sexual, marriage) as needed. Provide adequate literature on sex and health teaching for client.

Nursing Diagnosis: *Sexual Dysfunction related to loss of body part or physiologic limitations*

Explore prior sexual patterns. Explore alternatives. Provide resource material on self-help groups (e.g., Ostomy Association).

Suggest use of foreplay and lubricants to increase secretions as necessary. Provide literature and referrals.

Nursing Diagnosis: Risk for Impaired Elimination Pattern *related to parental knowledge deficit of toilet-training techniques*

Teach parents the importance of physiologic and psychological readiness in toilet training. Explain use of "potty chairs" and that bowel control precedes bladder control. Inform parents of the benefits of positive reinforcement and that nocturnal enuresis may persist up to the age of 4 to 5 years.

Nursing Diagnosis: Readiness for Enhanced Self-Health Management: Sexual Function

Sexual education is recommended in the early school years. Assess what child already knows and what he or she is ready to know.

Fourth to fifth grade: Interested in conception and birth

Fifth to sixth grade: Interested in their bodies and opposite sex changes. Education on birth control may be appropriate

---

because of early experimentation. Discuss normal development of secondary sexual characteristics and the normal psychological changes associated with puberty. The CDC now recommends administering the HPV vaccine at 11 to 12 years of age for boys and girls to prevent the human papillomavirus. It is a three-dose series. The first dose is given, with the second and third dose administered 2 to 6 months following the first dose. However, the vaccine may be administered between the ages of 9 and 26 years of age (CDC, 2012c).

Adolescent: Teach the importance of abstinence or use of condoms if currently sexually active. Explain that there are an estimated 19 million new cases of STDs reported yearly and 50,000 new HIV infections yearly in the United States, of which one half of all new STD including HIV infections are in people less than the age of 25 years and most are infected through sexual behavior (CDC, 2013c). The CDC (2013b) reports that HIV rates over several years have remained stable, except for a marked increase in young black gay men.

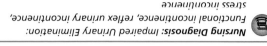

Nursing Diagnosis: Impaired Urinary Elimination: *Functional incontinence, reflex urinary incontinence, stress incontinence*

Explain to family how to decrease environmental barriers (offer bedpan frequently, provide proper lighting, ensure availability and proximity of commode) for functional incontinence. Teach client the cutaneous triggering mechanisms for reflex incontinence.

 Collaborative Problem: *Potential complication: Prostate hypertrophy*

Teach client about effects of normal enlargement of prostate on urination (frequency, dribbling, and nocturia). The American Cancer Society (2012) recommends men greater than 50 years of age and at average risk for the disease discuss with their healthcare provider the benefits and risks of having prostate cancer screening including yearly digital rectal exams and prostate-specific antigen (PSA) testing. The U.S. Preventive Services Task Force (2011) recommends against routine screening with PSA test for men in the United States population who do not have symptoms suggesting prostate cancer, regardless of age, race, or family history.

CHAPTER 23

Assessing Female Genitalia and Rectum

Structure and Function Overview

EXTERNAL GENITALIA

The external genitalia include the *vulva* that extends from the mons pubis to the anal opening. The *mons pubis*, a fat pad located over the symphysis pubis covered with pubic hair, protects the symphysis pubis during sexual intercourse. The *labia majora*, the two folds of skin that are composed of adipose tissue, sebaceous glands, and sweat glands, extend from the mons pubis to the perineum. The inner surface of the labia majora is pink, smooth, and moist.

Inside the labia majora is the *labia minora*, folds that join anteriorly at the clitoris and form a *prepuce* or hood and join posteriorly to form the *frenulum*. The labia minora contain sebaceous glands that produce lubrication for the vaginal area. The *clitoris*, located at the anterior end of the labia minora, is a small, cylindrical mass of erectile tissue and nerves. The skin folds of the labia majora and labia minora form a boat-shaped area or fossa called the *vestibule*. Located between the clitoris and the vaginal orifice is the *urethral meatus*. The openings of *Skene glands*, usually not visible, are on either side of the urethral opening and secrete mucus.

Below the urethral meatus is the *vaginal orifice*, covered by the hymen, a fold of membranous tissue that covers a part of the vagina. The *Bartholin glands*, located on both sides of vaginal not visible to the eye, secrete mucus (Fig. 23-1).

INTERNAL GENITALIA

The internal genital reproductive organs (Fig. 23-2) are the vagina, the uterus, the cervix, the fallopian tubes, and the ovaries. The *vagina*, about 10 cm long, extends up and slightly back toward the rectum from the vaginal orifice to the cervix. It allows the passage of menstrual flow, receives the penis during sexual intercourse, and serves as the birth canal during delivery. The *cervix* (or neck of the uterus) separates the upper end of the vagina from the isthmus of the uterus. The junction of the isthmus and the cervix forms the *internal os*, and the junction of the cervix and the vagina forms the *external os*. The cervix allows the entrance of sperm into the uterus, allows the passage of menstrual flow, and secretes mucus and prevents the entrance of vaginal bacteria. During childbirth,

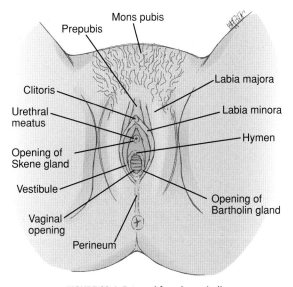

FIGURE 23-1 External female genitalia.

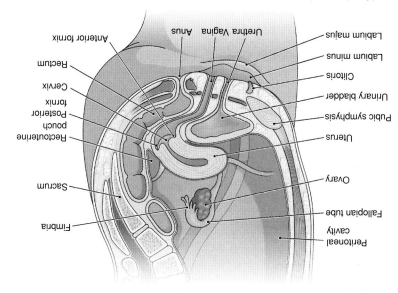

FIGURE 23-2 Internal female reproductive system and relationship to other pelvic structures including the rectum and anus.

the cervix can stretch to allow the passage of the fetus. The *uterus*, a pear-shaped organ, has two components: the *corpus* and the *cervix*. The corpus is divided into the fundus (upper portion), the body (central portion), and the isthmus (narrow lower portion). The uterus is usually situated in a forward position above the bladder at approximately a 45-degree angle to the vagina when standing. The *endometrium*, the myometrium, and the *peritoneum* are the three layers of the uterine wall. The endometrium, the inner mucosal layer, has glands that secrete an alkaline substance to keep the uterine cavity moist. A portion of the endometrium sheds during menses and childbirth. The myometrium is the middle layer functions to expel the products of conception. The peritoneum is the outer uterine layer that covers the uterus and separates it from the abdominal cavity. The *ovaries*, small oval-shaped organs, are on the lateral sides of the pelvic cavity and produce ova, estrogen, progesterone, and testosterone. The ovum travels from the ovary to the uterus through the fallopian tubes.

ANUS AND RECTUM

The *anal canal* begins at the anal sphincter and ends at the anorectal junction. It is 2.5 to 4 cm long. Within the anus are the two sphincters that hold the anal canal closed except when passing gas and feces. The *external sphincter* is composed of skeletal muscle and is under voluntary control. The *internal sphincter* is composed of smooth muscle and is under involuntary control by the autonomic nervous system. Just above the internal sphincter is the *anorectal junction*, the dividing point of the anal canal and the rectum. The rectum is lined with folds of mucosa, known as the columns of Morgagni, which contain arteries, veins, and visceral nerves. The *rectum* is the lowest portion of the large intestine and is approximately 12 cm long, extending from the end of the *sigmoid colon* to the anorectal junction. It enlarges above the anorectal junction and proceeds in a posterior direction toward the hollow of the sacrum and coccyx, forming the rectal ampulla. The inside of the rectum contains three inward foldings called the valves of Houston. The *peritoneum* lines the upper two thirds of the anterior rectum and dips down so that it may be palpated where it forms the *rectouterine pouch* in women.

Nursing Assessment

COLLECTING SUBJECTIVE DATA

Focus Questions

Last menstrual period? Length of cycle? Amount of blood flow? Associated symptoms? Age of menarche? Unpleasant odor?

Knowledge about toxic shock syndrome? Age of menopause if applicable? Hormone replacement therapy? Vaginal discharge? Pain, itching, or lumps in inguinal/groin area? Pain with intercourse? Difficulty urinating? Color or odor of urine? Difficulty controlling urine? Stress incontinence? Sexual performance? Activity? Change in libido? Fertility problems/concerns? History of gynecologic problems or sexually transmitted infections (STIs)? Pregnancies? Number of children? Chance of pregnancy now? History of family reproductive or genital cancer? Self-care: Monthly genital self-examinations? Cotton underwear? Wiping pattern after bowel movement? Douching—how often? Use of contraceptives? Number of sexual partners? Comfort level with talking with sexual partner? Fears related to sex? Tested for HIV (human immunodeficiency virus)? Tested for HPV (human papillomavirus)? Last Pap test? Received HPV vaccine?

Bowel pattern? Constipation? Diarrhea? Character of stools? Rectal itching or pain? Hemorrhoids? Rectal surgery? Last stool test for blood detection? Proctosigmoidoscopy? Last digital rectal exam by a primary care provider? History of polyps, colon, or rectal cancer? Use of laxatives, engagement in anal

sex? Usual diet? Amount of fiber? Exercise? Use of calcium supplements? Anal or rectal problems that have affected activities of daily living?

Risk Factors

Risk for cervical cancer related to sexually active female, HPV infection, first and frequent intercourse at young age, multiple sexual partners, history of STI, multiple births, history of no prior Pap exams, lower socioeconomic status, low level of education, poor hygiene especially with uncircumcised partner.

COLLECTING OBJECTIVE DATA

Equipment Needed

Some of the following equipment is depicted in Figure 23-3.

- Stool
- Light
- Speculum
- Water-soluble lubricant
- Cotton-tipped applicators

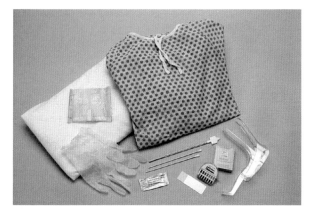

FIGURE 23-3 Some of the equipment needed for female genitalia examination.

- *Chlamydia* culture tube
- Culturette
- Test tube with water
- Sterile disposable gloves
- Ayre spatula (plastic)
- Endocervical cytobroom
- pH paper
- Feminine napkins
- Mirror

Physical Assessment

See Figures 23-1 and 23-2 for a review of the structures and the function of the female genitalia and anorectal structures. Maintain client privacy with a chaperone in the room. Wash hands, wear gloves, and make sure the equipment is between room and body temperature.

EXTERNAL GENITALIA

Ask the client to empty her bladder and lie on her back with head slightly elevated on a pillow. Knees should be bent and separated with feet resting on the bed. Adjust the light to provide good visualization of the genitalia.

ASSESSMENT PROCEDURE	NORMAL FINDINGS	ABNORMAL FINDINGS
Inspect **mons pubis**	Pubic hair is distributed in an inverted triangular pattern and there are no signs of infestation. (Amount and pattern of pubic hair varies with age and culture.)	Absence of public hair in the adult client is abnormal. Lice or nits (eggs) at the base of the public hairs indicate infestation with *pediculosis pubis*. This condition, commonly referred to as "crabs," is most often transmitted by sexual contact.
Inspect the **labia majora and perineum** for the following. • Lesions, swelling, excoriation	• Equal in size, free of lesions, swelling, and excoriation.	• Lesions seen in infectious disease; swelling and excoriation seen with scratching or self-treatment of the lesions (see Abnormal Findings 23-1, p. 533).
• Skin texture	• Smooth, loose skin	• Vesicles, warts, open sores
• Color	• Pink	• Blue, visible veins, shiny

ASSESSMENT PROCEDURE	**NORMAL FINDINGS**	**ABNORMAL FINDINGS**
Inspect the **labia minora, clitoris, urethral meatus, and vaginal opening** (Fig. 23-4). Using an examination glove, insert thumb and index or third finger between labia and separate. Inspect for lesions, excoriation, swelling, and discharge. 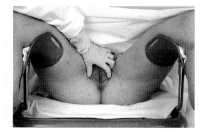 **FIGURE 23-4** Inspecting the labia minora, clitoris, urethral meatus, and vaginal opening.	The labia minora appear symmetric, dark pink, and moist. The clitoris is a small mound of erectile tissue, sensitive to touch. The normal size of the clitoris varies. The urethral meatus is small and slitlike. The vaginal opening is positioned below the urethral meatus. Its size depends on sexual activity or vaginal delivery. Clear, milky, serosanguineous discharge normal depending on the stage of menstrual cycle. A hymen may cover the vaginal opening partially or completely.	Asymmetric labia may indicate abscess. Lesions, swelling, and bulging in the vaginal opening are abnormal findings. Any purulent, irritating, foul-smelling discharge is abnormal and should be cultured. Excoriation may result from the client scratching or self-treating a perineal irritation. Urinary meatus not visible; located within or near the anterior surface of vaginal wall. Urinary meatus red, inflamed with perineal irritation.

Continued on following page

EXTERNAL GENITALIA (Continued)

ASSESSMENT PROCEDURE	NORMAL FINDINGS	ABNORMAL FINDINGS
Palpate the **posterior vaginal orifice** for the following.		
• Swelling	• None	• Present
• Lumps or nodules	• Smooth, soft tissue	• Hard, nonpliable tissue
Palpate **Bartholin glands.** If the client has labial swelling or a history of it, palpate Bartholin glands for swelling, tenderness, and discharge (Fig. 23-5). Place your index finger in the vaginal opening and your thumb on the labia majora. With a gentle pinching motion, palpate from the inferior portion of the posterior labia majora to the anterior portion. Repeat on the opposite side.	Bartholin glands are usually soft, nontender, and drainage-free.	Swelling, pain, and discharge may result from infection and abscess. If you detect a discharge, obtain a specimen to send to the laboratory for culture.

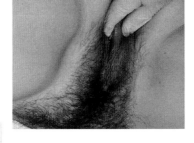

FIGURE 23-5 Technique for palpating Bartholin gland.

ASSESSMENT PROCEDURE	NORMAL FINDINGS	ABNORMAL FINDINGS
Palpate the **urethra**. If the client reports urethral symptoms or urethritis, or if you suspect inflammation of Skene glands, insert your gloved index finger into the superior portion of the vagina and milk the urethra from the inside, pushing up and out.	No drainage should be noted from the urethral meatus. The area is normally soft and nontender.	Drainage from the urethra indicates possible urethritis. Any discharge should be cultured. Urethritis may occur with infection with *Neisseria gonorrhoeae* or *Chlamydia trachomatis*.
Have the client strain down, and observe the **vaginal wall** for bulging.	Slight movement	Bulging of anterior wall may be a cystocele; bulging of posterior vaginal wall may indicate a rectocele; if cervix or uterus protrudes down, the client may have a uterine prolapse; if urine is produced, stress incontinence may be present (see Abnormal Findings 23-1, p. 533).

INTERNAL GENITALIA

ASSESSMENT PROCEDURE	NORMAL FINDINGS	ABNORMAL FINDINGS
Assess the **internal genitalia** • Determine the size of vaginal opening.	• Size varies with age, sexual history, vaginal deliveries	

Continued on following page

INTERNAL GENITALIA (Continued)

ASSESSMENT PROCEDURE	NORMAL FINDINGS	ABNORMAL FINDINGS
• Determine the position of cervix. Insert gloved index finger into the vagina.	• Anterior or posterior • Midline • Extends into the vagina 1–3 cm	
• With index finger in vagina, ask the client to squeeze around the finger to check vaginal musculature.	• Able to squeeze finger	• Inability to squeeze finger indicates decreased muscle tone.
• Separate the labia minora and ask the client to bear down.	No bulging No urinary discharge	Bulging of anterior wall may indicate cystocele. Bulging of posterior wall may indicate rectocele. If urine leaks out, the client may have stress incontinence.
Inspect the **cervix.** With the speculum inserted in position to visualize the cervix (Fig. 23-6), observe the following: • Cervix for color, size, position	• Surface of cervix smooth, pink, even • Pregnant clients bluish • Older women pale	• Asymmetric, reddened area, strawberry spots, white patches
• Cervical secretions	• Clear to opaque • Odorless • Nonirritating	• Discolored (gray, yellow, green) • Malodorous • Irritating

ASSESSMENT PROCEDURE	NORMAL FINDINGS	ABNORMAL FINDINGS

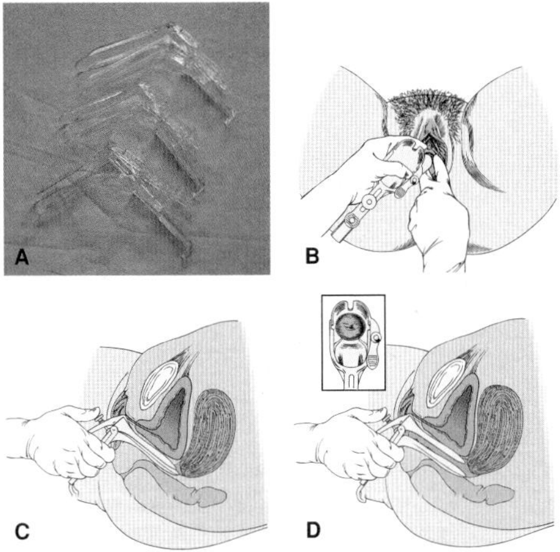

FIGURE 23-6 Speculum insertion for inspection of cervix. **A:** Select proper size speculum. **B:** Use right and middle Index finger to push the introitus down and open to relax muscle, while inserting the speculum blades downward at a 45 degree angle. **C:** Withdraw fingers once the blades pass fingers and switch to holding speculum with right hand. **D:** After the blades are fully inserted, open them by squeezing the handles together to view the full cervix.

Continued on following page

INTERNAL GENITALIA (Continued)

ASSESSMENT PROCEDURE	NORMAL FINDINGS	ABNORMAL FINDINGS
Inspect the **vagina.** Unlock the speculum and slowly rotate and remove it. Inspect the vagina as you remove the speculum. Inspect the vagina for color, surface, consistency, discharge, vaginal pH of secretions, using cotton swab on lateral or anterior (not posterior) vaginal wall. Touch swab to pH paper strip to test secretions.	• Pink, moist, smooth without lesions, irritations, or malodorous discharge • pH: 3.8–4.2	• Reddened area • Lesions • Malodorous discharge • <3.8 • >4.2–6: consider bacterial vaginosis, sexual intercourse (pH of semen ↑). • >6: consider trichomoniasis.
• Obtain Tissue Specimens for analysis. See Assessment Guide 23-1, p. 531.		
• Cervical os	• Small, round if nulliparous • Horizontal slit if parous	• Lesions • Erosions

BIMANUAL EXAMINATION

Tell the client you are going to perform a manual examination. Apply water-soluble lubricant to gloved middle and index fingers of your dominant hand. Stand and place your nondominant hand on the client's lower abdomen. Next insert index and middle fingers into the vagina.

ASSESSMENT PROCEDURE	NORMAL FINDINGS	ABNORMAL FINDINGS
Apply pressure to the posterior vaginal wall; wait for relaxation of vaginal opening before palpating (Fig. 23-7).	Vaginal wall is smooth without tenderness.	Tenderness may indicate infection.

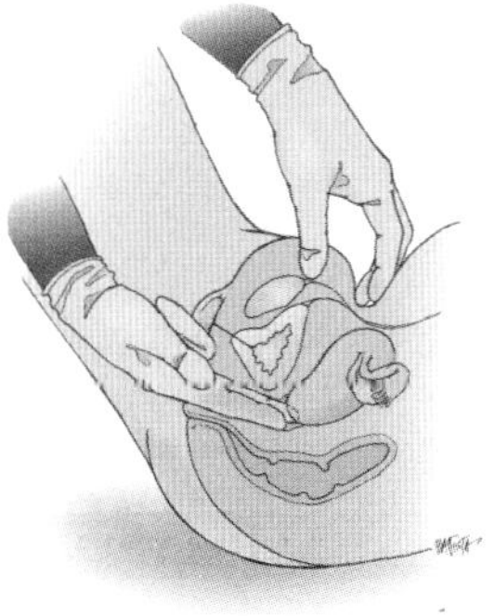

FIGURE 23-7 Palpating the vaginal walls.

Continued on following page

BIMANUAL EXAMINATION (Continued)

ASSESSMENT PROCEDURE	NORMAL FINDINGS	ABNORMAL FINDINGS
Palpate the cervix.		
Advance the fingers to the cervix; palpate for the following:	• Feels firm and soft like the tip of the nose	• Hardness and immobility may indicate cancer.
• Contour		• Pain with movement (and chandelier sign) may indicate infection.
• Consistency		
• Mobility		
• Tenderness		
Palpate the uterus.		
Move the fingers intravaginally into the opening above the cervix. Apply pressure with the hand resting on the abdomen. Squeeze the uterus between the two hands (Fig. 23-8).		• An enlarged uterus above the level of the pubis is abnormal.
		• Irregular shape may indicate abnormality.

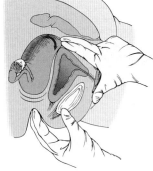

FIGURE 23-8 Palpating the uterus.

ASSESSMENT PROCEDURE	NORMAL FINDINGS	ABNORMAL FINDINGS
Note uterine: • Size • Position • Shape • Consistency		
Palpate the **ovaries**.		
Slide your intravaginal fingers toward the left ovary in the left lateral fornix and place your abdominal hand on the left lower abdominal quadrant. Press your abdominal hand toward your intravaginal fingers and attempt to palpate the ovary (Fig. 23-9).	Ovaries are approximately $3 \times 2 \times 1$ cm (or the size of a walnut) and almond-shaped.	Enlarged size, masses, immobility, and extreme tenderness are abnormal and should be evaluated.
Slide your intravaginal fingers to the right lateral fornix and attempt to palpate the right ovary. Note size, shape, consistency, mobility, and tenderness.	Ovaries are firm, smooth, mobile, and somewhat tender on palpation.	Ovaries that are palpable 3–5 years after menopause are also abnormal.

Continued on following page

BIMANUAL EXAMINATION (Continued)

ASSESSMENT PROCEDURE	NORMAL FINDINGS	ABNORMAL FINDINGS

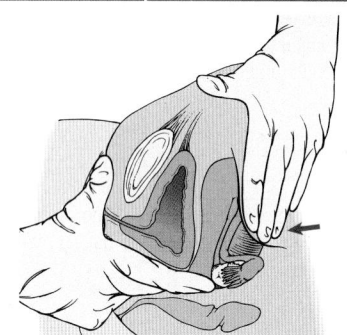

FIGURE 23-9 Palpating the ovaries.

Withdraw your intravaginal hand and inspect the glove for secretions.	A clear, minimal amount of drainage appearing on the glove from the vagina is normal.	Large amounts of colorful, frothy, or malodorous secretions are abnormal.
Perform the **rectovaginal examination**.		

ASSESSMENT PROCEDURE	NORMAL FINDINGS	ABNORMAL FINDINGS
Explain that you will perform a rectovaginal examination. Forewarn the client that she may feel uncomfortable as if she wants to move her bowels, but that she will not. Encourage her to relax. Change the glove on your dominant hand and lubricate your index and middle fingers (Fig. 23-10).	• The rectovaginal septum is normally smooth, thin, movable, and firm. The posterior uterine wall is normally smooth, firm, round, movable, and nontender.	• Masses, thickened structures, immobility, and tenderness are abnormal.

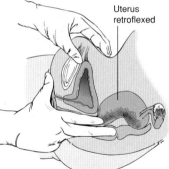

FIGURE 23-10 Hands positioned for rectovaginal examination.

Continued on following page

BIMANUAL EXAMINATION (Continued)

ASSESSMENT PROCEDURE	NORMAL FINDINGS	ABNORMAL FINDINGS
Ask the client to bear down and insert your index finger into the vaginal orifice and your middle finger into the rectum. While pushing down on the abdominal wall with your other hand, palpate the internal reproductive structures through the anterior rectal wall. Withdraw your vaginal finger and continue with the rectal examination.		

ANUS AND RECTUM

The most frequently used position for examining the anus and rectum is the left lateral position, which allows adequate inspection and palpation of the anus, rectum, and prostate client comfort. Drape the client's torso and legs. Ask the client to lie on the left side, with the buttocks as close to the edge of the examining table as possible, and to bend the right knee. Support the leg on a pillow if needed and provide a pillow for the head. Another method is to perform the anus and rectum exam while the client stands and bends over the examining table with her hips flexed. Use the position best for the particular client and promotion of comfort (see Fig. 22-7 on p. 496 in Chapter 22). The rectum will be able to be examined only to a certain point with the examiner's finger. If an exam of the upper rectum and sigmoid colon is necessary, refer the client for a sigmoidoscopy.

ASSESSMENT PROCEDURE	NORMAL FINDINGS	ABNORMAL FINDINGS
Inspect the **perianal area**. Spread the client's buttocks and inspect the anal opening and surrounding area for the following: • Lumps • Ulcers • Lesions • Rashes • Redness • Fissures • Thickening of the epithelium	Anal opening is hairless, moist, and tightly closed. The surrounding perianal area is free of redness, lumps, ulcers, lesions, or rashes.	Lesions may indicate sexually transmitted diseases, cancer, or hemorrhoids. A thrombosed external hemorrhoid appears swollen. It is itchy, painful, and bleeds when the client passes stool. A previously thrombosed hemorrhoid appears as a skin tag that protrudes from the anus.
Ask the client to perform Valsalva maneuver by straining or bearing down. Inspect the anal opening for any bulges or lesions.	No bulging or lesions appear.	Bulges of red mucous membrane may indicate a rectal prolapse. Hemorrhoids or an anal fissure may also be seen.
Inspect the **sacrococcygeal area** for color, hair, and texture.	Smooth, free of hair, and redness	Red, swollen area covered by a small tuft of hair located in the lower sacrum suggests the presence of a pilonidal cyst.

Continued on following page

ANUS AND RECTUM (Continued)

ASSESSMENT PROCEDURE	NORMAL FINDINGS	ABNORMAL FINDINGS
Palpate the **anus.** Explain to the client what you are going to do. Explain that the client may feel like her bowels will move. With one hand, gently separate the buttocks so the rectum is exposed. Lubricate gloved index finger and ask the client to bear down. Then place the pad of your index finger on the anal opening.	Sphincter relaxes.	Sphincter tightens, preventing further examination.
Assess **sphincter tone.**	Can close sphincter around gloved finger	Poor tone may be a result of spinal cord injury, previous surgery, trauma, prolapsed rectum, sexual abuse. Tightened sphincter may be the result of anxiety, scarring, inflammation.
Palpate for **tenderness, nodules, and hardness.**	Normally smooth, nontender, without nodules or hardness	Tenderness indicates hemorrhoids, fistula, fissure; nodules indicate polyps, cancer; hardness indicates scarring, cancer.

ASSESSMENT PROCEDURE	NORMAL FINDINGS	ABNORMAL FINDINGS
Palpate the **rectum**. Insert finger farther into the rectum. Turn finger clockwise, then counterclockwise. Note tenderness irregularities, nodules, and hardness.	The rectal mucosa is normally soft, smooth, nontender, and free of nodules.	Hardness and irregularities may be from scarring or cancer. Nodules may indicate polyps or cancer.
Inspect the **stool**. Withdraw your gloved finger. Inspect any fecal matter on your glove. Assess the color and test the feces for occult blood. Provide the client with a towel to wipe the anorectal area.	Stool is normally semisolid, brown, and free of blood.	Black stool seen in upper gastrointestinal bleeding, gray or tan stool results from the lack of bile pigment, yellow stool suggests steatorrhea (increased fat content). Blood in stool may indicate cancer of the rectum or colon. An endoscopic examination of the colon should be performed if blood is detected.

ASSESSMENT GUIDE 23-1 Obtaining Tissue Specimens for Analysis

Some methods for obtaining female tissue specimens follow.

Papanicolaou (Pap) Smear
Liquid-based technology has improved the accuracy of findings to test for human papillomavirus (HPV) and determine the HPV type. The specimen for the Pap smear is obtained using a wooden spatula,

cotton swab, or brush and placed in the preservative solution slide (Lab Tests Online, 2012).

Obtaining an Ectocervical and Endocervical Specimen
This procedure is performed on nonpregnant clients. This combined procedure uses a special cytobroom to collect *both* endocervical and

Continued on following page

ASSESSMENT GUIDE 23-1 Obtaining Tissue Specimens for Analysis (Continued)

ectocervical cells. 1. Insert cytobroom into the cervical os rotating cytobroom in a full circle five times, collecting cells from squamoco-lumnar junction and cervical surface. 2. Withdraw cytobroom. 3. Swish cytobroom in the preservative solution by pushing cytobroom into the bottom of the vial 10 times, forcing the bristles apart. Swirl cytobroom vigorously to further release material. 4. Discard the cytobroom. 5. Tighten cap on preservative and send to laboratory.

Obtaining an Ectocervical Specimen
1. Insert one end of plastic spatula into the cervical os. 2. Press down rotating spatula, scraping cervix and transformation zone (squamoco-lumnar junction) in a full circle. 3. Withdraw spatula. 4. Rinse spatula in preservative solution by swishing spatula vigorously in vial 10 times. 5. Discard spatula.

Obtaining an Endocervical Specimen
1. Insert endocervical brush into cervical os rotating brush one half turn in one direction gently to minimize possible bleeding. 2. With-draw brush. 3. Rinse brush in preservative solution by rotating device in solution 10 times while pushing against vial wall. Swirl brush vigorously to further release material. 4. Discard brush. 5. Tighten

cap on solution. 6. Record client's name and date on vial to send to laboratory.

Vaginal Specimen
1. Select appropriate-sized warmed speculum testing on patient's leg for comfortable temperature.
2. Insert speculum at 45-degree angle, rotate, and open when com-pletely inserted.
3. Obtain a specimen of vaginal fluid from the posterior fornix.
4. On a glass slide, place a drop of sodium chloride (NaCl) and a drop of potassium hydroxide (KOH) on separate ends of the slide.
5. Mix small amount of vaginal fluid with each solution and apply coverslip (APGO, 2008).

Culture Specimens: Gonorrhea and Chlamydia
Specimens for gonorrhea or *Chlamydia* cultures are obtained if you suspect the client has these sexually transmitted diseases. The exact procedures for gathering and preparing the specimens vary according to each laboratory's policy.
    http://www.cdc.gov/vaccines/vpd-vac/hpv/vac-faqs.htm

| ABNORMAL FINDINGS | 23-1 | Abnormalities of the External Genitalia and Vaginal Opening |

When assessing the female genitalia, the nurse will see various abnormal lesions on the external genitalia as well as abnormal bulging in the vaginal opening. Some common findings appear below.

SYPHILITIC CHANCRE

Syphilitic chancres often first appear on the perianal area as silvery white papules that become superficial red ulcers. Syphilitic chancres are painless. They are sexually transmitted and usually develop at the site of initial contact with the infecting organism.

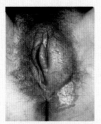

Chancre typical of syphilis. (Courtesy of Upjohn Co.)

GENITAL WARTS

Genital warts, caused by the human papillomavirus (HPV), are moist, fleshy lesions on the labia and within the vestibule. They are painless and believed to be sexually transmitted.

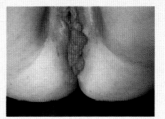

Genital warts. (Courtesy Reed & Carnrick Pharmaceuticals.)

Continued on following page

ABNORMAL FINDINGS   23-1   Abnormalities of the External Genitalia and Vaginal Opening (Continued)

GENITAL HERPES SIMPLEX

The initial outbreak of herpes may have many small, painful ulcers with erythematous base. Recurrent herpes lesions are usually not as extensive.

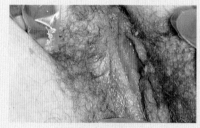

Small, painful, red-based, ulcer-like lesions of herpes simplex virus, type 2. (© 1992. Science Photo Library/CMSP.)

CYSTOCELE

A cystocele is a bulging in the anterior vaginal wall caused by thickening of the pelvic musculature. As a result, the bladder, covered by vaginal mucosa, prolapses into the vagina.

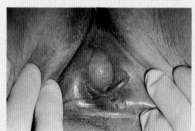

Cystocele. (© 1995. Science Photo Library/CMSP.)

ABNORMAL FINDINGS 23-1 Abnormalities of the External Genitalia and Vaginal Opening (Continued)

RECTOCELE

A rectocele is a bulging in the posterior vaginal wall caused by weakening of the pelvic musculature. Part of the rectum covered by the vaginal mucosa protrudes into the vagina.

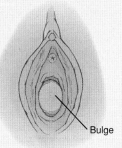

Rectocele.

UTERINE PROLAPSE

Uterine prolapse occurs when the uterus protrudes into the vagina. It is graded according to how far it protrudes into the vagina. In first-degree prolapse, the cervix is seen at the vaginal opening; in second-degree prolapse, the uterus bulges outside of vaginal openings; in third-degree prolapse, the uterus bulges completely out of the vagina.

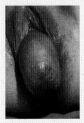

Prolapsed uterus. (© 1991, Michael English, MD/CMSP.)

Hamilton, B., & Ventura, S. (2012). Birth rates for U.S. teenagers reach historic lows for all ages and ethnic groups. NCHS Data Brief, no. 89. Available at http://www.cdc.gov/nchs/data/databriefs/db89.pdf.

PEDIATRIC VARIATIONS

Focus Questions

During puberty: Development of secondary sexual characteristics? Previous education on sexual development and activities? Use of contraceptives? Type? Age of menarche? Frequency of menstrual periods? Amount of flow? Pain? Irregularities? Attitude toward menstrual cycle?

Physical Assessment

Inspection and palpation of external genitalia constitute the *total* genitourinary assessment until puberty. Assessment of the level of sexual development usually begins at approximately age 11 years. This determination involves the assessment of secondary characteristics associated with sexual maturity. Table 23-1 summarizes the timing of sexual development for girls.

GERIATRIC VARIATIONS

• Due to decreased natural vaginal lubrication, make sure that instruments are well lubricated. If there is vaginal stenosis, only one gloved finger may be needed for the bimanual examination. If the older person has arthritis, a mild analgesic or anti-inflammatory medicine may be taken to ease comfort for exam positioning.

• Bladder capacity decreases to 250 mL owing to periurethral atrophy.

• Pubic hair becomes thin and sparse.

• Mons pubis is smaller with flatter labia due to thinner skin and decreased fat deposits.

• Clitoris decreases in size.

• Estrogen production decreases, causing atrophy of the vaginal mucosa.

• Decrease in size and elasticity of labia; constriction of vaginal opening.

• Diminished vaginal secretions and decreased elasticity of vaginal walls.

• Shortened and narrowed vaginal vault.

• Vaginal walls and cervix pale pink that shrinks in size.

• Uterus is smaller and firmer.

• Nonpalpable ovaries.

• It is recommended to discontinue screening for cervical cancer, or offering the option for patients to discontinue screening, after age 65 or 70, provided there is documented evidence of adequate past screening with normal Pap smears and are not otherwise at high risk for cervical cancer (ACS, 2012/2013; USPSTF, 2012a).

TABLE 23-1 Tanner's Sexual Maturity Rating: Female Pubic Hair Growth and Breast Development

Developmental Stage	Pubic Hair	Breast
Stage 1	Prepubertal: no pubic hair; fine vellus hair	Prepubertal: elevation of nipple only
Stage 2	Sparse, long, straight, downy hair	Breast bud stage; elevation of breast and nipple as small mound, enlargement of areolar diameter

Continued on following page

TABLE 23-1 Tanner's Sexual Maturity Rating: Female Pubic Hair Growth and Breast Development (Continued)

Developmental Stage	Pubic Hair	Breast
Stage 3 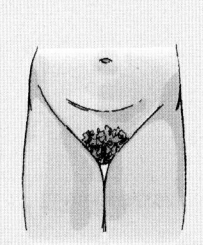	Darker, coarser, curly; sparse over mons pubis	Enlargement of the breasts and areola with no separation of contours 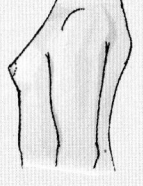
Stage 4	Dark, curly, and abundant on mons pubis; no growth on medial thighs	Projection of areola and nipple to form secondary mound above level of breast 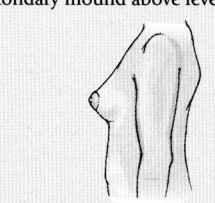

TABLE 23-1 Tanner's Sexual Maturity Rating: Female Pubic Hair Growth and Breast Development (Continued)

Developmental Stage	Pubic Hair	Breast
Stage 5	Adult pattern of inverse triangle; growth on medial thighs	Adult configuration; projection of nipple only, areola receded into contour of breast

CULTURAL VARIATIONS

Female genitalia are mutilated in pubertal rites in some cultures. Examples involve removal of the clitoris, removal of part of the inner or outer labia, and/or stitching together of the labia with only a small opening for urination and menstrual flow. In some cultures, women shave or pluck their pubic hair.

POSSIBLE COLLABORATIVE PROBLEMS—RISK OF

Bladder perforation
Urinary tract infection
Pelvic inflammatory disease
Genitalia ulcers or lesions
Obstruction of urethra
Hemorrhage

Hormonal imbalances
Renal failure
Renal calculi
Hypermenorrhea
Polymenorrhea

Teaching Tips for Selected Nursing Diagnoses and Collaborative Problems

Nursing Diagnosis: Readiness for Enhanced Urinary Elimination and Reproductive Pattern

Teach client to drink eight glasses of fluid per day and to limit intake of alcohol, caffeine, and carbonated beverages. Teach client to avoid bubble baths and scented tissue that may irritate urethra. Teach female client to wear cotton underwear and to wipe perineum from front to back when cleansing.

Nursing Diagnosis: Risk for Infection (STD) related to unprotected intercourse with multiple partners

Teach early warning signs and symptoms. Discuss methods of prevention (limit to one uninfected partner and use of condoms) and modes of transmission. Routine screening for infection is recommended during pelvic exam 3 years after onset of sexual activity for sexually active women less than 21, and annually for those 21 and older (but for those 30 to 64 with 3 years of normal results, screening can be reduced to every 2 to 3 years) (ACOG, 2013).

Nursing Diagnosis: Ineffective Health Maintenance related to a lack of knowledge of birth control methods

Teach alternate forms of birth control, proper use of methods, and advantages and disadvantages of each. Discuss the importance of increasing vitamin B_6 and folic acid in the diet because of malabsorption of these vitamins while taking birth control pills. Instruct on use of alternate birth control for 3 months after discontinuing the pill to re-establish menstrual cycle before attempting to conceive.

Nursing Diagnosis: Readiness for Enhanced Health Maintenance during Menopause

Inform client that pregnancy may still occur during early menopausal years. Instruct to consume calcium 1,200 mg/day along with a well-balanced diet (NIH, 2011a). Explain that water-soluble lubricant may be used for vaginal dryness if intercourse is painful. Explain ways to help client cope with hot flashes (e.g., use of cool clothing, fans, showers, cool drinks; avoidance of red wine, aged cheeses, and chocolate—these contain tyramine, which can trigger hot flashes). .

***Nursing Diagnosis: Ineffective Health Maintenance** related to knowledge deficit of need for pelvic examinations, Pap smears, and colorectal screening*

Explain procedure. Teach relaxation. Approach sexuality as a normal part of activities of daily living. Prepare adolescent girl for first pelvic examination. ACOG (2010a) recommends that women who have been sexually active for 3 years or are 21 years old should have a Pap test with cytology every year. For a woman 30 years or older who has had three or more consecutive satisfactory and normal annual examinations, the Pap test may be performed every 2 to 3 years at the physician's discretion. Most women 70 years and older who have had three or more consecutive normal Pap tests and most who have had total hysterectomies do not need continued screening, unless their mothers received DES while pregnant with them. Women at high risk for endometrial cancer (major risk factors—weak immune system, estrogen replacement therapy, tamoxifen, early menarche, late menopause, never having children, and history of failure to ovulate; other risk factors—infertility, diabetes, gallbladder disease, hypertension, and obesity) should have an endometrial tissue sample at menopause and thereafter at the physician's discretion (ACS, 2012/2013). For colorectal cancer and polyps beginning at age 50, one of the following should be done to screen for polyps or cancer: Flexible sigmoidoscopy every 5 years, or Colonoscopy every 10 years, or Double-contrast barium enema every 5 years, or CT colonography (virtual colonoscopy) every 5 years. If the test is positive, a colonoscopy should be done (ACS, 2012/2013).

***Nursing Diagnosis:** Readiness for enhanced bowel elimination pattern related to lack of exercise regimen, poor dietary habits*

Teach the importance of balanced diet high in fiber, regular exercise pattern, and adequate water/fluid intake.

***Nursing Diagnosis: Sexual Dysfunction** related to partner communication and deficient knowledge of psychological and physical health and sexual performance*

Teach effects and benefits of exercise. Explore communication with partner. Refer to counselor (psychiatric, sexual, marriage) as needed. Provide adequate literature on sex and health teaching for client.

Nursing Diagnosis: Sexual Dysfunction related to loss of body part or physiologic limitations (e.g., dyspareunia with aging)

Explore prior sexual patterns. Explore alternatives. Provide resource material on self-help groups (e.g., Ostomy Association, Reach for Recovery). Suggest use of foreplay and lubricants to increase secretions as necessary. Provide literature and referrals.

Nursing Diagnosis: Risk for Impaired Elimination Pattern related to parental knowledge deficit of toilet-training techniques

Teach parents the importance of physiologic and psychological readiness in toilet-training. Explain the use of "potty chairs" and that bowel control precedes bladder control. Inform parents of the benefits of positive reinforcement and that nocturnal enuresis may persist up to age 4 to 5 years.

Nursing Diagnosis: Readiness for Enhanced Sexual Function

Sexual education is recommended in the early school years. Assess what child already knows and what he or she is ready to know.

Fourth to fifth grade: Interested in conception and birth.

Fifth to sixth grade: Interested in their bodies and opposite sex changes. Education on birth control may be appropriate because of early experimentation. Discuss normal development of secondary sexual characteristics and the normal psychological changes associated with puberty. The CDC now recommends administering the HPV vaccine at 11 to 12 years of age for boys and girls to prevent the human papillomavirus. It is a three-dose series. The first dose is given, with the second and the third dose administered 2 and 6 months following the first dose. The vaccine may be administered between the ages of 9 and 26 (CDC, 2012).

Adolescent: Teach the importance of abstinence or use of condoms and/or methods of birth control if sexually active. Explain that there are an estimated 19 million new cases of STDs reported yearly and 50,000 new HIV infections yearly in the United States, of which one half of all new STDs including HIV infections are in people less than age 25 and most are infected through sexual behavior (CDC, 2013b, 2013d).

The teenage birth rate in the United States was 34.4 births per 1,000 women 15 to 19 years of age in 2010 (CDC, 2012e). Advise that teens who are pregnant are at greater risk for complications during pregnancy and after delivery. Some of these complications include elevated blood pressure, sexually transmitted infections, preterm labor, premature birth, low birth weight, delivery complications, postpartum depression, and feelings of loneliness and isolation.

 Nursing Diagnosis: *Impaired Urinary Elimination: functional incontinence, reflex urinary incontinence, stress incontinence*

Explain to family how to decrease environmental barriers (offer bedpan frequently, provide proper lighting, ensure availability and proximity of commode) for functional incontinence. Teach client cutaneous triggering mechanisms for reflex incontinence. Teach client Kegel exercises to strengthen pelvic floor muscles (i.e., tightening of buttocks and practicing starting and stopping stream) for stress incontinence.

Assessing Childbearing Women

The body experiences many anatomic/physiologic changes during pregnancy. Findings in a physical assessment that would be considered abnormal in the nonpregnant client may be a result of pregnancy and not an abnormal state. In this chapter, the physical changes that occur in a woman as a result of pregnancy are identified as *normal variations.* Changes that are not a result of pregnancy or that represent an abnormal state during pregnancy are identified as *devia-*

tions from normal. Fetal assessment will also be discussed, noting normal variations along with deviations from normal for the fetus.

For the sake of brevity, those systems described previously will not be repeated. Only variations of pregnancy will be noted. For procedures, the reader is referred to sections describing assessment of specific body systems. Assessment of the newborn is covered in Chapter 25.

Prenatal Maternal and Fetal Assessment

This chapter is divided into three sections: Prenatal Maternal and Fetal Assessment, Intrapartum Maternal and Fetal Assessment, and Postpartum Maternal Assessment.

During pregnancy, physical assessment should be performed every month for the first 27 weeks, every 2 weeks from week 28 to week 36, and then every week. More frequent examinations may be indicated for pregnancies at risk.

COLLECTING SUBJECTIVE DATA

Ask the following *focus questions.*

Past pregnancies: Age in years of pregnancy? Outcome of each pregnancy? Number of living children? Complications? Length of labor? Type of delivery? Years since last pregnancy? Current pregnancy: First day of LMP? Estimated due date? Confirmed by ultrasound? Problems during pregnancy? Nausea? Vomiting? Cramping or bleeding? Planned pregnancy? Date of first prenatal visit? Prenatal education? Concurrent medical conditions? Current medications? Date of initial fetal movement? Has the fetus has been active?

COLLECTING OBJECTIVE DATA

Equipment Needed

See Chapters 9 to 22 for the equipment needed for the specific body system to be assessed for the maternal assessment. The following equipment are needed for the prenatal fetal assessment.

- Bed or examination table
- Drape
- Pillow
- Paper centimeter tape measure
- Fetoscope or Doppler

Physical Assessment

PRENATAL MATERNAL AND FETAL ASSESSMENT		
ASSESSMENT PROCEDURE	**NORMAL FINDINGS**	**ABNORMAL FINDINGS**
Assess the following: • Age	• Ideal childbearing years: 18–35	• Younger than 18 or older than 35; advanced maternal age increases risk of genetic abnormalities such as Down syndrome; increased risk of complications to mother and baby with age extremes.
• Maternal history	• Uncomplicated maternal/neonatal history. Determine gravida/para status (see Box 24-1, p. 556).	• Premature labor and/or delivery; pregnancy-induced hypertension; previous abortion or tubal pregnancy
• Weight	• Prenatal weight gain: Determine weight gain by the prepregnancy body mass index (BMI). Underweight women (BMI < 19.8): 12.7–18.1 kg (28–40 lb); women of normal weight (BMI 19.8–26): 11.3–15.9 kg (25–35 lb); overweight women (BMI > 26–29): 6.8–11.3 kg (15–25 lb); obese women (BMI > 29): 6.8 kg (15 lb) (Fig. 24-1).	• Prepregnant weight <45.4 or >90.7 kg (<100 or >200 lb); sudden gain of more than 0.91 kg (2 lb) per week may be seen in pregnancy-induced hypertension (PIH); weight loss or failure to gain weight.

Continued on following page

PRENATAL MATERNAL AND FETAL ASSESSMENT (Continued)

ASSESSMENT PROCEDURE	NORMAL FINDINGS	ABNORMAL FINDINGS

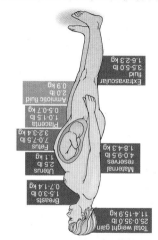

Total weight gain
25.0–35.0 lb
11.4–15.9 kg

Breasts
1.5–3.0 lb
0.7–1.4 kg

Uterus
2.5 lb
1.1 kg

Maternal
reserves
4.0–9.5 lb
1.8–4.3 kg

Fetus
7.0–7.5 lb
3.2–3.4 kg

Placenta
1.0–1.5 lb
0.5–0.7 kg

Amniotic fluid
2.0 lb
0.9 kg

Extravascular
fluid
3.5–5.0 lb
1.6–2.3 kg

FIGURE 24-1 Distribution of weight gain during pregnancy.

ASSESSMENT PROCEDURE	NORMAL FINDINGS	ABNORMAL FINDINGS
	First trimester: 0.91–1.81 kg (2–4 lb)	
	Second trimester: 4.99 kg (11 lb) (0.45 kg [1 lb] per week)	
	Third trimester: 4.99 kg (11 lb) (0.45 kg [1 lb] per week)	
• Blood pressure	• Range of 90–139/60–89 mm Hg; falls during second trimester, prepregnant level first and third trimesters.	• ≥140/90 mm Hg or increase of 30 mm Hg above baseline systolic or 15 mm Hg above baseline diastolic taken with client in side-lying position; increased levels are seen with PIH.
• Pulse	• 60–90 beats/minute; may increase 10–15 beats/minute higher than prepregnant levels	• Irregularities; persistently <60 or >100 beats/minute at rest
• Behavior	• *First trimester:* Tired, ambivalent. *Second trimester:* Introspective, energetic *Third trimester:* Restless, preparing for baby, labile moods (the father may experience some of these same behaviors).	• Denial of pregnancy, withdrawal, depression, psychosis

Continued on following page

PRENATAL MATERNAL AND FETAL ASSESSMENT (Continued)

ASSESSMENT PROCEDURE	NORMAL FINDINGS	ABNORMAL FINDINGS
Observe skin color	Linea nigra, striae gravidarum (see Fig. 24-2); chloasma (Fig. 24-3); spider nevi	Pale, yellowing changes of the skin as seen with liver diseases

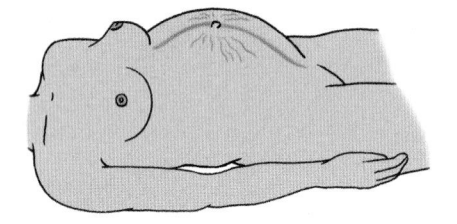

FIGURE 24-2 Pregnancy pigmentation: Abdominal midline (linea nigra) and striae gravidarum. Dark-haired, brown-skinned women are more prone to pregnancy pigmentation.

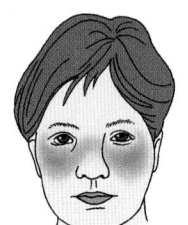

FIGURE 24-3 Marked chloasma of pregnancy.

Assess head and neck		Facial edema, headache
• Nose	• Nasal stuffiness, nosebleeds	• Ulceration of mucosa, yellow, green drainage.
• Eyes	No changes in exam or vision.	Blurred vision and visual spots are symptoms of PIH.
• Neck	• Slight enlargement of thyroid	• Nodules or marked enlargement, asymmetry of thyroid gland as seen with thyroid disease

ASSESSMENT PROCEDURE	NORMAL FINDINGS	ABNORMAL FINDINGS
Assess cardiovascular system • Heart	• Short systolic blowing murmurs	• Progressive dyspnea, palpitations, markedly decreased activity tolerance may be seen with cardiac diseases
• Blood volume	• Increases throughout pregnancy; peaks at 32–34 weeks, reaching 30–50% above prepregnancy levels	Monitor women with heart disease closely due to the high cardiac demands during pregnancy. Shortness of breath, chest pain, heart failure, etc.
Assess peripheral vascular system	Late pregnancy: Dependent edema, varicose veins, supine hypotension	Perineal varicosities; calf pain may be related to deep vein thrombosis; generalized edema; diminished pedal pulses
Assess respiratory system	Increased anteroposterior diameter, thoracic breathing, slight hyperventilation, shortness of breath in late pregnancy especially with activity/walking	Dyspnea may be seen in patients with cardiac disease and/or lung diseases such as asthma
Assess breasts	Increased size and nodularity, tenderness, prominent vascularization, darkening of nipples and areola, colostrum in third trimester (Fig. 24-4)	Localized redness; localized pain and warmth; erythemic streaks are commonly seen with mastitis; inverted nipples may cause difficulty for breastfeeding infants

Continued on following page

PRENATAL MATERNAL AND FETAL ASSESSMENT (Continued)

ASSESSMENT PROCEDURE	NORMAL FINDINGS	ABNORMAL FINDINGS

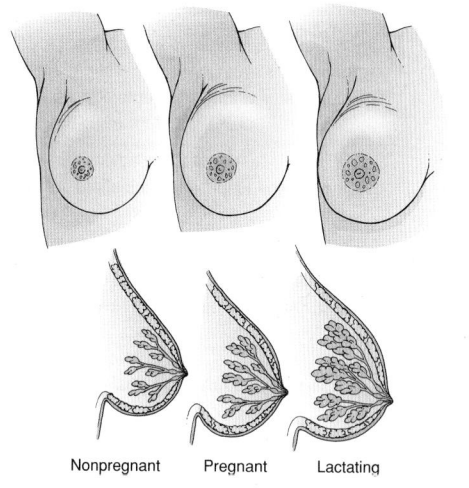

Nonpregnant   Pregnant   Lactating

FIGURE 24-4 Breast changes during pregnancy.

ASSESSMENT PROCEDURE	NORMAL FINDINGS	ABNORMAL FINDINGS
Assess gastrointestinal system	Nausea and vomiting, increased saliva, heartburn, bloating, constipation	Severe epigastric pain is seen with PIH; severe nausea and vomiting may be seen during the first trimester with hyperemesis gravidarum
Assess genitourinary–reproductive systems	Urinary frequency in first and third trimesters, increased pigmentation of vulva and vagina, increased vaginal discharge	Flank pain, dysuria, oliguria, proteinuria, purulent vaginal discharge, vaginal bleeding
Assess musculoskeletal system	Relaxation of pelvic joints: "Waddling" gait; increased lumbar curve, backache, diastasis recti, leg cramps	Generalized weakness, back pain, difficulty walking, joint pain
Assess neurologic system	Cranial nerves II–XII intact	Hyperactive reflexes, positive clonus seen with PIH
Assess prenatal labs/immunizations	Lab work within normal limits; recent influenza immunization for women who are pregnant during influenza season	Hepatitis positive, rubella nonimmune, HIV positive, anemia, positive drug screen, positive testing for sexually transmitted infections, gestational diabetes, positive antibody screen for Rh-negative antibody screen

Continued on following page

PRENATAL MATERNAL AND FETAL ASSESSMENT (Continued)

ASSESSMENT PROCEDURE	NORMAL FINDINGS	ABNORMAL FINDINGS
Palpate and measure the uterine fundal height. Using both hands, gently palpate the outline of the fetus and the top of the uterus (fundus). Using the centimeter tape, measure from the top of the symphysis pubis to the top of the uterine fundus (Fig. 24-5). Take fundal height measurement and multiply by 8/7 (this equals weeks of gestation; McDonald's rule: Fundal height (cm) × 8/7 = gestation of pregnancy in weeks). **Auscultate fetal heart rate (FHR).** With Doppler or fetoscope, listen for fetal heartbeat. Locate fundus; begin listening halfway between the fundus and the pubis. Work outward in widening circles until a beating sound is heard. Compare with the maternal pulse. If different, count fetal heart rate for 1 full minute.	Accurate within 2 weeks until 36 weeks (Fig. 24-6). Obesity or extremes in height may alter findings. Fundal height measures greater than dates with multiple gestations (twins, triplets, etc.)	Lag in progression may indicate problems with fetal development and/or oligohydramnios commonly seen with congenital abnormalities. Sudden increase in fundal height size may also indicate fetal abnormalities.

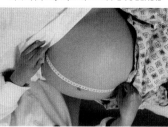

FIGURE 24-5 Measuring the fundal height.

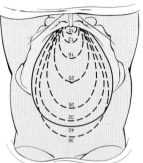

FIGURE 24-6 Approximate height of fundus at various weeks of gestation.

ASSESSMENT PROCEDURE	NORMAL FINDINGS	ABNORMAL FINDINGS
Assess for the following: • Presence	• Audible at 10–12 weeks' gestation with fetal Doppler; audible at 15–20 weeks' gestation with fetoscope	• Absence of fetal heart tones after the 20th week of gestation indicates intrauterine fetal demise
• Rate	• Very rapid initially; gradually slows to 120–160 beats/minute at term; increased rate with fetal movement; during fetal sleep cycle, FHR may be in the 110–120 range	• <120 beats/minute with activity and not in sleep cycle; no change or decrease in FHR with movement may indicate fetal distress
• Rhythm	• Regular	• A marked variance or variance of <5 beats/minute may indicate fetal distress
Inspect abdomen for shape and contour of the fetus. With the client supine and head slightly elevated on a pillow, inspect abdomen for shape and contour of the fetus. *Note: During the second and third trimesters, time spent in the supine position should be minimal. This position puts the weight of the fetus and uterus on the aorta and obstructs blood flow.*	*First trimester:* Unable to palpate fetal parts. *Second trimester:* Early trimester may be difficult to palpate body parts. *Third trimester:* Lower abdomen/distal—palpate to identify fetal head (feels firm with palpation), buttocks (feels soft with palpation). Palpate lateral sides of abdomen—fetal back (palpates as smooth, no bony prominences palpated), fetal parts (arms, fists, legs, feet may be palpated as small, firm bony prominences).	Abdomen: (distal) Should palpate as firm, bony prominence, fetal head, vertex presentation. Palpation of soft prominence, high probability of breech presentation.

CULTURAL VARIATIONS

- Rh-negative blood is rare in nonwhite groups.
- Dizygotic twinning is higher in blacks than whites or Asians.

BOX 24-1   GRAVIDA/PARA STATUS

Determine patient's gravida/para status.

- **Gravida:** Total number of pregnancies.
- **Para:** Number of pregnancies that have delivered at 20 weeks' gestation or greater.
- **Term gestation:** Delivery of pregnancy 38–42 weeks.
- **Preterm gestation:** Delivery of pregnancy after 20 weeks and before the start of 38 weeks' gestation.
- **Abortion:** Termination of pregnancy (miscarriage) prior to the 20th week of gestation.
- **Living:** Number of living children.

Example:

G # P T Pt Ab L

G 4 P 2 1 1 3

This represents a patient who has been pregnant four times: two term deliveries, one preterm delivery, one miscarriage, and three children living.

POSSIBLE COLLABORATIVE PROBLEMS—RISK OF

- Bleeding disorder of pregnancy
- Hyperemesis gravidarum
- Spontaneous abortion
- Ectopic pregnancy
- Placenta previa
- Abruptio placentae
- Pregnancy-induced hypertension
- Gestational diabetes
- Pre-existing medical conditions
- Hyperglycemia/hypoglycemia
- Hypertension
- Dehydration
- Renal disease
- Cardiac conditions

Teaching Tips for Selected Nursing Diagnoses

Nursing Diagnosis: Risk for Ineffective Therapeutic Regimen Management during pregnancy

Inform client of normal variations during the prenatal period. Also inform the client of those abnormal symptoms to be reported immediately. Encourage the client to write down questions; provide time to discuss them. Instruct the client on methods to cope with normal variations (e.g., nausea and vomiting). Encourage attendance at prenatal classes and appropriate reading material. Prenatal health care must begin in the first trimester of pregnancy (Healthy People 2020, 2012a).

Nursing Diagnosis: Risk for Imbalanced Nutrition: Less Than Body Requirements related to increased metabolism and fetal demands

Diet should be selected from basic five food groups, with an additional 300 calories per day over recommended daily allowances. A balanced diet should provide all essential nutrients during pregnancy except folic acid and iron. These should be supplemented throughout pregnancy, because adequate amounts are closely related to fetal well-being and pregnancy outcome.

Nursing Diagnosis: Disturbed Body Image related to effects of physical changes during pregnancy

An exercise program started early in pregnancy and continued throughout will help maintain muscle tone and facilitate a return to prepregnant size after delivery. Exercise has the added benefit of creating a feeling of well-being and satisfaction. Exercise programs should be approved by the obstetrician prior to initiation. In general, those activities practiced prior to pregnancy can be continued unless they have a potential of causing physical harm to mother and baby.

Allow the client to express her feelings about body changes, and reassure her that most changes are reversible or minimized after delivery. Emphasize positive changes.

Nursing Diagnosis: Readiness for Enhanced Parenting

Beginning education on growth and development of fetus and infant early in pregnancy can provide an opportunity for prospective parents to anticipate and understand development and expected patterns of developmental skill mastery.

Nursing Diagnosis: Readiness for Enhanced Infant Nutrition

The decision to breast- or bottle-feed the infant is usually made prior to or during pregnancy. Providing factual information with an opportunity for questions and answers early in pregnancy will facilitate a decision best suited to the client's needs and lifestyle.

Intrapartum Maternal and Fetal Assessment

During the intrapartum period, an initial physical assessment should be done on admission to the labor room, and findings should be compared with those of the prenatal period. The order of the assessment will vary based on the presenting signs of labor.

COLLECTING SUBJECTIVE DATA

History of prenatal care? Gravida? Para? Age? Estimated date of confinement (EDC)? Are contractions occurring? If so, when did contractions begin? Rupture of membranes? Color of vaginal fluid? Vaginal bleeding and amount? Frequency and duration of contractions? Is fetal movement present? Has there been a decrease in fetal movement? If so, when was fetal movement last noted? Problems with this pregnancy? Duration and outcome of previous labors? Childbirth preparation? Blood type and Rh status? Concurrent disease?

COLLECTING OBJECTIVE DATA

Equipment Needed

- Bed with pillow
- Sterile examination glove
- Lubricant
- Electronic fetal monitor or Doppler
- Nitrazine paper
- Reflex hammer

Physical Assessment

INTRAPARTUM MATERNAL AND FETAL ASSESSMENT

ASSESSMENT PROCEDURE	NORMAL FINDINGS	ABNORMAL FINDINGS
Abdomen		

Have the client completely undress except for gown. Place the client in a supine position with head slightly elevated. Knees and hips should be flexed with feet resting on mattress. *Note: Examination with the client in this position should be performed as rapidly as possible to prevent supine hypotension or fetal compromise.*

With the client on back and head slightly elevated, place fingertips on fundus. During a contraction, the fundus becomes firm. The client should relate when she feels a contraction begins and when it ends. Time seconds from beginning to end of contractions (duration). Calculate elapsed time from beginning of one contraction to beginning of another (frequency). Do this for several contractions in sequence to determine regularity. During contraction, gently push in on uterus with fingertips and note the degree to which uterus indents (intensity). A large amount of subcutaneous tissue over the uterus may interfere with accurate assessment of intensity. Palpate several contractions in a row. To palpate bladder, gently push in on abdomen directly above symphysis pubis and release. Note the degree of resistance met.

Inspect abdomen for the following:
- Uterine size (see Fig. 24-6, p. 554)

- Uterine shape

	NORMAL FINDINGS	ABNORMAL FINDINGS
	• Large variation; fundus just below xiphoid process	• Uterus small or large for gestational age may indicate fetal malformations
	• Fetal outline longitudinal	• Fetal outline horizontal indicates the presentation of the baby may be transverse or breech

Continued on following page

INTRAPARTUM MATERNAL AND FETAL ASSESSMENT (Continued)

ASSESSMENT PROCEDURE	NORMAL FINDINGS	ABNORMAL FINDINGS
Palpate uterus for the following:		
• Frequency of contractions	• As labor progresses, contractions gradually get closer together, in a regular pattern progressing to every 2–3 minutes; may be less frequent during second stage	• Irregular pattern; more frequent than every 2 minutes may cause placental insufficiency for the fetus to get sufficient oxygenation during labor
• Duration of contractions	• Gradually increases to 60–90 seconds as labor progresses	• No increase; duration >90 seconds may deplete fetal oxygenation reserves
• Intensity of contractions	• Gradually become stronger, uterus feels firm (rock-like); internal pressure monitor 40–60 mm Hg	• No increase; pressure <60 mm Hg is seen with hypertonic contractions

Note: Contraction frequency and duration may be monitored with an electronic fetal monitor tocodynamometer. Initial assessment of contraction frequency and duration may be performed by palpation. Accurate intensity can only be determined with an intrauterine pressure catheter.

| Palpate above symphysis pubis for the **bladder** | Soft, spongy | Bouncy, full, distended is seen with overdistention of the bladder |

FHR

Locate FHR (see Prenatal Maternal and Fetal Assessment section) and apply external fetal monitor ultrasound transducer or Doppler. Monitor FHR every 5 minutes during the second stage of labor. Monitor high-risk pregnancies with ruptured amniotic fluid membranes with internal electrodes to assess fetal well-being accurately.

ASSESSMENT PROCEDURE	NORMAL FINDINGS	ABNORMAL FINDINGS
Monitor FHR for the following: • Baseline rate (must be determined by a 10-minute strip) • Baseline variability (measurable only with internal fetal electrode) • Periodic changes	• 120–160 beats/minute • 5–25 beats/minute • Periodic acceleration (increased FHR with fetal movement, stimulation, or contractions); early-onset deceleration (mirrors contraction and occurs in late first stage and second stage of labor)	• <120 or >160 beats/minute for a 10-minute period may indicate fetal distress • <5 beats/minute for longer than 20 minutes and not associated with maternal medication • Periodic deceleration; decreased FHR occurs with contractions; repetitive variable decelerations are seen with cord compression; late decelerations are seen in fetal distress; prolonged or slow return to baseline and associated loss of variability may be seen in fetal distress

Perineum

With the client supine, have her rest her feet on the bed with knees and hips flexed. Instruct the client to relax and separate knees. If discharge is noted, obtain specimen to assess for ruptured membranes with nitrazine paper.

Observe perineum for the following: • Lesions	• None	• Vesicles could indicate genital herpes; genital warts, open sores may be seen with sexually transmitted infections.

Continued on following page

INTRAPARTUM MATERNAL AND FETAL ASSESSMENT (Continued)

ASSESSMENT PROCEDURE	NORMAL FINDINGS	ABNORMAL FINDINGS
• Discharge	• Bloody mucus; clear or milky fluid; amniotic fluid will turn nitrazine paper blue	• Bright red blood is seen with placenta previa; purulent fluid; green or brown fluid may indicate meconium stool in utero, which puts the fetus at risk for meconium aspiration at delivery. Lubricant or blood may give a false-positive result with nitrazine paper.
• Swelling	• May be present in second stage of labor	• Present before second stage of labor
• Shape	• As fetal head descends, perineum flattens and bulges	• Fetal hand or foot visible with the presenting part indicates a compound presentation, which may occur with the occiput or breech presentation; loop of umbilical cord visible on the perineum puts the fetus at high risk for prolapse cord and requires immediate cesarean section
• Fetal parts	• Occiput becomes visible during second stage of labor	

ASSESSMENT PROCEDURE	NORMAL FINDINGS	ABNORMAL FINDINGS
Cervix and Fetal Presenting Part		

Have the client separate knees, and instruct her to relax perineum. Put on sterile examination glove, and lubricate index and middle fingers. Gently insert fingers into vagina and palpate cervix and fetal presenting part. Insert finger between cervix and the presenting part, and rotate entire circumference of cervix. This examination should be performed on admission and thereafter only when behavior and contraction pattern indicate progression of labor.

Palpate cervix for the following:		
• Position	• In early labor, cervix may be in posterior vaginal vault; it becomes more anterior as labor progresses	
• Effacement	• *Primipara:* Effacement before dilatation	• Swelling of part or all of cervix occurs when the patient begins pushing before the cervix is completely dilated
	Multipara: Effacement and dilatation simultaneous	
• Dilatation (in cm)	• *Primipara:* Average 1 cm per hour; may be slower in early phase	• Failure to progress with active labor longer than 24 hours; complete dilatation in <3 hours of labor
	Multipara: Average 1.5 cm per hour	
Palpate presenting part of the fetus for the following:		
• Amniotic membrane	• If intact, can be felt over presenting part; may rupture prior to or during labor	

Continued on following page

INTRAPARTUM MATERNAL AND FETAL ASSESSMENT (Continued)

ASSESSMENT PROCEDURE	NORMAL FINDINGS	ABNORMAL FINDINGS
• Presentation	• Cephalic; should feel skull, suture lines, and one or both fontanelles (Fig. 24-7); caput succedaneum may mask landmarks	• Breech: Soft tissue, anus, or testicles; other small parts such as hands and feet

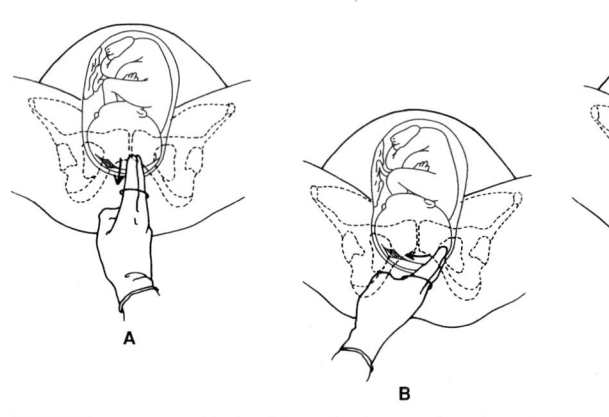

FIGURE 24-7 Assessment of fetal position and station. **A:** Palpate the sagittal suture and assess station. **B:** Identify posterior fontanelle. **C:** Identify anterior fontanelle.

ASSESSMENT PROCEDURE	NORMAL FINDINGS	ABNORMAL FINDINGS
• Position	• Cephalic; posterior fontanelle felt in anterior position, anterior fontanelle in posterior position	• Anterior fontanelle in anterior position; fontanelles in transverse position
• Station (Fig. 24-8)	• *Primipara:* 0 station; gradually descends during second stage *Multipara:* May be −1 station or higher at onset of labor	• Failure to descend to 0 station during first stage of labor; failure to descend during second stage with pushing longer than 2 hours is seen in failure to progress, which requires cesarean section

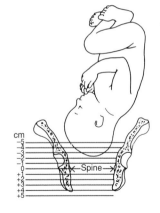

FIGURE 24-8 Measuring station of the fetal head while it is descending.

Continued on following page

INTRAPARTUM MATERNAL AND FETAL ASSESSMENT (Continued)

ASSESSMENT PROCEDURE	NORMAL FINDINGS	ABNORMAL FINDINGS
• Umbilical cord	• Not palpable	• May feel loop or pulsations in the umbilical cord, which requires immediate cesarean section

Note: If painless, bright red vaginal bleeding occurs, vaginal examination should be omitted. If fetal gestational age is less than 34 weeks and membranes have ruptured with no evidence of labor, vaginal examination should be omitted.

Face, Extremities, and Behavior

With client in semi-Fowler position, observe face, hands, legs, and feet. Also assess client's mood.

Observe client's face for the following.		
• Color	• Pink	• Red, pale
• Edema	• None	• Periorbital edema
Observe extremities for the following.		
• Color	• Pink	• Pale, blue seen with cyanosis
• Swelling	• Dependent in ankles	• Swelling in the tibia or hands, not relieved by elevating
Percuss extremities for reflexes and clonus.	See Chapter 22 for normal findings.	Hyperreflexia or clonus seen in PIH

ASSESSMENT PROCEDURE	NORMAL FINDINGS	ABNORMAL FINDINGS
Auscultate BP every hour or more often as indicated. With the client in a side-lying position, auscultate blood pressure (BP) between contractions.	BP <140/90 mm Hg. May see BP increase during contractions.	BP ≥140/90 mm Hg or increase of 30 mm Hg systolic or 15 mm Hg diastolic over prenatal baseline seen in PIH
Observe for behavior changes: • Early labor (1–4 cm) • Active labor (4–7 cm) • Transition (7–10 cm)	• Excited, happy • Cooperative; increased dependence on support person • Irritable, inner focused, hopeless	• Irrational • Uncooperative, psychotic • Confused

POSSIBLE COLLABORATIVE PROBLEMS—RISK OF

- Preeclampsia/eclampsia
- Bleeding disorders
- Placenta previa
- Abruptio placentae
- Uterine rupture
- Fetal malpresentation

- Fetal distress
- Labor dystocia
- Cephalopelvic disproportion
- Premature labor
- Fetal malposition

Teaching Tips for Selected Nursing Diagnoses

Nursing Diagnosis: Acute pain related to uterine contractions

Instruct and demonstrate relaxation techniques. Provide feedback on muscle relaxation. Offer encouragement and support.

vomiting. Consider antiemetics for persistent vomiting. Monitor for dehydration or decreased placental perfusion. Administer intravenous fluids as indicated.

Postpartum Maternal Assessment

The postpartum period begins with the delivery of the placenta and lasts an average of 6 weeks, during which time all body systems return to prepregnant levels. Some changes are rapid and others occur over time. During the first 24 hours many changes occur and frequent assessment is essential.

Changes occurring as an expected part of postpartum recovery are identified as *Normal Findings*. See Chapter 3 for a more detailed description of technique for assessing various body systems. See Chapter 25 for assessment of the newborn.

COLLECTING SUBJECTIVE DATA

Problems during pregnancy? Labor—induction, augmentation, length of labor? Gravida, para? Method of delivery? Size of baby? Anesthesia/analgesia? Concurrent disease and/or chronic conditions.

Provide comfort measures such as gentle massage; temperature control; clean, dry, and wrinkle-free linens; ice chips or lip lubricant. The laboring woman should be encouraged to assume varying positions of comfort and to ambulate unless complications contraindicate this. Provide analgesics as needed.

Nursing Diagnosis: Fear related to unfamiliar environment, pain, and concern for fetal well-being

Orient to surroundings. Provide short and simple explanation for all procedures and encourage questions.

Provide evidence of fetal well-being (monitor data). Encourage support person to stay with the client. The client should not be left alone during active labor.

Nursing Diagnosis: Risk for Fluid Volume Deficit related to increased muscle activity, increased respiratory rate, nausea and vomiting, and decreased gastric motility or absorption

Offer small amounts of fluids such as ice chips or popsicles. Avoid solid foods that are difficult to digest and often promote

COLLECTING OBJECTIVE DATA

POSTPARTUM MATERNAL ASSESSMENT

ASSESSMENT PROCEDURE	NORMAL FINDINGS	ABNORMAL FINDINGS
Monitor the following: • Temperature	• 38 °C (100.4 °F) in first 24 hours	• Higher than 38 °C (100.4 °F) in first 24 hours or 38 °C (100.4 °F) and above on any 2 of the first 10 days postpartum seen in puerperal infection
• Blood pressure	• No change from prepregnant levels	• PIH can occur up to 48 hours postpartum; persistent elevation of blood pressure from PIH beyond 48 hours
• Pulse	• Bradycardia (50–70 beats/minute) for 6–10 days	• Tachycardia; pre-existing hypertension may be difficult to control; postural hypotension may occur when assuming the upright position after delivery
• Weight	• Initial 4.53–5.44 kg (10–12 lb) loss; 4.53–9.07 kg (10–20 lb) loss in next 6–8 weeks	
• Behavior	• *First 2–3 days postpartum:* Preoccupied with food and sleep; passive and dependent	• Psychosis is noted when patient is unable to care for herself and newborn

Continued on following page

POSTPARTUM MATERNAL ASSESSMENT (Continued)		
ASSESSMENT PROCEDURE	**NORMAL FINDINGS**	**ABNORMAL FINDINGS**
	• *After 2–3 days postpartum:* Increased interest in control of body functions, mothering skills; gradually includes others in social circle; transient depression, let down feeling, cries easily	• Failure to assume maternal role; prolonged depression; unrealistic expectations of newborn

Breast

With client in supine or semi-Fowler position, inspect breasts. Gently palpate all quadrants of each breast.

Inspect and palpate the breasts in non-nursing mothers for the following:		
• Size	• May be enlarged initially; will gradually return to prepregnant size	• Full, engorged breasts
• Shape	• May sag	
• Color	• May have striae	• Localized redness, tenderness, pain may be seen with mastitis
• Tenderness	• Soft	• Full, tender
• Texture	• Nodular	• Lumps, masses may be seen with clogged breast ducts

ASSESSMENT PROCEDURE	NORMAL FINDINGS	ABNORMAL FINDINGS
Inspect and palpate the breasts in nursing mothers for the following: • Size • Texture • Nipples • Discharge • Tenderness • Texture • Hardened area, most often in upper, outer quadrant, indicates clogged milk ducts and/or mastitis	• Enlarged • Increased nodularity • Everted, tender • Colostrum, thin milk, may leak between feedings • Full, slightly tender • Small lumps	• Heat, localized pain • Blisters, cracked, bleeding • Purulent, bloody discharge may indicate infection • Painful breasts are seen with mastitis

Abdomen

Place client in a supine position with knees extended and head slightly elevated on a pillow. For palpation, have the client empty bladder and assume supine position. Place one hand over lower abdomen above symphysis pubis to support uterus. With the fingertips of the other hand, locate the fundus. Start in the midline, slightly above the umbilicus, and press in and down. Work fingers gradually down toward the symphysis pubis until the fundus of the uterus is located. It should feel like a firm, round ball, similar to a grapefruit. Measure the distance above or below the umbilicus in fingerbreadths (Figs. 24-9 and 24-10). If the uterus is not firm, gently massage until firm, and then gently push down on fundus and observe for expression of clots from the vagina.

Continued on following page

POSTPARTUM MATERNAL ASSESSMENT (Continued)		
ASSESSMENT PROCEDURE	**NORMAL FINDINGS**	**ABNORMAL FINDINGS**

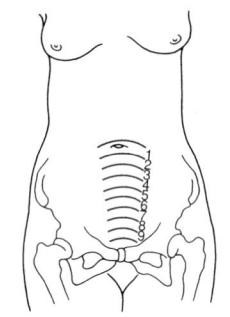

FIGURE 24-9 Involution of the uterus. The height of the fundus decreases about 1 fingerbreadth (approximately 1 cm) each day.

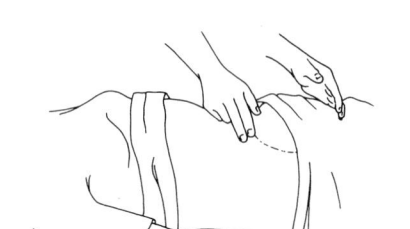

FIGURE 24-10 Measurement of the descent of the fundus. The fundus is located 2 fingerbreadths below the umbilicus.

Inspect abdomen for the following:
- Size

- Color

- Texture

- Uterus visible, outlined unless obese; gradually recedes to prepregnant size with exercise
- Striae dark red or purple; recede to silvery or white and become smaller
- Loose and flabby

- Distention seen when patient is unable to void and bladder becomes distended
- Yellow, pale

- Dry, cracked

ASSESSMENT PROCEDURE	NORMAL FINDINGS	ABNORMAL FINDINGS
Palpate uterine fundus for the following: • Location	• Midline	• Deviated to left or right could indicate a distended bladder
• Consistency	• Firm; boggy to firm with massage; smooth surface	• Boggy; does not stay firm after massage may indicate uterine atony and/or retained placental fragments
• Height	• Halfway between umbilicus and symphysis immediately after delivery; within 12 hours, at the umbilicus or 1 cm above; descends 1 cm per day	• More than 1 cm above umbilicus; failure to descend
• Expression of clots	• Small clots or increased flow with massage	• Large clots; continuous trickle of bright red blood with firm fundus indicates an unrepaired laceration

Face and Extremities

To inspect the face and extremities, the supine position is preferred. Adequate light must be available. With legs extended, gently palpate calves. Place one hand on knee, and gently dorsiflex each foot. Pregnancy-related seizures can occur for up to 48 hours postpartum. Reflexes should be assessed for hyperreflexia and clonus during this time. See Chapter 22 for technique.

Continued on following page

POSTPARTUM MATERNAL ASSESSMENT (Continued)

ASSESSMENT PROCEDURE	NORMAL FINDINGS	ABNORMAL FINDINGS
Inspect face for the following:		
• Color	• Petechiae after prolonged second stage of labor	• Paleness may be seen with anemia
• Edema	• None	• Periorbital
Inspect extremities for the following.		
• Color	• Pink; red tones visible under dark pigmentation	• Dusky, mottled color indicates decreased oxygenation
• Edema	• Slight pedal edema	• Pitting edema, edema of hands seen with PIH
• Tenderness	• Calves may have generalized muscle tenderness	• Calf with localized tenderness or pain seen with deep vein thrombosis
• Texture	• Smooth	• Knots or lumps in calf
• Homans sign	• Negative (no pain in calf)	• Positive (pain in calf) may indicate deep vein thrombosis

Bladder

Have the client void within 4 hours after delivery or sooner if there are bleeding problems during the immediate postpartum period.

To palpate the bladder, have the client empty supine position. Palpate for bladder above the symphysis pubis. If unable to void within 4 hours after delivery or if the bladder is full, empty the bladder with a catheter.

ASSESSMENT PROCEDURE	NORMAL FINDINGS	ABNORMAL FINDINGS
Inspect voiding for the following: • Amount • Color	• 200 mL or more each voiding; diuresis of greater than 2,000 mL in first 24 hours • Yellow, clear; may be mixed with lochia	• Less than 100 mL per voiding; unable to void • Dark, cloudy, bloody urine may indicate urinary tract infection
Palpate bladder	Nonpalpable	Spongy mass in lower abdomen

Perineum

Have the client turn to side and flex upper leg. Place one hand on upper buttock and gently separate so that perineum is visible.

Inspect perineum for the following: • Approximation of episiotomy • Color • Swelling • Lochia	• Skin edges meet • Pink to red • Generalized swelling for 12–24 hours • *Color: Days 1–3:* Rubra (dark red); small clots may also be expelled *Days 4–10:* Serosa (pinkish red) *Days 11–20:* Alba (creamy yellow)	• Skin edges gape • Purple, mottled • Localized swelling with increased pain indicates hematoma • More than eight peripads per day or saturated pad in 1 hour seen in postpartum hemorrhage; purulent, large clots; return to dark red after several days

Continued on following page

POSTPARTUM MATERNAL ASSESSMENT (Continued)		
ASSESSMENT PROCEDURE	NORMAL FINDINGS	ABNORMAL FINDINGS
	Amount: Days 1–10: Vaginal discharge requires 6–10 pads per day (moderate flow).	
	Days 11–20: Decreased amount of vaginal discharge still requires pad change (less than 6–8 pads per day).	
• Odor • Hemorrhoids	• None; musky scent • Small, nontender	• Foul odor with bacterial infections • Swollen, painful

POSSIBLE COLLABORATIVE PROBLEMS—RISK OF

- Urinary retention
- Breast engorgement/abscess
- Preeclampsia/eclampsia
- Hemorrhage
- Uterine atony
- Hematoma
- Cervical/vaginal lacerations
- Retained placenta
- Infections
- Exacerbation of pre-existing medical conditions
- Heart conditions
- Hypertension
- Hyperglycemia
- Hypoglycemia

Teaching Tips for Selected Nursing Diagnoses

Nursing Diagnosis: Disturbed Sleep Pattern related to fatigue and increased need for sleep

All teaching sessions should be brief and reinforced with written information about infant care and self-care (e.g., care of breasts). Encourage mother to sleep when baby sleeps. Advise mother to avoid strenuous activities until 6-week postpartum physical examination. Enlist help of other family members.

Nursing Diagnosis: Readiness for Enhanced Infant Care and Self-Care

Demonstrate infant care and allow time for mother to practice. A follow-up phone call or home visit can assist in evaluation and reinforcement of information taught. Include father whenever possible.

Nursing Diagnosis: Readiness for Enhanced Family Coping related to addition of family member and role changes

Discuss plans for incorporating new member into family. Offer suggestions to decrease sibling jealousy. Explore plans for infant care, division of labor, and changes in activities of daily living.

Nursing Diagnosis: Risk for Impaired Parent/Infant Attachment related to unrealistic expectations of self

Discuss normal growth and development of infant; emphasize things infant can do. Provide early and continued contact of infant and parents to maximize bonding. Teach parents the skills needed to meet infant's physical and psychological needs.

Nursing Diagnosis: Impaired Parenting related to inadequate skills, unrealistic expectation of infant, stress, lack of adequate support

Be aware of risk factors for child abuse/neglect that may be evident during postpartal period. Explore resources available to parents, and make appropriate referrals for follow-up or support groups.

Nursing Diagnosis: Ineffective Breastfeeding related to lack of knowledge

Clarify misconceptions, and provide instructions or proper technique. Assist with first feedings and problems such as soreness or difficulty latching on to breasts, etc.

Nursing Diagnosis: Ineffective Infant Feeding Pattern related to sluggish sucking and difficulty latching onto nipple

May use nipple with larger hole. Hold infant in upright position during feeding. Burp infant often (after every 14.8–29.6 mL [0.5–1 oz]). Infant needs frequent feedings with careful monitoring of intake and weight gain. May need to teach parents gavage feedings. If so, infant will attempt to nurse at each feeding and be gavage-fed remaining formula/breast milk.

Nursing Diagnosis: Interrupted Breastfeeding related to change in daily routine lifestyle

To continue breast milk supply, mother should pump breasts at intervals similar to infant feeding patterns. Milk letdown is optimal immediately after infant contact. Mother should be relaxed and have privacy. If possible, both breasts should be emptied at each feeding. Increased fluid consumption is needed for milk production. Discuss methods to enhance milk production if deficient. To terminate breastfeeding, mother should avoid any stimulation of breasts. Encourage use of good support bra. Painful engorgement may be alleviated with analgesics and intermittent ice packs to breasts.

CHAPTER 25

Assessing Newborns and Infants

A newborn, or neonate, is the term used to describe a child from birth to 28 days old. An infant refers to a child between the ages of 28 days and 1 year.

Nursing Assessment of the Newborn and Infant

Nursing assessment of the newborn and infant consists of collecting subjective and objective data. The nurse interviews the parents or primary caretaker of the newborn or infant to collect subjective data. The nurse will perform an initial newborn physi-

cal assessment right at the time of birth; subsequent physical assessments of the newborn and infant are performed at regular intervals throughout the first year of life.

COLLECTING SUBJECTIVE DATA

- *Prenatal history:* Gravida? Para? Estimated date of confinement (EDC)? Gestational age? Maternal history? Risk factors? Prenatal exposure to drugs? Complications? Blood type? Maternal testing?
- *Labor and delivery history:* Date, time, type of delivery? Prolonged labor? Narcotics? Time of rupture of membranes? Intrapartum complications? Shoulder dystocia?

COLLECTING OBJECTIVE DATA

- *Delivery history:* Apgar scores? Respiratory effort? Resuscitation efforts? Medications? Procedures performed? Evidence of injury? Void? Stool?
- *Social history:* Parent interaction? Significant others? Cultural variations? Type of infant feeding? Male circumcision requested?

Equipment Needed

- Gloves
- Stethoscope
- Tape measure

Physical Assessment

At birth, the newborn will undergo an *initial assessment*. This special assessment is performed to evaluate the following.

- Apgar Score
- Vital Signs
- Measurements
- Gestational Age
- Newborn Reflexes

These assessments are performed in order to evaluate the newborn's transition from intrauterine life and to detect any health concerns that may require prompt intervention. The *initial assessment* is performed immediately after birth, while the infant is supine under a radiant warmer with the temperature probe attached to the abdomen.

Subsequent physical assessments of the infant are performed using the guide provided below. Physical assessment of the infant is a complete head-to-toe examination that also includes developmental screening.

INITIAL NEWBORN ASSESSMENT

ASSESSMENT PROCEDURE	NORMAL FINDINGS	ABNORMAL FINDINGS
Apgar Score		
Assign Apgar scores at 1 and at 5 minutes after delivery. The Apgar score is an assessment of infant's ability to adapt to extrauterine life. Assess the following.	The score is 8 to 10. See Table 25-1 for Apgar scoring.	<8 points may indicate poor transition from intrauterine into extrauterine life.
Auscultate **apical pulse.**	>100 beats/minute	<100 beats/minute indicates bradycardia; absent heart beat indicates fetal demise.
Inspect chest and abdomen for **respiratory effort.**	Crying	Absent, slow, irregular respirations
Stroke **back or soles of feet.**	Crying	Delayed neurologic function may be seen in grimace, no response.
Inspect **muscle tone** by extending legs and arms. Observe degree of flexion and resistance in extremities.	Extremities flexed, active movement	Moderate degree of flexion, limp may indicate neurologic deficits.
Inspect body and extremities for **skin color.**	Full body pink, acrocyanosis	Cyanosis, pale

Continued on following page

INITIAL NEWBORN ASSESSMENT (Continued)

ASSESSMENT PROCEDURE	NORMAL FINDINGS	ABNORMAL FINDINGS
Vital Signs		
Monitor **axillary temperature.**	36.38–37.2 °C (97.5–99 °F)	<36.38 °C (<97.5 °F): hypothermia, which may indicate sepsis >37.2 °C (>99 °F): hyperthermia (Consider infection or improper monitoring of temperature probe.)
Inspect and auscultate **lung sounds.**	Easy, nonlabored, clear lungs bilaterally	Labored breathing, nasal flaring, rhonchi, rales, retractions, grunting
Monitor **respiratory rate.**	Rate: 30–60 breaths/minute	Rate <30 or >60 breaths/minute is seen with respiratory distress.
Auscultate **apical pulse.**	Regular 120–160 beats/minute (100 sleeping, 180 crying)	Irregular <100 or >180 beats/minute may indicate cardiac abnormalities.

ASSESSMENT PROCEDURE	NORMAL FINDINGS	ABNORMAL FINDINGS
Measurements		
Weigh newborn unclothed using a newborn scale (Fig. 25-1).	2,500–4,000 g	<2,500 g >4,000 g

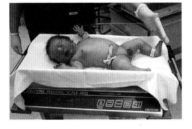

FIGURE 25-1 Weighing the newborn.

Measure **length**.	44–55 cm	<44 cm >55 cm
Measure **head circumference**.	33–35.5 cm	<33 cm >35.5 cm
Measure **chest circumference**.	30–33 cm (1–2 cm < head)	<30 cm >33 cm

Continued on following page

INITIAL NEWBORN ASSESSMENT (Continued)

ASSESSMENT PROCEDURE	NORMAL FINDINGS	ABNORMAL FINDINGS

Gestational Age

Assess the newborn's gestational age within 4 hours after birth to identify any potential age-related problems that may occur within the next few hours. Examine the newborn's neuromuscular and physical maturity. After examination, use the Ballard Scale to rate the gestational age (Fig. 25-2 and Fig. 25-3).

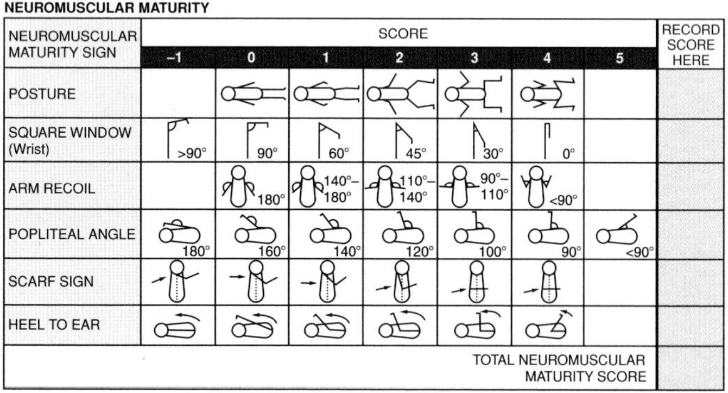

NEUROMUSCULAR MATURITY

NEUROMUSCULAR MATURITY SIGN	SCORE						RECORD SCORE HERE
	−1	0	1	2	3	4	5
POSTURE							
SQUARE WINDOW (Wrist)	>90°	90°	60°	45°	30°	0°	
ARM RECOIL		180°	140°–180°	110°–140°	90°–110°	<90°	
POPLITEAL ANGLE	180°	160°	140°	120°	100°	90°	<90°
SCARF SIGN							
HEEL TO EAR							
					TOTAL NEUROMUSCULAR MATURITY SCORE		

FIGURE 25-2 New Ballard Scale. Used to rate neuromuscular maturity of gestational age.

ASSESSMENT PROCEDURE	NORMAL FINDINGS	ABNORMAL FINDINGS

PHYSICAL MATURITY

PHYSICAL MATURITY SIGN	SCORE							RECORD SCORE HERE
	-1	0	1	2	3	4	5	
SKIN	sticky, friable, transparent	gelatinous, red, translucent	smooth, pink, visible veins	superficial peeling and/or rash, few veins	cracking pale areas, rare veins	parchment, deep cracking, no vessels	leathery, cracked, wrinkled	
LANUGO	none	sparse	abundant	thinning	bald areas	mostly bald		
PLANTAR SURFACE	heel-toe 40–50 mm:–1 <40 mm:–2	>50 mm no crease	faint red marks	anterior transverse crease only	creases ant. 2/3	creases over entire sole		
BREAST	impercep-tible	barely perceptible	flat areola no bud	stippled areola 1–2 mm bud	raised areola 3–4 mm bud	full areola 5–10 mm bud		
EYE-EAR	lids fused loosely: –1 tightly: –2	lids open pinna flat stays folded	sl. curved pinna; soft; slow recoil	well-curved pinna; soft but ready recoil	formed and firm instant recoil	thick cartilage, ear stiff		
GENITALS (Male)	scrotum flat, smooth	scrotum empty, faint rugae	testes in upper canal, rare rugae	testes descending, few rugae	testes down, good rugae	testes pendulous, deep rugae		
GENITALS (Female)	clitoris prominent and labia flat	prominent clitoris and small labia minora	prominent clitoris and enlarging minora	majora and minora equally prominent	majora large minora small	majora cover clitoris and minora		
						TOTAL PHYSICAL MATURITY SCORE		

SCORE
Neuromuscular ___
Physical ___
Total ___

MATURITY RATING

Score	Weeks
-10	20
-5	22
0	24
5	26
10	28
15	30
20	32
25	34
30	36
35	38
40	40
45	42
50	44

GESTATIONAL AGE (weeks)
By dates ___
By ultrasound ___
By exam ___

FIGURE 25-3 New Ballard Scale. Used to rate physical maturity of gestational age.

Continued on following page

INITIAL NEWBORN ASSESSMENT (Continued)		
ASSESSMENT PROCEDURE	**NORMAL FINDINGS**	**ABNORMAL FINDINGS**
Assess **neuromuscular maturity** (see Fig. 25-2, p. 584) by performing each of the following with the newborn in the supine position.		
Inspect **posture** (with newborn undisturbed)	• Arms and legs flexed	• Arms and legs limp, extended away from body seen with premature infants
Assess for **square window:** bend wrist toward ventral forearm until resistance is met. Measure angle (Fig. 25-4).	• 0–30 degrees • Premature infants may have square window measurement of >30 degrees.	

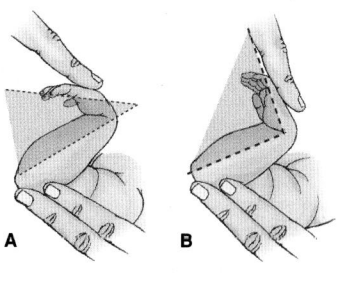

FIGURE 25-4 Square window sign. **A:** Term infant. **B:** Preterm infant.

ASSESSMENT PROCEDURE	NORMAL FINDINGS	ABNORMAL FINDINGS
Test **arm recoil**: bilaterally flex elbows up with hands next to shoulders and hold approximately 5 seconds; extend arms down next to side, release; observe elbow angle and recoil.	• Elbow angle <90 degrees, rapid recoil to flexed state	• Elbow angle >110 degrees, delayed recoil seen in premature infants
Assess **popliteal angle**: flex thigh on top of abdomen; push behind ankle and extend lower leg up toward head until resistance is met; measure angle behind knee.	• <100 degrees	• >100 degrees
Assess for **scarf sign**: Lift arm across chest toward opposite shoulder until resistance is met; note location of elbow in relation to middle of chest (Fig. 25-5).	• Elbow position less than midline of chest	• Elbow position midline of chest or greater, toward opposite shoulder seen in premature infants

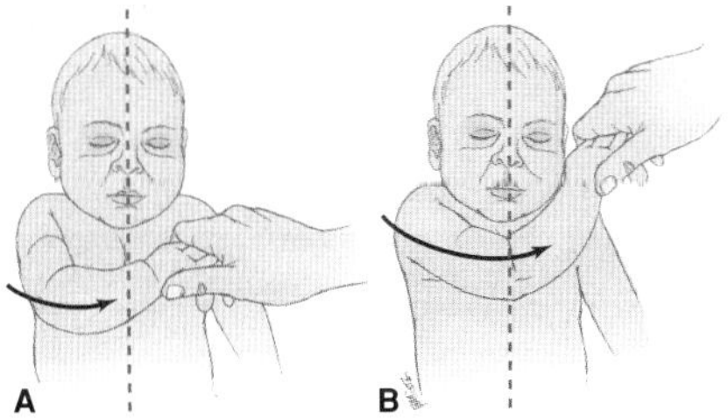

FIGURE 25-5 Scarf sign. **A:** Term infant. **B:** Preterm infant.

Continued on following page

INITIAL NEWBORN ASSESSMENT (Continued)

ASSESSMENT PROCEDURE	NORMAL FINDINGS	ABNORMAL FINDINGS
Perform **heel to ear test.** Pull leg toward ear on same side, keeping buttocks flat on bed; inspect popliteal angle and proximity of heel to ear.	• Popliteal angle <90 degrees, heel distal from ear	• Popliteal angle <90 degrees, heel proximal to ear seen in premature infants
Assess **physical maturity** (see Fig. 25-3, p. 585) by performing the following:		
• Inspect skin.	• Parchment, few or no vessels on abdomen, cracking in ankle area	• Translucent, visible veins; rash; leathery, wrinkled skin seen in postmature infants
• Inspect for lanugo.	• Thinning, balding on back, shoulders, knees	• Abundant amount of fine hair on face seen in premature infants
• Inspect plantar surface of feet for creases.	• Creases on anterior two thirds or entire sole	• Anterior transverse crease on sole only, no creases; fewer creases indicate prematurity.
• Inspect and palpate breast tissue with middle finger and forefinger; measure bud in millimeters.	• Raised areola, full areola	• Absence of bud tissue, bud <3 mm seen in premature infants
• Observe ear cartilage in upper pinna for curving. Fold pinna down toward side of head and release; observe recoil of ear.	• Pinna well curved, cartilage formed, instant recoil	• Pinna slightly curved, slow recoil seen in premature infants

ASSESSMENT PROCEDURE	NORMAL FINDINGS	ABNORMAL FINDINGS
• Inspect genitals.		
Male: Observe scrotum for rugae and palpate position of testes.	• *Male:* Deep rugae; testes positioned down in scrotal sac	• *Male:* Decreased presence of rugae; testes positioned in upper inguinal canal
Female: Observe labia majora, labia minora, and clitoris.	*Female:* Labia majora cover labia minora and clitoris.	*Female:* Labia majora and labia minora equally prominent, clitoris prominent seen with premature infants
Determine **score rating:** Use Figures 24-2 and 24-3, pp. 584–585. Mark the boxes that most closely represent each observation.		
• Add the total scores from both tables.	• Total score: 35–45 points	• Total score: <35 points or >45 points
• Using Figure 25-2, p. 584, plot total score in column on right-hand side of page; this score corresponds to the number in weeks on the maturity rating scale; circle the number of weeks.	• Gestational age: 38–42 weeks	• Gestational age: <38 or >42 weeks

Continued on following page

INITIAL NEWBORN ASSESSMENT (Continued)		
ASSESSMENT PROCEDURE	**NORMAL FINDINGS**	**ABNORMAL FINDINGS**
• Using gestational weeks assessed, plot weight, length, and head circumference on the growth charts found in Appendix 8 and record classification of newborn on Figure 25-6	• 10th to 90th percentile is appropriate for gestational age (AGA).	• Less than the 10th percentile (small for gestational age); greater than the 90th percentile (large for gestational age)

CLASSIFICATION OF INFANT*	Weight	Length	Head Circ.
Large for Gestational Age (LGA) (>90th percentile).			
Appropriate for Gestational Age (AGA) (10th to 90th percentile)			
Small for Gestational Age (SGA) (<10th percentile)			

*Place an "X" in the appropriate box (LGA, AGA, or SGA) for weight, for length, and for head circumference.

FIGURE 25-6 Classification of infant for gestational age.

Newborn Reflexes		
Assess newborn reflexes. See Chapter 21.	Infantile reflexes are present when appropriate and are symmetric (see Chapter 21)	Presence of newborn reflexes beyond the time they are expected to disappear.

TABLE 25-1 **APGAR Score**

	Scores 0	Scores 1	Scores 2
Heart Rate	Absent	<100 beats/minute	>100 beats/minute
Respiratory Rate	Absent	Slow, irregular	Good lusty cry
Reflex Irritability	No response	Grimace, some motion	Cry, cough
Muscle Tone	Flaccid, limp	Flexion of extremities	Active flexion
Color	Cyanotic, pale	Pink body, acrocyanosis	Pink body, pink extremities

SUBSEQUENT INFANT PHYSICAL ASSESSMENT

ASSESSMENT PROCEDURE	NORMAL FINDINGS	ABNORMAL FINDINGS
General Appearance and Behavior		
Observe general appearance. Observe hygiene. Note interaction with parents and yourself (and siblings if present). Note also facies (facial expressions) and posture.	Child appears stated age; is clean, has no unusual body odor, and clothing is in good condition and appropriate for climate. Child is alert, active, responds appropriately to stress of the situation. Child is appropriately interactive for age, seeks comfort from parent; appears happy. Newborn's arms and legs are in flexed position.	Note any facies that indicate acute illness, respiratory distress. Flaccidity or rigidity in newborn may be from neurologic damage, sepsis, or pain. Poor hygiene and clothes may indicate neglect, poverty. Infant does not appear stated age (mental retardation, abuse, neglect).

Continued on following page

SUBSEQUENT INFANT PHYSICAL ASSESSMENT (Continued)

ASSESSMENT PROCEDURE	NORMAL FINDINGS	ABNORMAL FINDINGS
Developmental Assessment		
Screen for cognitive, language, social, and gross and fine motor developmental delays in the beginning of the physical assessment in infants. Growth and development of the newborn/infant may be assessed using the Denver Developmental Screening Test. This test is used to guide the nurse to the appropriate developmental milestones for the child's gross motor, language, fine motor, and personal social development.	Infant meets normal parameters for age, see Appendix 5. Gross and fine motor skills should be appropriate for the child's developmental age.	Child lags in earlier stages. Gross and fine motor skills that are inappropriate for developmental age and lack of head control by age 6 months may indicate cerebral palsy.
Vital Signs		
Assess temperature. Use rectal or axillary routes in infants less than 6 months of age. The tympanic and temporal arterial routes may be used in infants older than 6 months (see Chapter 6 for detailed information on measuring temperature in infants).	Normal axillary temperature ranges from 36.3–37.3 °C (97.4–99.3 °F). Normal rectal, tympanic and temporal arterial temperature is 37.8 °C (100.2 °F) or less.	Temperature may be altered by exercise, stress, crying, environment, diurnal variation (highest between 4 and 6 PM). Both hyperthermic and hypothermic conditions are noted in infants.

ASSESSMENT PROCEDURE	NORMAL FINDINGS	ABNORMAL FINDINGS
Note apical pulse rate. Count the pulse for a full minute.	Awake and resting rates vary with the age of the child (see Chapter 6). For a newborn to 1-month-old child it should be 120–160 beats/minute. When crying, the heart rate may increase up to 180 beats/minute. Rate decreases gradually with age. At 6 months to 1 year, rate is approximately 110 beats/minute.	Pulse may be altered by medications, activity, and pain as well as pathologic conditions. Bradycardia (<100 beats/minute) in an infant is usually an ominous finding. Tachycardia may also indicate cardiac/respiratory problems or sepsis.
Assess respiratory rate and character. Measure respiratory rate and character in infants by observing abdominal movements.	In newborns up to 3 months of age: Rate is 30–50 breaths/minute. In infants greater than 3 months of age: Rate is 20–30 breaths/minute. Breathing is unlabored; lung sounds clear. Newborns are obligatory nose breathers.	Respiratory rate and character may be altered by medications, positioning, fever, activity as well as pathologic conditions. Retractions, see-saw respirations, apnea >15 seconds, grunting, nasal flaring, stridor, rale, tachypnea >60 breaths/minute should be further evaluated for respiratory distress.

Continued on following page

SUBSEQUENT INFANT PHYSICAL ASSESSMENT (Continued)

ASSESSMENT PROCEDURE	NORMAL FINDINGS	ABNORMAL FINDINGS
Measure length. Determine infant's height by measuring the recumbent length. Fully extend the body, holding the head in midline and gently grasping the knees and pushing them downward until the legs are fully extended and touching the table. If using a measuring board, place the head at the top of the board and the heels firmly at the bottom. Without a board, use paper under the infant and mark the paper at the top of the head and bottom of the heels. Then measure the distance between the two points. Plot height measurement on an appropriate age-and-gender-specific growth chart.	See the growth charts in Appendix 8 for normal findings.	Significant deviation from normal in the growth charts would be considered abnormal.
Measure weight. Measure weight on an appropriately sized beam scale with nondetectable weights. Weigh an infant lying or sitting on a scale that measures to the nearest 14.1 g (0.5 oz) or 10 g. Weigh an infant naked. Plot weight measurement on age- and gender-appropriate growth chart.	See the growth charts in Appendix 8 for normal findings.	Deviation from the wide range of normal weights is abnormal. See Appendix 8 and compare differences.

ASSESSMENT PROCEDURE	NORMAL FINDINGS	ABNORMAL FINDINGS
Determine **head/chest circumference.** Measure **head circumference (HC)** or occipital frontal circumference (OFC) at every physical examination for infants and toddlers up to 2 years of age.	HC (OFC) measurement should fall between the 5th and 95th percentiles and should be comparable to the child's height and weight percentiles.	Abnormal circumference of head include <29 cm and >34 cm. HC (OFC) not within the normal percentiles may indicate pathology. Those greater than 95% may indicate macrocephaly. Those under the 5th percentile may indicate microcephaly.

Skin, Hair, and Nails

Assess for **skin color, odor, and lesions.** 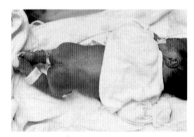 **FIGURE 25-7** Mongolian spots.	Skin color ranges from pale white with pink, yellow, brown, or olive tones to dark brown or black. Skin is without strong odor and lesion free. Common variations: Acrocyanosis (sluggish perfusion of peripheral circulation); Harlequin sign (one side of the body turns red; the other side is pale); Mottling (general red/white discoloration of skin caused by chilling); Mongolian spots (Fig. 25-7); Petechiae or bruising on the presenting part (due to rapid pressure and release with delivery); Physiologic	Yellow skin may indicate jaundice or passage of meconium in utero secondary to fetal distress. Jaundice within 24 hours after birth is pathologic and may indicate hemolytic disease of the newborn. Blue skin suggests cyanosis, pallor suggests anemia, and redness suggests fever, irritation. Ecchymoses in various stages or in unusual locations or circular burn areas suggest child abuse. Petechiae, lesions, or rashes may indicate blood disorders or neurologic disorders.

Continued on following page

SUBSEQUENT INFANT PHYSICAL ASSESSMENT (Continued)

ASSESSMENT PROCEDURE	NORMAL FINDINGS	ABNORMAL FINDINGS

Palpate for **texture, temperature, moisture, turgor, and edema.**

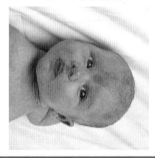

FIGURE 25-8 Stork bites.

Skin soft, warm and slightly moist. Vernix caseosa (cheesy, white substance that is found on the skin, especially in skin folds) is a common finding; it eventually absorbs into the skin. Skin turgor should have quick recoil. Edema may be present around the eyes and genitalia of the newborn.

Jaundice; Birthmarks; Milia; Erythema toxicum; Telangiectatic nevi (stork bites) (Fig. 25-8); Café au lait < 1.5 cm; Benign hemangioma (including Port wine stain, Strawberry mark)

Abnormal skin lesions include:
Café au lait spots: if there are 6 or more hyperpigmented macules, greater than 1.5 cm diameter, it may indicate neurofibromatosis, an inherited neurocutaneous disease.

Pallor, ruddy complexion, and jaundice should be further evaluated for cardiac anomalies, blood disorders.

ASSESSMENT PROCEDURE	NORMAL FINDINGS	ABNORMAL FINDINGS
Inspect and palpate **hair**. Observe for distribution, characteristics, and presence of any unusual hair on body.	Hair is normally lustrous, silky, strong, and elastic. Lanugo, fine, downy hair that covers parts of the body, such as the shoulders, back and sacral area, may be seen in the newborn or young infant.	Dirty, matted hair may indicate neglect. Tufts of hair over spine may indicate spina bifida occulta.
Inspect and palpate **nails**. Note color, texture, shape, and condition of nails.	Nails extend to end of fingers or beyond; are well-formed.	Blue nail beds indicate cyanosis. Yellow nail beds indicate jaundice. Blue-black nail beds suggest a nail bed hemorrhage.

Head, Neck, and Cervical Lymph Nodes

Inspect and palpate the **head**. Note shape and symmetry. In newborns, inspect and palpate the condition of fontanelles and sutures (Fig. 25-9).	Head is normocephalic and symmetric. In newborns, the head may be oddly shaped from molding (overriding of the sutures) during	A very large head is found with hydrocephalus.

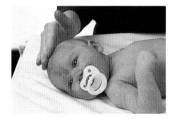

FIGURE 25-9 Palpating the anterior fontanelle. (Photo by B. Proud.)

Continued on following page

SUBSEQUENT INFANT PHYSICAL ASSESSMENT (Continued)

ASSESSMENT PROCEDURE	NORMAL FINDINGS	ABNORMAL FINDINGS

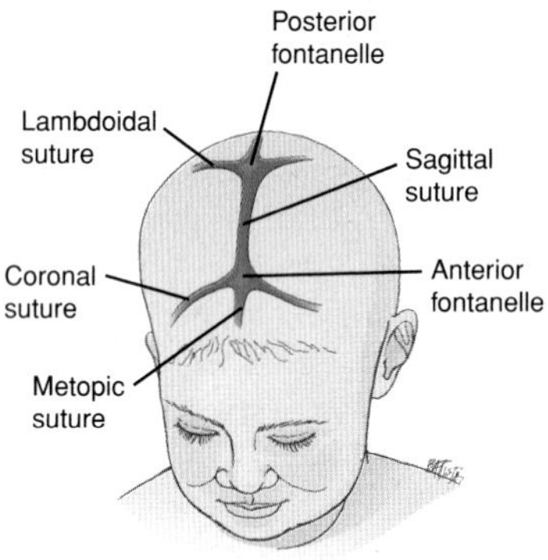

FIGURE 25-10 The infant head.

ASSESSMENT PROCEDURE

vaginal birth. The diamond-shaped anterior fontanelle measures about 4–5 cm at its widest part. The triangular posterior fontanelle measures about 0.5–1 cm at its widest part and it should close at 2 months of age (Fig. 25-10).

A common variation is caput succedaneum (Fig. 25-11A).

NORMAL FINDINGS

Bulging fontanelle indicates increased cranial pressure. Microcephaly is seen with infants who have been exposed to congenital infections.

Premature closure of sutures (craniosynostosis) may result in caput succedaneum (edema from trauma), which crosses the suture line, and cephalohematoma (bleeding into the periosteal space), which does not extend across the suture line (Fig. 25-11B).

ABNORMAL FINDINGS

An oddly shaped head is found with premature closure of sutures (possibly genetic). One-sided flattening of the head suggests prolonged positioning on one side.

A third fontanelle between the anterior and posterior fontanelle is seen with Down syndrome.

ASSESSMENT PROCEDURE	NORMAL FINDINGS	ABNORMAL FINDINGS

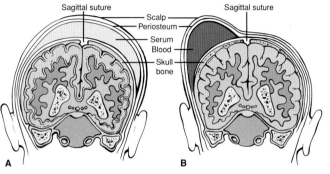

FIGURE 25-11 A: Caput succedaneum. **B:** Cephalohematoma.

Test **head control, head posture, range of motion.**

Full range of motion—up, down, and sideways—is normal.

Infants should have head control by 4 months of age.

Hyperextension is seen with opisthotonos or significant meningeal irritation.

Limited range of motion may indicate torticollis (wryneck).

Continued on following page

SUBSEQUENT INFANT PHYSICAL ASSESSMENT (Continued)

ASSESSMENT PROCEDURE	NORMAL FINDINGS	ABNORMAL FINDINGS
Inspect and palpate **the face.** Note appearance, symmetry, and movement. Palpate the parotid glands for swelling.	Face is normally proportionate and symmetric. Movements are equal bilaterally. Parotid glands are normal size.	Unusual proportions (short palpebral fissures, thin lips, and wide and flat philtrum, which is the groove above the upper lip) may be hereditary or they may indicate specific syndromes such as Down syndrome and fetal alcohol syndrome. Unequal movement may indicate facial nerve paralysis. Abnormal facies may indicate chromosomal anomaly.
Inspect and palpate **the neck.** Palpate the thyroid gland and the trachea. Also inspect and palpate the cervical lymph nodes for swelling, mobility, temperature, and tenderness. *Note: The thyroid is very difficult to palpate in an infant because of the short, thick neck.*	The neck is usually short with skin folds between the head and shoulder during infancy. The isthmus is the only portion of the thyroid that should be palpable. The trachea is midline. Lymph nodes are usually nonpalpable in infants. Clavicles are symmetrical and intact.	Implications of some abnormal findings include the following: • Short, webbed neck suggests anomalies or syndromes such as Down syndrome. • Distended neck veins may indicate difficulty breathing. • Enlarged thyroid or palpable masses suggest a pathologic process.

ASSESSMENT PROCEDURE	NORMAL FINDINGS	ABNORMAL FINDINGS
		• Shift in tracheal position from midline suggests a serious lung problem (e.g., foreign body or tumor). • Crepitus when clavicle palpated along with decreased movement in arm of that side may indicate fractured clavicle.
Eyes		
Inspect the **external eye.** Note the position, slant, and epicanthal folds of the external eye.	Inner canthus distance approximately 2.5 cm, horizontal slant, no epicanthal folds. Outer canthus aligns with tips of the pinnae.	Wide-set position (hypertelorism), upward slant, and thick epicanthal folds suggest Down syndrome. "Sun-setting" appearance (upper lid covers part of the iris) suggests hydrocephalus.
Observe **eyelid placement, swelling, discharge, and lesions.**	Eyelids have transient edema, absence of tears.	Eyelid inflammation may result from infection. Swelling, erythema, or purulent discharge may indicate infection or blocked tear ducts.
		Purulent discharge seen with sexually transmitted infections (gonorrhea, chlamydia).

Continued on following page

SUBSEQUENT INFANT PHYSICAL ASSESSMENT (Continued)

ASSESSMENT PROCEDURE	NORMAL FINDINGS	ABNORMAL FINDINGS
Inspect the **sclera and conjunctiva** for color, discharge, redness, and lacerations.	Sclera and conjunctiva are clear and free of discharge, lesions, redness, or lacerations. Small subconjunctival hemorrhages may be seen in newborns.	Yellow sclera suggests jaundice, blue sclera may indicate osteogenesis imperfecta ("brittle bone disease").
Observe the **iris and the pupils.**	Typically the iris is blue in light-skinned infants and brown in dark-skinned infants; permanent color develops within 9 months. Brushfield spots (white flecks on the periphery of the iris) may be normal in some infants. Pupils are equal, round, and reactive to light and accommodation (PERRLA).	Brushfield spots may indicate Down syndrome. Sluggish pupils indicate a neurologic problem. Miosis (constriction) indicates iritis or narcotic use or abuse. Mydriasis (pupillary dilation) indicates emotional factors (fear), trauma, or certain drug use.
Inspect the **eyebrows and eyelashes.**	Eyebrows should be symmetric in shape and movement. They should not meet midline. Eyelashes should be evenly distributed and curled outward.	Sparseness of eyebrows or lashes could indicate skin disease.

ASSESSMENT PROCEDURE	NORMAL FINDINGS	ABNORMAL FINDINGS
Perform **visual acuity tests.** Assess visual acuity by observing infant's ability to gaze at an object.	Visual acuity is difficult to test in infants; test by observing the infant's ability to fix on and follow objects. Normal visual acuity is as follows: • Birth: 20/100 to 20/400 • 1 year: 20/200 By 4 weeks of age, the infant should be able to fixate on objects. By 6–8 weeks, eyes should follow a moving object. By 3 months, the infant is able to follow and reach for an object.	Children with a one-line difference between eyes should be referred for ophthalmology exam.
Perform **extraocular muscle tests.** Hirschberg test: Shine light directly at the cornea while the infant looks straight ahead.	In the Hirschberg test, the light reflects symmetrically in the center of both pupils. Light causes pupils to vasoconstrict bilaterally and blink reflex occurs. Blink reflex also occurs as an object is brought toward the eyes. By 10 days of age, when turning the head, the infant's eyes should follow the position of the head.	Unequal alignment of light on the pupils in the Hirschberg test signals strabismus. Doll's eye reflex is an abnormal reflex that occurs when the eyes do not follow or adjust to movement of head.

Continued on following page

SUBSEQUENT INFANT PHYSICAL ASSESSMENT (Continued)

ASSESSMENT PROCEDURE	NORMAL FINDINGS	ABNORMAL FINDINGS
Perform **ophthalmoscopic examination.** The procedure is the same as for adults. Distraction is preferred over the use of restraint, which is likely to result in crying and closed eyes. Careful ophthalmoscopic examination of newborns is difficult without the use of mydriatic medications.	Red reflex is present. This reflex rules out most serious defects of the cornea, aqueous chamber, lens, and vitreous humor. When visualized, the optic disc appears similar to an adult's. A newborn's optic discs are pale; peripheral vessels are not well developed.	Absence of the red reflex indicates cataracts. Papilledema is unusual in children of this age owing to the ability of the fontanelles and sutures to open during increased intracranial pressure. Disc blurring and hemorrhages should be reported immediately. Abnormal findings include congenital defects, such as cataracts.

Ears

Inspect **external ears.** Note placement, discharge, or lesions of the ears.	Top of pinna should cross the eye-occiput line and be within a 10-degree angle of a perpendicular line drawn from the eye-occiput line to the lobe. No unusual structure or markings should appear on the pinna.	Low-set ears with an alignment greater than a 10-degree angle suggest retardation or congenital syndromes, such as Down syndrome. Abnormal shape may suggest renal disease process, which may be hereditary. Preauricular skin tags or sinuses suggest other anomalies of ears, or the renal system.

ASSESSMENT PROCEDURE	NORMAL FINDINGS	ABNORMAL FINDINGS
Inspect **internal ear.** The internal ear examination requires using an otoscope. The nurse should always hold the otoscope in a manner that allows for rapid removal if the child moves. Have the caregiver hold and restrain the infant. Because an infant's external canal is short and straight, pull the pinna down and back.	No excessive cerumen, discharge, lesions, excoriations, or foreign body in external canal. Amniotic fluid/vernix may be present in canal of the ear of newborn. Tympanic membrane is pearly gray to light pink with normal landmarks. Tympanic membranes redden bilaterally when child is crying or febrile.	Presence of foreign bodies or cerumen impaction. Purulent discharge may indicate otitis externa or presence of foreign body. Purulent, serous discharge suggests otitis media. Bloody discharge suggests trauma, and clear discharge may indicate cerebrospinal fluid leak. Perforated tympanic membrane may also be noted.
Hearing acuity. Routine newborn hearing screening is performed in most newborn nurseries 24–48 hours after birth or prior to discharge. In the infant, test hearing acuity by noting the reaction to noise. Stand approximately 30.48 cm (12 in) from the infant and create a loud noise (e.g., clap hands, shake/squeeze a noisy toy).	A newborn will exhibit the startle (Moro) reflex and blink eyes (acoustic blink reflex) in response to noise. Older infant will turn head.	Audiometry results outside normal range suggest hearing deficit. No reactions to noise may indicate a hearing deficit.

Continued on following page

SUBSEQUENT INFANT PHYSICAL ASSESSMENT (Continued)

ASSESSMENT PROCEDURE	NORMAL FINDINGS	ABNORMAL FINDINGS
Mouth, Throat, Nose, and Sinuses		
Inspect **mouth and throat.** Note the condition of the lips, palates, tongue, and buccal mucosa.	Epstein pearls, small yellow-white retention cysts on the hard palate and gums, are common in newborns and usually disappear in the first weeks of life. In infants, a sucking tubercle (pad) from the friction of sucking may be evident in the middle of the upper lip.	White discharge noted on the tongue or buccal mucosa is thrush.

Cleft lip and/or palate are congenital abnormalities.

Excessive salivation, unable to tolerate feedings may indicate esophageal atresia. |
| Observe the **condition of the gums.** When teeth appear, count teeth and note location. | Gums appear pink and moist. Teeth may begin erupting at 4–6 months. Teeth develop in sequential order. By 10 months, most infants have two upper and two lower central incisors. | Abnormal findings include lesion and edema. |
| Inspect **nose and sinuses.** To inspect the nose and sinuses in infants push up the tip of the nose and shine a light into each nostril. Observe the structure and patency of the nares, discharge, tenderness, and any color or swelling of the turbinates. | Nose is midline in face, septum is straight, and nares are patent. No discharge or tenderness is present. Turbinates are pink and free of edema. | Choanal atresia is blockage of the posterior nares in the newborn. If the blockage is bilateral, the newborn is at risk for acute respiratory distress. Immediate referral is necessary. Deviated septum may be congenital or caused by injury. Foul discharge from one nostril may indicate a foreign body. |

ASSESSMENT PROCEDURE	NORMAL FINDINGS	ABNORMAL FINDINGS
Note: Infants are obligatory nose breathers. Consequently obstructed nasal passages may precipitate serious health conditions, making it very important to assess the patency of the nares in the newborn. If, after suctioning fluid and mucus from the nares, you suspect obstruction, insert a small-lumen catheter into each nostril to assess patency.		
Thorax		
Inspect the **shape of the thorax**.	Infant's thorax is smooth, rounded, and symmetric.	Abnormal shapes of the thorax include pectus excavatum and pectus carinatum.
Observe **respiratory effort**, keeping in mind newborns and young infants are obligatory nose breathers.	Respirations should be unlabored and regular in all ages except for immediate newborn period when respirations are irregular (see "Vital Signs" section). Some newborns, especially the premature, have periodic irregular breathing, sometimes with apnea (episodes when breathing stops) lasting a few seconds. This is a normal finding if bradycardia does not accompany irregular breathing.	Retractions (suprasternal, sternal, substernal, intercostal) and grunting suggest increased inspiratory effort, which may be due to airway obstruction. Periods of apnea that last longer than 15 seconds and are accompanied by bradycardia may be a sign of a cardiovascular or CNS disease. Nasal flaring, tachypnea, and see-saw movement of chest indicate respiratory distress.

Continued on following page

SUBSEQUENT INFANT PHYSICAL ASSESSMENT (Continued)

ASSESSMENT PROCEDURE	NORMAL FINDINGS	ABNORMAL FINDINGS
Auscultate for **breath sounds and adventitious sounds.** If a newborn lung sounds seem noisy, auscultate the upper nostrils.	Breath sounds may seem louder and harsher in young children because of their thin chest walls. No adventitious sounds should be heard although transmitted upper airway sounds may be heard on auscultation of thorax.	Diminished breath sounds suggest respiratory disorders such as pneumonia or atelectasis. Stridor (inspiratory wheeze) is a high-pitched, piercing sound that indicates a narrowing of the upper tracheobronchial tree. Expiratory wheezes indicate narrowing in the lower tracheobronchial tree. Rhonchi and rales (crackles) may indicate a number of respiratory diseases such as pneumonia, bronchitis, or bronchiolitis.
Breasts		
Inspect and palpate **breasts.** Note shape, symmetry, color, tenderness, discharge, lesions, and masses.	Newborns may have enlarged and engorged breasts with a white liquid discharge resulting from the influence of maternal hormones. This condition resolves spontaneously within days.	A palpable mass of the breast is abnormal. The newborn or infant may have extra nipples noted on the chest or abdomen called supernumerary nipples.

ASSESSMENT PROCEDURE	NORMAL FINDINGS	ABNORMAL FINDINGS
Heart		
Inspect and palpate the **precordium.** Note lifts, heaves, apical impulse.	The apical pulse is at the 4th intercostal space (ICS) until the age of 7 years, when it drops to the 5th. It is to the left of the midclavicular line (MCL) until age 4.	A systolic heave may indicate right ventricular enlargement. Apical impulse that is not in proper location for age may indicate cardiomyopathy, pneumothorax, or diaphragmatic hernia.
Auscultate **heart sounds.** Listen to the heart. Note rate and rhythm of apical impulse, S_1, S_2, extra heart sounds, and murmurs. Keep in mind that sinus arrhythmia is normal in infants. Heart sounds are louder, higher pitched, and of shorter duration in infants. A split S_2 at the apex occurs normally in some infants and S_3 is a normal heart sound in some children. A venous hum also may be normally heard in children.	Normal heart rates are cited in the "Vital Signs" section above. Innocent murmurs, which are common throughout childhood, are classified as systolic; short duration; no transmission to other areas; grade III or less; loudest in pulmonic area (base of heart); low-pitched, musical, or groaning quality that varies in intensity in relation to position, respiration, activity, fever, and anemia. No other associated signs of heart disease should be found.	Murmurs that do not fit the criteria for innocent murmurs may indicate a disease or disorder. Extra heart sounds and variations in pulse rate and rhythm also suggest pathologic processes.

Continued on following page

SUBSEQUENT INFANT PHYSICAL ASSESSMENT (Continued)

ASSESSMENT PROCEDURE	NORMAL FINDINGS	ABNORMAL FINDINGS
Abdomen		
Inspect the shape of the abdomen.	In infants, the abdomen shape is cylindrical, round, soft.	A scaphoid (boat-shaped; i.e., sunken with prominent rib cage) abdomen may result from malnutrition or dehydration. Distended abdomen may indicate pyloric stenosis.
Inspect **umbilicus**. Note color, discharge, evident herniation of the umbilicus.	Umbilicus is pink, no discharge, odor, redness, or herniation. Cord should demonstrate three vessels (two arteries and one vein). Remnant of cord should appear dried 24–48 hours after birth.	Inflammation, discharge, and redness of umbilicus suggest infection. Diastasis recti (separation of the abdominal muscles) is seen as midline protrusion from the xiphoid to the umbilicus or pubis symphysis. This condition is secondary to immature musculature of abdominal muscles and usually has little significance. As the muscles strengthen, the separation resolves on its own.

ASSESSMENT PROCEDURE	NORMAL FINDINGS	ABNORMAL FINDINGS
		A bulge at the umbilicus suggests an umbilical hernia, which may be seen in newborns; many disappear by the age of 1 year (Fig. 25-12).
		Abnormal insertion of cord, discolored cord, or two-vessel cord could indicate genetic abnormalities; however, these are also seen in newborns without abnormalities.

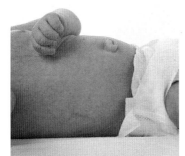

FIGURE 25-12 Umbilical hernia.

| Auscultate **bowel sounds.** Follow auscultation guidelines for adult clients provided in Chapter 22. | Bowel sounds present 30–60 minutes after birth. Normal bowel sounds occur every 10–30 seconds. They sound like clicks, gurgles, or growls. | Marked peristaltic waves almost always indicate a pathologic process such as pyloric stenosis. |

Continued on following page

SUBSEQUENT INFANT PHYSICAL ASSESSMENT (Continued)

ASSESSMENT PROCEDURE	NORMAL FINDINGS	ABNORMAL FINDINGS
Palpate for **masses and tenderness.** Palpate abdomen for softness or hardness.	Abdomen is soft to palpation and without masses or tenderness.	A rigid abdomen is almost always an emergent problem. Masses or tenderness warrants further investigation. Hirschsprung disease could also be considered, especially with suprapubic mass palpable.
Palpate **liver.** Palpate the liver the same as you would for adults (see Chapter 22).	Liver is usually palpable 1–2 cm below the right costal margin. *Note: It is difficult to palpate in the newborn.*	An enlarged liver with a firm edge that is palpated more than 2 cm below the right costal margin usually indicates a pathologic process.
Palpate **spleen.** Palpate the spleen the same as you would for adults.	Spleen tip may be palpable during inspiration. The spleen is difficult to palpate in the newborn.	Enlarged spleen is usually indicative of a pathologic process.
Palpate **kidneys.** Palpate the kidneys the same as you would for adults.	The tip of the right kidney may be palpable during inspiration.	Enlarged kidneys are usually indicative of a pathologic process.
Palpate **bladder.** Palpate the bladder the same as you would for adults.	Bladder may be slightly palpable in infants and small children. The newborn voids within first 24 hours after birth. No urinary output beyond 48 hours after birth	An enlarged bladder is usually due to urinary retention but may be due to a mass.

ASSESSMENT PROCEDURE	NORMAL FINDINGS	ABNORMAL FINDINGS
Male Genitalia		
Inspect **penis and urinary meatus.** Inspect the genitalia, observing size for age and any lesions.	Penis is normal size for age, and no lesions are seen. Diaper rash, however, is a common finding in infants. The foreskin is retractable in uncircumcised child. Urinary meatus is at tip of glans penis and has no discharge or redness. Penis may appear small in large for gestational age (LGA) boys because of overlapping skinfolds. For circumcised boys, the site is dry with minimal swelling and drainage.	An unretractable foreskin in a child older than 3 months suggests phimosis. Paraphimosis is indicated when the foreskin is tightened around the glans penis in a retracted position. Hypospadias, urinary meatus on ventral surface of glans, and epispadias, urinary meatus on dorsal surface of glans, are congenital disorders.
Inspect and palpate **scrotum and testes.** To rule out cryptorchidism, it is important to palpate for testes in the scrotum in infants.	Scrotum is free of lesions. Testes are palpable in scrotum with the left testicle usually lower than the right. Testes are equal in size, smooth, mobile, and free of masses. If a testicle is missing from the scrotal sac but the scrotal sac appears well developed, suspect physi-ologic cryptorchidism. The testis has originally descended into the scrotum but has moved	Absent testicle(s) and atrophic scrotum suggest true cryptorchidism (undescended testicles). This suggests that the testicle(s) never descended. This condition occurs more frequently in preterm than term infants because testes descend at 8 months of gestation. It can lead to testicular atrophy and infertility, and increases the risk for testicular cancer.

Continued on following page

SUBSEQUENT INFANT PHYSICAL ASSESSMENT (Continued)		
ASSESSMENT PROCEDURE	**NORMAL FINDINGS**	**ABNORMAL FINDINGS**
	back up into the inguinal canal because of the cremasteric reflex and the small size of the testis. You should be able to milk the testis down into the scrotum from the inguinal canal. This normal condition subsides at puberty.	Hydroceles are common in infants. They are a collection of fluid along the spermatic cord within the scrotum that can be transilluminated. They usually resolve spontaneously.
		A scrotal hernia is usually caused by an indirect inguinal hernia that has descended into the scrotum. It can usually be pushed back into the inguinal canal. This mass will not transilluminate.
Inspect and palpate **inguinal area for hernias.** Observe for any bulge in the inguinal area. Using your pinky finger, palpate up the inguinal canal to the external inguinal ring if a hernia is suspected.	No inguinal hernias are present.	A bulge in the inguinal area or palpation of a mass in the inguinal canal suggests an inguinal hernia. Indirect inguinal hernias occur most frequently in children.

ASSESSMENT PROCEDURE	NORMAL FINDINGS	ABNORMAL FINDINGS
Female Genitalia		
Inspect **external genitalia**. Note labia majora, labia minora, vaginal orifice, urinary meatus, and clitoris.	Labia majora and minora are pink and moist. Newborn's genitalia may appear prominent because of influence of maternal hormones. Bruises and swelling may be caused by breech vaginal delivery. Pseudomenstruation (blood-tinged discharge), smegma (cheesy white discharge) of the sebaceous gland. Reddish, orange, pink-tinged urine or stained on diaper may also be normal due to uric acid crystals.	Enlarged clitoris in newborn combined with fusion of the posterior labia majora suggests ambiguous genitalia.
Anus and Rectum		
Inspect the **anus**. The anus should be inspected in infants. Spread the buttocks with gloved hands; note patency of anal opening, presence of any lesions and fissures, and condition and color of perianal skin.	The anal opening should be visible and moist. Meconium is passed within 24–48 hours after birth. Perianal skin should be smooth and free of lesions. Perianal skin tags may be noted.	Imperforate anus (no anal opening) should be referred. No passage of meconium stool could indicate no patency of anus or cystic fibrosis. Pustules may indicate secondary infection of diaper rash.

Continued on following page

SUBSEQUENT INFANT PHYSICAL ASSESSMENT (Continued)

ASSESSMENT PROCEDURE	NORMAL FINDINGS	ABNORMAL FINDINGS
Musculoskeletal		
Assess **arms, hands, feet, and legs.** Note symmetry, shape, movement, and positioning of the feet and legs. Perform neurovascular assessment.	Five fingers and toes on each extremity, no webbing, normal palmar creases. Bilateral movement with full ROM in arms and legs. Legs have equal length, normal position of feet.	Short, broad extremities, hyperextensible joints, and palmar simian crease may indicate Down syndrome. Polydactyly (extra digits) and syndactyly (webbing) are sometimes found in children with mental retardation. Fixed-position (true) deformities do not return to normal position with manipulation. Meta-tarsus varus is inversion (a turning inward that elevates the medial margin) and adduction of the forefoot. Talipes varus is adduction of the forefoot and inversion of the entire foot. Talipes equinovarus (clubfoot) is indicated if foot is fixed in the following position: adduction of forefoot, inversion of entire foot, and equinus (pointing downward) position of entire foot.

ASSESSMENT PROCEDURE	NORMAL FINDINGS	ABNORMAL FINDINGS
Assess for **congenital hip dysplasia.** Assessing for hip dysplasia is an important aspect of the physical examination for infants. The assessment should be performed at each visit until the child is about 1 year old. (Several tests are described below.)	Symmetrical bilateral gluteal folds and full hip abduction are normal findings.	Unequal gluteal folds and limited hip abduction are signs of congenital hip dysplasia.
Begin by assessing the symmetry of the gluteal folds. Also assess hip abduction using the maneuvers below.		
Perform Ortolani maneuver to test for congenital hip dysplasia. With the infant supine, flex infant's knees while holding your thumbs on midthigh and your fingers over the greater trochanters; abduct the legs, moving the knees outward and down toward the table.	Negative Ortolani sign is normal.	Positive Ortolani sign: A click heard along with feeling the head of the femur slip in or out of the hip.
Perform Barlow maneuvers. With the infant supine, flex the infant's knees while holding your thumbs on midthigh and your fingers over the greater trochanters; adduct legs until thumbs touch.	Negative Barlow sign is normal.	Positive Barlow sign: A feeling of the head of the femur slipping out of the hip socket (acetabulum).

Continued on following page

SUBSEQUENT INFANT PHYSICAL ASSESSMENT (Continued)

ASSESSMENT PROCEDURE	NORMAL FINDINGS	ABNORMAL FINDINGS
Assess **spinal alignment.** Observe spine and posture.	No spinal openings. In newborns, the spine is flexible and rounded in infants younger than 3 months old (Fig. 25-13).	Opening in spinal column, pilonidal dimple could indicate spina bifida or other spinal abnormalities. In newborns, flaccid or rigid posture is considered abnormal. In older infants, abnormal posture suggests neuromuscular disorders such as cerebral palsy.

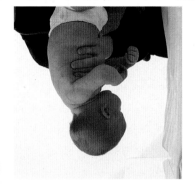

FIGURE 25-13 The spine is rounded in infants less than the age of 3 months.

ASSESSMENT PROCEDURE	NORMAL FINDINGS	ABNORMAL FINDINGS
Assess **joints.** Note range of motion, swelling, redness, and tenderness.	Full range of motion and no swelling, redness, or tenderness.	Limited range of motion, swelling, redness, and tenderness indicate problems ranging from mild injuries to serious disorders.
Assess **muscles.** Note size and strength. (For example, can the infant bear weight on her legs?)	Muscle size and strength should be adequate for the particular age and should be equal bilaterally.	Inadequate muscle size and strength for the particular age indicate neuromuscular disorders such as muscular dystrophy.
Neurologic System		
Assess the newborn's and infant's **cry, responsiveness, and adaptation.**	The newborn's and infant's cries are lusty and strong; responds appropriately to stimuli and quiets to soothing when held in the en face position.	Inappropriate response to stimuli suggests CNS disorders or problems. An inability to quiet to soothing and gaze aversion is seen in "cocaine babies." Infantile reflexes present when inappropriate, absent, or asymmetric may indicate a CNS problem.
Test **deep tendon and superficial reflexes** (see Chapter 21).	Infantile reflexes are present when appropriate and are symmetric.	Absence or marked intensity of these reflexes, asymmetry may demonstrate pathology.
Test **motor function.** See Developmental Assessment section in the beginning of the subsequent infant physical assessment.		

POSSIBLE COLLABORATIVE PROBLEMS—RISK OF

- Elevated bilirubin levels
- Infection
- Circumcision
- Nosocomial
- Bacterial

Teaching Tips for Selected Nursing Diagnoses

*Nursing Diagnosis: **Ineffective Breathing Pattern** related to transient alteration in lung expansion*

Monitor respiratory status every 30 minutes × 4 until stable, then per protocol. Auscultate breath sounds per protocol. Promote oxygenation and fluid drainage by placing infant on side; use postural drainage with head of bed slightly lower than body. Have suction equipment ready for use.

*Nursing Diagnosis: **Risk for Suffocation, Sudden Infant Death Syndrome (SIDS)** related to newborn status and mother's lack of knowledge of safe infant positioning in bed*

Healthy infants should be placed on their back, using a firm sleep surface, when putting them to sleep (Task Force on Sudden Infant Death Syndrome, 2011).

*Nursing Diagnosis: **Ineffective Thermoregulation** related to newborn decrease in body fat and cool environment*

Assess temperature every 30 minutes × 4, then per protocol. Maintain temperature at 36.4 to 37.3 °C (97.6 to 99.2 °F). Keep infant temperature probe attached properly to skin to ensure reading probe accurately. Monitor for signs and symptoms of cold stress. Keep infant warm and dry. Postpone bath until temperature is stable. Apply cap to head and extra blankets to infant if temperature <36.4 °C (97.6 °F). Teach parents mechanisms of heat loss: radiation, convection, conduction, evaporation. Teach techniques used to prevent cold stress and to maintain or increase infant temperature (e.g., dress, cap, blanket wrap, cuddle). Teach parents correct procedure in taking newborn axillary temperature, reading thermometer, interpreting results.

*Nursing Diagnosis: **Imbalanced Nutrition**: less than body requirements related to low maternal pregnancy weight gain and infant's poor feeding pattern*

Review prenatal history, looking for maternal risk factors such as gestational diabetes. Assess for hypoglycemia, checking blood glucose values at birth and at 1 hour of age or per hospital protocol. Weigh infant on admission and daily. Auscultate bowel sounds every shift. Assess for rooting/sucking behaviors. Initiate breast-bottle-feeding at birth and on demand for breastfeeding and per hospital protocol for bottlefeeding. Record frequency, amount, and length of feeding. If regurgitation occurs, note frequency and amount. Monitor newborn stools/voids and record per shift. Observe for feeding problems (refusal to eat, regurgitation, gagging, difficulty swallowing, difficulty with latching onto breast, etc.). Evaluate neonate after feeding for satisfaction of feeding. Observe parents/newborn for feeding problems; encourage questions and problem solving for parents regarding feeding difficulties or concerns.

CHAPTER 26

Assessing Older Adults

Common physical findings in older adult clients have been identified throughout the preceding body system chapters. Advancing age places a person at greater risk for chronic illness and disability. It is not, however, the physiologic changes of aging alone that warrant a special approach to assessment of the older adult client. Many older adults are healthy, active, and independent despite these normal physical changes in their bodies. It is, rather, that advancing age has a tendency to place a person at greater risk for chronic illness and disability. The term "frail elderly" describes the vulnerability of the "old-old" (generally

mideighties, nineties, and centenarians) to be in poorer health, to have more chronic disabilities, and to function less independently. Loss of physiologic reserve is the main reason that older adults are more likely to be sick and disabled.

Older Adult Nursing Assessment

When the physiology of advanced age is combined with comorbidity, assessment is complicated. In fact, the signs and symptoms of illness often present differently in the oldest-old. Adverse events or adverse drug effects in this population often include falls, confusion, incontinence, generalized weakness, and lethargy. These complications are referred to as geriatric syndromes and are more common signs and symptoms of illness in the very old than are the more common manifestations of illness in younger adults such as fever, pain, and abnormal lab values. The population at greatest risk for developing atypical presentation are the very old who also have cognitive or functional impairment, multiple comorbidities, and who are being treated with multiple medications (Micelli & Mezey, 2007).

Knowing the older person's usual daily pattern and functional level is the best baseline against which to compare assessment data.

COLLECTING SUBJECTIVE DATA

Be sensitive to the older person's need to be respected and acknowledged. Always begin the interview by addressing an older person as "Mr.," "Mrs.," or "Ms.," or with an appropriate title such as "Reverend" or "Doctor." If the older person is too lethargic, agitated, or medically unstable to respond, family or professional caregivers should be queried with regard to how current cognition and behavior compares with the client's prior level of function.

Mental status: History of falls, weakness, incontinence, confusion, sleep difficulties, or loss of appetite? Social and economic resources? Current living environment including any isolation, physical barriers, or neglect? Changes in your memory? Anger or inability to control your frustrations?

Falls: Use of assistive devices to walk or for balance? Lightheaded or dizzy when getting up from chair or bed? Difficulty getting up out of bed or from sitting in a chair? Stiffness and soreness inhibit ability to move about? Feel like legs are going to "give way" or weak?

Weakness: Fatigue and dyspnea: Daily activities and exercise? Leg pain, cramping, aching, fatigue, or weakness in the calf? Change in energy level and effects on daily activities? Shortness of breath and relationship to activities? Sweating, cough, and production?

Weakness: Nutrition and hydration: Daily nutrition and habits? Change in weight or appetite? A screening tool (36-hour food diary or Mini-Nutritional Assessment) may be helpful in identifying those at risk for being malnourished. Anorexia? Choking? Amount of fluid intake? Pneumococcal vaccine?

Urinary incontinence: Leakage, difficulty starting stream, dribbling, nighttime medications? (Male) Do you have difficulty starting a stream of urine? Frequency? Nighttime frequency? Dribbling?

Bowel elimination: Problems with bowel elimination? Change in bowel habits? Blood in stools? Narcotics?

Pain: Pain, discomfort, aching, or soreness? Relieved by rest or aggravated with activity? If the older adult is nonverbal and demented, routinely evaluate behaviors such as grimacing, striking out, moaning, and agitation to identify pain as well as to evaluate the degree to which the pain is being relieved (Box 26-1).

COLLECTING OBJECTIVE DATA

Equipment Needed

The following items will be needed for assessing the functional capacity of the frail elderly adult.
• Newspaper or book and lamplight for vision testing.
• Lemon slice or mint for sense of smell test.

BOX 26-1   ASSESSMENT OF PAIN IN OLDER ADULT CLIENTS WITH OR WITHOUT COGNITIVE IMPAIRMENT

Baricek (2010) lists tools and behaviors for assessing pain in older adults with and without cognitive impairment.

To assess pain in the *cognitively impaired older adult*, consider the following indicators of pain:
• Medical diagnoses known to commonly cause pain such as arthritis, osteoporosis, fractures, cancer, and history of back pain.
• Pain history and use of analgesics.
• Family or professional caregiver reports of possible pain.
• Behavioral patterns of aggressiveness or resisting care.

In addition, observe behaviors that may indicate pain: facial expressions (frowning, grimacing); vocalization (crying, groaning); change in body language (rocking, guarding); rubbing on specific areas of body; behavioral change (refusing to eat, alteration in usual patterns); physiologic change (blood pressure, heart rate); and physical change (skin tears, pressure areas). A good pain assessment scale to use for the older adult with cognitive impairment is the Faces Pain Scale—Revised (FPS-R) (Flaherty, 2008) (see Chapter 7).

To assess pain in the older adult *without* cognitive impairment, use one of the three following pain assessment tools: Visual Analog Scale (VAS), the Verbal Numerical Rating Scale (VNRS), or the categorical rating scale using words such as "none (0)," "mild (1)," "moderate (2)," or "severe (3)." The VNRS has been shown to be the best scale for assessing pain in older adults with no cognitive impairment. See Chapter 7 for more details of pain assessment scales.

- Pudding or food of pudding consistency and spoon for swallowing examination. A teacup may also be used.
- Food and fluid diary sheets or forms.
- Two or three pillows for client comfort and positioning.
- Straight-backed chair for "Get Up and Go" test.

Physical Assessment

ASSESSMENT PROCEDURE	NORMAL FINDINGS/VARIATIONS	ABNORMAL FINDINGS
Measure client's height and weight, noting weight changes, appetite changes and problems with swallowing or chewing. **Review laboratory values** (complete blood count and levels of vitamin B_{12}, cholesterol, albumin, and prealbumin).	Antral cells and intestinal villi atrophy, and gastric production of hydrochloric acid decreases with age. Chronic diseases such as cancer and arthritis are associated with increases in inflammatory chemicals that can cause anorexia and fatigue. A certain degree of anorexia also always accompanies pain—especially chronic pain.	Indicators of malnutrition include the following: • Client weighs <80% of ideal body weight. • Client has had 10% loss in body weight over past 6 months or 5% loss in body weight over past month. **Note:** *Suspect drug toxicity in clients taking medications such as digoxin, theophylline, quinidine, or antibiotics if client reports nausea, diarrhea, or sudden and severe appetite loss.* Hemoglobin level is <12 g/dL. Hematocrit is <35%. Vitamin B_{12} level is <100 µg/mL. Indicators of poor nutritional status include serum cholesterol level <160 mg/dL; serum albumin level <3.5 g/dL; prealbumin level <19.5 hg/dL.

Continued on following page

ASSESSMENT PROCEDURE	NORMAL FINDINGS/VARIATIONS	ABNORMAL FINDINGS
Evaluate hydration status as you would evaluate nutritional status. Begin with accurate serial measurements of weight, careful review of laboratory test findings (serial serum sodium level, hematocrit, osmolality, BUN level, and urine-specific gravity), and a 2- to 3-day diary of fluid intake and output.	Normal findings include stable weight and stable mental status. *Note: Increases over time in laboratory values may be indicators of deteriorating hydration (even though values may be within normal limits).*	Sudden weight loss; fever; dry, warm skin; furrowed, swollen, and red tongue; decreased urine output; lethargy and weakness are all signs of dehydration. An acute change in mental status (particularly confusion), tachycardia, and hypotension may indicate severe dehydration, which may be precipitated by certain medications such as diuretics, laxatives, tricyclic antidepressants, or lithium.

SKIN AND HAIR

PROCEDURE	NORMAL FINDINGS/VARIATIONS	ABNORMAL FINDINGS
Inspect and palpate skin lesions. Wear gloves while palpating lesions (flat, raised, palpable or nonpalpable; color, size, and exudates).	Despite decrease in total number of melanocytes, hyperpigmentation occurs in sun-exposed skin (neck, face, and arms). Environmental exposure and diminished immunity increase risk of skin cancer and cutaneous infections such as ringworm, candidal infections of mouth, vagina, and nail beds. This risk is increased in diabetes mellitus, malnutrition, steroid, or antibiotic use.	Abnormal findings include the following: • Irregularly shaped lesion or scaly, elevated lesion (squamous cell carcinoma). • Actinic keratoses, round or irregularly shaped tan, scaly lesions that may bleed or be inflamed (premalignancy). • Waxy or raised lesion, especially on sun-exposed areas (basal cell carcinoma).

PROCEDURE	NORMAL FINDINGS/VARIATIONS	ABNORMAL FINDINGS
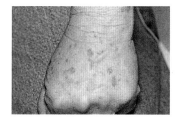 **FIGURE 26-1** Solar lentigines are very common on aging skin.	Normal variations include the following: • Lentigines: Hyperpigmentation in sun-exposed areas appears as brown, pigmented, round or rectangular patches, often called liver spots (Fig. 26-1). • Venous lakes: Reddish vascular lesions on ears or other facial areas resulting from dilation of small, red blood vessels. • Skin tags: Acrochordons, flesh-colored pedunculated lesions. • Seborrheic keratoses: Tan, brown, or reddish, flat lesions commonly found on fair-skinned people in sun-exposed areas. • Cherry angiomas: Small, round, red spots. • Senile purpura: Vivid purple patches (lesion should not blanch to touch).	• Herpes zoster vesicles (shingles) draining clear fluid or pustules atop an erythematous base following a clear linear pattern and accompanied by pain. More than half of elderly with shingles will have neuralgia that persists after resolution of the skin lesions. • Pinpoint-sized, red-purple, nonblanchable petechia (common sign of platelet deficiency). • Large bruises may result from anticoagulant therapy, a fall, renal or liver failure, or elder abuse.

Continued on following page

SKIN AND HAIR (Continued)

PROCEDURE	NORMAL FINDINGS/VARIATIONS	ABNORMAL FINDINGS
Note color, texture, integrity, and moisture of skin and sensitivity to heat or cold. *Note: Pinching skin is not an accurate test of turgor in older adults.*	Somewhat transparent, pale skin with an overall decrease in body hair on lower extremities. Dry skin is common. Elastic collagen is gradually replaced with more fibrous tissue and loss of subcutaneous tissue. Skin may wrinkle and tent when pinched.	Torn skin (possibly the result of abrasive tape used to hold bandages or tubes in place). Extremely thin, fragile skin (friable skin) with excessive purpura (possibly from corticosteroid use). Dry, warm skin, furrowed tongue, and sunken eyes due to dehydration (especially with decreased urinary output, increased serum sodium, BUN, and creatinine levels, increased osmolality, and hematocrit values, tachycardia; and mental confusion). Sudden heat or cold intolerance could be signs of thyroid dysfunction. Decreased vascularity and diminished neurologic response to temperature changes and atrophy of eccrine sweat glands increase risk of hyperthermia and hypothermia.

PROCEDURE	NORMAL FINDINGS/VARIATIONS	ABNORMAL FINDINGS
Inspect and palpate hair, scalp, and nails.	Loss of pigmentation causes graying of scalp, axillary, and pubic hair.	Patchy or asymmetric hair loss is abnormal.
	Mild hair growth on upper lip of women may appear as a result of decreased estrogen to testosterone ratio. Toenails usually thicken while fingernails often become thinner. Both usually become yellowish and dull.	

HEAD AND NECK

ASSESSMENT PROCEDURE	NORMAL FINDINGS/VARIATIONS	ABNORMAL FINDINGS
Inspect head and neck for symmetry and movement. Observe facial expression (Fig. 26-2).	Atrophy of face and neck muscles.	Abnormalities include the following:
	Reduced range of motion (ROM) of head and neck.	• Asymmetry of mouth or eyes possibly from Bell palsy or stroke (cerebral vascular accident; CVA).
	Shortening of neck due to vertebral degeneration and development of "buffalo hump" at the top of cervical vertebrae.	• Marked limitation of movement or crepitation in back of neck from cervical arthritis.
		• Involuntary facial or head movements from an extrapyramidal disorder such as Parkinson disease or some medications.

Continued on following page

HEAD AND NECK (Continued)		
ASSESSMENT PROCEDURE	**NORMAL FINDINGS/VARIATIONS**	**ABNORMAL FINDINGS**

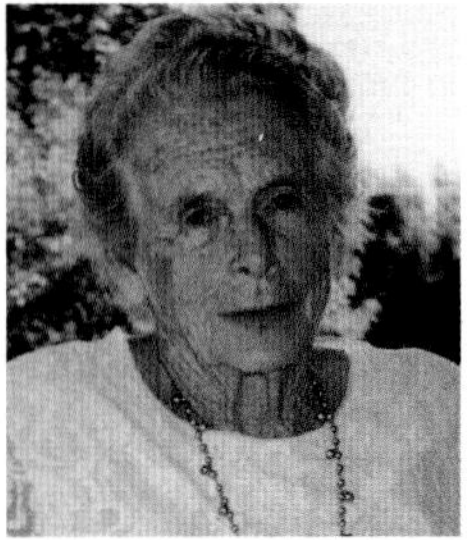

FIGURE 26-2 Observe facial expression.

MOUTH AND THROAT		
ASSESSMENT PROCEDURE	**NORMAL FINDINGS/VARIATIONS**	**ABNORMAL FINDINGS**
Inspect the gums and buccal mucosa for color, consistency, and odor.	Slight decrease in saliva production.	Saliva-depressing medications include antihistamines, antipsychotics, and antihypertensives, and any drug with anticholinergic side effects may promote dental caries and increase risk of pneumonia.

ASSESSMENT PROCEDURE	NORMAL FINDINGS/VARIATIONS	ABNORMAL FINDINGS
		Foul-smelling breath may indicate periodontal disease.
		Whitish or yellow-tinged patches in mouth or throat may be candidiasis from use of steroid inhalers or antibiotics.
If the client is wearing dentures, inspect them for fit. Then ask the client to remove them for the rest of the oral examination.	Resorption of gum ridge commonly results in poorly fitting dentures. Tooth surfaces may be worn from prolonged use.	Loose-fitting dentures or inability to close mouth completely may also be the result of a significant weight gain or loss.
Examine the tongue. Observe symmetry and size.	Tongue pink and moist.	A swollen, red, and painful tongue may indicate vitamin B or riboflavin deficiency.
Observe the client swallowing food or fluids.	Mild decrease in swallowing ability.	Coughing, drooling, pocketing, or spitting out food are all possible signs of dysphagia. A drooping mouth, chronic congestion, or a weak or hoarse voice (especially after eating or drinking) suggests dysphagia.
Depress the posterior third of the tongue and note gag reflex.	Gag reflex may be slightly sluggish.	Absence of a gag reflex may be the result of a neurologic disorder.

Continued on following page

NOSE AND SINUSES

ASSESSMENT PROCEDURE	NORMAL FINDINGS/VARIATIONS	ABNORMAL FINDINGS
Inspect the nose for color and consistency.	Nose and nasal passages are not inflamed, and skin and mucous membranes are intact.	Edema, redness, swelling, or clear drainage, which may indicate allergies or rhinitis.
	Nose may seem more prominent on face because of loss of subcutaneous fat. Nasal hairs are coarser.	**Note:** *Relocation into a newly constructed residential or long-term care facility should be investigated further as a possible cause of allergic or nonallergic rhinitis due to exposure of new carpet, fiberboard, or paint fumes.*
Evaluate the sense of smell. Have the client close the eyes and smell a common substance, such as mint, lemon, or soap.	Slightly diminished sense of smell and ability to detect odors.	Client cannot identify strong odor. This may cause a decrease in appetite and may be a safety concern.
Test nasal patency by asking the client to breathe while blocking one nostril at a time.	Breathes with reasonable ease.	Client reports feeling of inadequate intake of air with respirations that may result from nasal polyps, a deviated septum, or allergic or infectious rhinitis or sinusitis.

ASSESSMENT PROCEDURE	NORMAL FINDINGS/VARIATIONS	ABNORMAL FINDINGS
Palpate the frontal and maxillary sinuses for consistency and to elicit possible pain. **Note:** *Older adult clients with nasogastric feeding tubes are at increased risk for sinusitis related to the obstruction.*	No lesions or pain.	Client reports pain and dryness; inflammation is evident. **Note:** *Older clients may self-treat sinus pain and/or nasal congestion with decongestants and antihistamines, which may further dry the nasal passages and prevent normal sinus drainage.*

EYES AND VISION

ASSESSMENT PROCEDURE	NORMAL FINDINGS/VARIATIONS	ABNORMAL FINDINGS
Inspect eyes, eyelids, eyelashes, and con-junctiva. Also observe eye and conjunctiva for dryness, redness, tearing, or increased sensitivity to light and wind.	Skin around the eyes becomes thin, and wrinkles appear normally with age. Stretched skin in eyelid may produce feeling of heaviness and a tired feeling. In lower eyelid, "bags" form. Excessive stretching of lower eyelid may cause it to droop downward, which keeps it from shutting completely and can cause dryness, redness, or sensitivity to light and wind. Eyes feel irritated or "scratchy."	A turning in of the lower eyelid (entropion) is more common and causes the eyelashes to touch the conjunctiva and cornea. Severe entropion may result in an ulcerous corneal infection. Abnormalities in blinking may result from Parkinson disease; dull or blank staring may be a sign of hypothyroidism.

Continued on following page

EYES AND VISION (continued)

ASSESSMENT PROCEDURE	NORMAL FINDINGS/VARIATIONS	ABNORMAL FINDINGS
Inspect the cornea and lens. Also ask the client when he or she last had an eye and vision examination. **Note:** *To detect glaucoma, tonometry should be performed every 1–2 years on everyone older than 35 years of age. Elevated intraocular pressure indicates the need for referral to an ophthalmologist and confirmation with applanation tonometry.*	An arcus senilis, a cloudy or grayish ring around the iris, and decreased pigment in iris are age-related changes. The lens loses elasticity, which results in decreased ability to change shape (presbyopia). A loss of transparency in the crystalline lens of the eyes is a natural part of aging process. Exposure to sunlight, smoking, and inherited tendencies increases risk.	Cataracts most commonly affect people after age 55 and result in a yellowish or brownish discoloration of the lens. Common symptoms include painless blurring of vision, glare and halos around lights, poor night vision, colors that look dull or brownish. A thickening of the bulbar conjunctiva that grows over the cornea (called pterygium) may interfere with vision.
Inspect the pupils. With a penlight or similar device, test pupillary reaction to light.	Overall decrease in size of pupil and ability to dilate in dark and constrict in light may occur with advanced age; this results in poorer night vision and decreased tolerance to glare.	An irregularly shaped pupil may indicate removal of a cataract. Asymmetric response may be due to a neurologic condition.

ASSESSMENT PROCEDURE	NORMAL FINDINGS/VARIATIONS	ABNORMAL FINDINGS
Test vision. Ask the client to read from a newspaper or magazine. Use only room lighting for the initial reading. Use task lighting for a second reading. Ask about changes in vision, trouble with night vision, or differences in vision with left versus right eye. Also ask client about small specks or "clouds" that move across the field of vision.	Impaired near vision is indicative of presbyopia (farsightedness), a common finding in older adults. Also common are slight decreases in peripheral vision and difficulty in differentiating blues from greens. *Note: Older adults generally require two to three times more diffuse and task lighting.* With aging, tiny clumps of gel may develop within the eye. These are referred to as "floaters." They should occur occasionally and not increase significantly in frequency.	A significant decrease in central vision, to the extent needed for activities of daily living, may signal a *cataract* in one or both eyes. *Macular degeneration* (thin membrane in the center of the retina) is suspected if the client has difficulty in seeing with one eye (Box 26-2). The disorder almost always becomes bilateral. Related abnormal findings include blurry words in the center of the page or door frames that do not appear straight. This condition should be referred and evaluated. A noticeable loss of vision—including cloudiness, distortion of familiar objects, and occasionally blind spots or floaters—is a common symptom of *diabetic retinopathy*. New floaters or an increase in frequency of floaters associated with flashes of light may be a sign of *retinal detachment* and requires immediate referral to prevent blindness (see Box 26-2).

BOX 26-2   AGE-RELATED ABNORMALITIES OF THE EYE

Common age-related abnormalities of the eye include glaucoma, macular degeneration, retinal detachment, and diabetic retinopathy.

GLAUCOMA

The client with glaucoma is usually symptom-free. In older adults, diabetes and atherosclerosis are conditions that increase the risk of glaucoma. The disorder is caused by increased pressure that can destroy the optic nerve and cause blindness if not treated properly. An acute form of glaucoma can occur at any age and is a true medical emergency because blindness can result in a day or two without treatment. Rainbow-like halos or circles around lights, severe pain in the eyes or forehead, nausea, and blurred vision may occur with the acute form of glaucoma.

MACULAR DEGENERATION

Macular degeneration, a gradual loss of central vision, is caused by aging and thinning of the micro-thin membrane in the center of the retina called the macula. Additional risk factors include sunlight exposure, family history, and white race. Most cases begin to develop after age 50, but damage may be occurring for months to years before symptoms occur. Peripheral vision is not affected, and the condition may occur initially in only one eye. Only about 10% of all age-related macular degeneration leaks occur in the small blood vessels in the retinal pigment epithelium. This type accounts for the most serious loss of vision.

RETINA DETACHMENT

Retinal detachment occurs at a greater frequency with aging as the vitreous pulls away from its attachment to the retina at the back of the eye, causing the retina to tear in one or more places. A retinal detachment is always a serious problem. Blindness will result if the detachment is not treated.

DIABETIC RETINOPATHY

Many older adults have diabetes, which can lead to cataracts, glaucoma, and diabetic retinopathy. Of those with diabetes mellitus, about 90% will develop diabetic retinopathy to some degree. The more serious of the two forms of the disease, proliferative diabetic retinopathy, occurs most often among those who have had diabetes for more than 25 years. People with the advanced form of the disease usually experience a noticeable loss of vision, including cloudiness, distortion of familiar objects, and, occasionally, blind spots or floaters. If not treated, diabetic retinopathy will lead to connective scar tissue, which over time can shrink, pulling on the retina and resulting in a retinal detachment. In the early stages of the milder form of the disease, background diabetic retinopathy, the person may be unaware of problems because the loss of sight is usually gradual and mainly affects peripheral vision.

EARS AND HEARING

ASSESSMENT PROCEDURE	NORMAL FINDINGS	ABNORMAL FINDINGS
Inspect the external ear. Observe shape, color, and hair growth. Also look for lesions or drainage.	Hairs may become coarser and thicker in the external ear, especially in men. Earlobes may elongate and pinna increases in length and width.	Inflammation, drainage, or swelling may be from infection.
Perform an otoscopic examination to determine quantity, color, and consistency of cerumen.	Cerumen production decreases leading to dryness and tendency toward accumulation.	Hard, dark brown cerumen signals impaction of the auditory canal that commonly causes a conductive hearing loss.
		A darkened hole in the tympanic membrane indicates perforation or scarring.
Perform the *voice–whisper test*, a functional examination to detect (conversational) hearing loss. Instruct the client to put a hand over one ear and to repeat the sentence you say. Stand approximately 60.96 cm (2 ft) away from the client and whisper a sentence. *Note: If you are facing the client, hold your hand close to your mouth so the client cannot read your lips.*	The inability to hear high-frequency sounds (presbycusis) or to discriminate a variety of simultaneous sounds and soft consonant sounds or background noises is due to degeneration of hair cells of inner ear.	Inability to hear the whispered sentence indicates a hearing deficiency and the need to refer the client to an audiologist for testing. *Note: Raising one's voice to someone with presbycusis usually only makes it more difficult for them to hear. Speaking more slowly will usually lower the frequency and be more therapeutic.*

Continued on following page

THORAX AND LUNGS

ASSESSMENT PROCEDURE	NORMAL FINDINGS/VARIATIONS	ABNORMAL FINDINGS
Inspect shape of thorax. Note respiratory rate, rhythm, and quality of breathing.	Decreased elasticity of alveoli causes lungs to recoil less during expiration, loss of resilience that holds thorax in a contracted position, and loss of skeletal muscle strength in thorax and abdomen. Decreased vital capacity, increased residual volume, and slight barrel chest are noted.	Respiratory rate >25 breaths/minute may signal a pulmonary infection, other respiratory diseases such as COPD, congestive heart failure, pulmonary embolus, or metabolic acidosis (Williams, 2009).
	Increased reliance on diaphragmatic breathing and increased work of breathing.	Respiratory rate of <16 breaths/minute may be a sign of neurologic impairment, which may lead to aspiration pneumonia. Significant loss of aerobic capacity and dyspnea with exertion is usually due to disease, exposure over a lifetime to pollutants, smoke, or severe or prolonged lack of exercise.
Percuss lung tones. Use the same technique as you would in a younger adult.	Resonant, except in the presence of structural changes such as kyphosis or a slight barrel chest, when hyperresonance may occur.	Consolidation of infection will cause dullness to percussion; alveolar retention of air, as occurs in emphysema, results in hyperresonance.

ASSESSMENT PROCEDURE	NORMAL FINDINGS/VARIATIONS	ABNORMAL FINDINGS
		Note: *Pneumonia is the most common cause of infection-related deaths in older adults. It seldom presents as the classic triad of cough, fever, and pleuritic pain. Instead subtle changes such as an increase in respiratory rate and sputum production, confusion, loss of appetite, and hypotension are more likely to be the presenting symptoms (Fitzpatrick, Fulmer, Wallace, & Flaherty, 2000).*
Auscultate lung sounds as you would in a younger adult. **Note:** *Lung expansion may be diminished in older adults. It may be necessary to emphasize taking deep breaths with the mouth open during the exam. This may be very difficult for those with dementia.*	Vesicular sounds should be heard over all areas of air exchange.	Breath sounds may be distant over areas affected by kyphosis or the barrel chest of aging. Rales and rhonchi are heard only with diseases, such as pulmonary edema, pneumonia, or restrictive disorders. Diminished breath sounds, wheezes, crackles, rhonchi that do not clear with cough, and egophony are signs of consolidation.

Continued on following page

HEART AND BLOOD VESSELS

ASSESSMENT PROCEDURE	NORMAL FINDINGS/VARIATIONS	ABNORMAL FINDINGS
Blood Pressure		
Take blood pressure to detect actual or potential orthostatic hypotension and, therefore, the risk for falling.	An older adult's baroreceptor response to positional changes is slightly less efficient. A slight decrease in blood pressure may occur.	More than 10 mm Hg drop in systolic or diastolic pressure and an increase in heart rate of 20 beats or more per minute indicate orthostatic hypotension. A serious consequence is the potential for lightheadedness and dizziness, which may precipitate hip fracture or head trauma from a fall. *Note: Some sources of orthostatic hypotension include medications, such as antihypertensives, diuretics, and drugs with anticholinergic side effects (anxiolytics, antipsychotics, hypnotics, tricyclic antidepressants, and antihistamines).*

ASSESSMENT PROCEDURE	NORMAL FINDINGS/VARIATIONS	ABNORMAL FINDINGS
Measure pressure with the client in lying, sitting, and standing positions. Also measure pulse rate. Have the client lie down for 5 minutes; take the pulse and blood pressure; at 1 minute, take blood pressure and pulse after client is sitting and again at 1 minute after client stands. If dizziness occurs, instruct client to sit a few minutes before attempting to stand up from a supine or reclining position.	Blood pressure increases as elasticity decreases in arteries with proportionately greater increase in systolic pressure resulting in a widening of pulse pressure. **Note:** *Any client with blood pressure >160/90 mm Hg should be referred to the health care provider for follow-up.*	A sudden and increasingly widened pulse pressure, especially in combination with other neurologic abnormalities and a change in mental status is a classic sign of increased intracranial pressure (which in older adult clients may be due to a hemorrhagic stroke or hematoma).

Exercise Tolerance

Measure activity tolerance. Evaluate, either by reviewing results of stress testing or by observing the client's ability to move from a sitting to a standing position or to flex and extend fingers rapidly.	The maximal heart rate with exercise is less than in a younger person. The heart rate will also take longer to return to its pre-exercise rate. Rise in pulse rate should be no greater than 10–20 beats/minute. The pulse rate should return to the baseline rate within 2 minutes.	A rise in pulse rate >20 beats/minute and a rate that does not return to baseline within 2 minutes is an indicator of exercise intolerance. Cardiac dysrhythmias as determined by stress testing are also indicative of exercise intolerance.

Continued on following page

HEART AND BLOOD VESSELS (Continued)

ASSESSMENT PROCEDURE	NORMAL FINDINGS/VARIATIONS	ABNORMAL FINDINGS
Note: Poor lower body strength, especially in the ankles, may impair the ability of the frail older adult to rise from a chair to a standing position. Poor upper body strength, especially in the shoulders, may impede the ability to push up from a bed or chair or to extend and flex fingers.		
Pulses		
Determine adequacy of blood flow by palpating the arterial pulses in all locations (carotid, brachial, radial, femoral, popliteal, posterior tibial, and dorsalis pedis) for strength and quality. *Note: Palpate carotid arteries gently and one side at a time to avoid stimulating vagal receptors in the neck, dislodging existing plaque, or causing syncope or a stroke.*	Proximal pulses may be easier to palpate due to loss of supporting tissue. However, distal lower extremity pulses may be more difficult to feel or even nonpalpable. The dorsalis pedis pulse is congenitally absent in approximately 2 % of adults (Miller, 2010).	Insufficient or absent pulses are a likely indication of arterial insufficiency. Partially obstructed blood flow increases the risk of ulcers and infection; completely obstructed blood flow is a medical emergency requiring immediate intervention to prevent gangrene and possible amputation.

ASSESSMENT PROCEDURE	NORMAL FINDINGS/VARIATIONS	ABNORMAL FINDINGS
Arteries and Veins		
Auscultate the carotid, abdominal, and femoral arteries.	No unusual sounds should be heard.	A bruit is abnormal, and the client needs a prompt referral for further care because of the high risk of stroke (CVA) from a carotid embolism or an abdominal or femoral aneurysm.
Evaluate arterial and venous sufficiency of extremities. Elevate the legs above the level of the heart and observe color, temperature, size of the legs, and skin integrity.	Hair loss with advanced age (cannot be used singly as an indicator of arterial insufficiency).	Leg pain associated with walking, burning or cramping, duskiness or mottling when the leg is in a dependent position; paleness with elevation; cool, thin, shiny skin; thickened, brittle nails; and diminished pulses are signs of arterial insufficiency.
Inspect and palpate veins while client is standing.	Prominent, bulging veins are common. Varicosities are considered a problem only if ulcerations, signs of thrombophlebitis, or cords are present. Cords are nontender; palpable veins having a rubber tubing consistency.	Unilateral warmth, tenderness, and swelling may be indications of thrombophlebitis.

Continued on following page

HEART AND BLOOD VESSELS (Continued)

ASSESSMENT PROCEDURE	NORMAL FINDINGS/VARIATIONS	ABNORMAL FINDINGS
Heart		
Inspect and palpate the precordium.	The precordium is still and without thrills, heaves, or visible, palpable pulsations (noted exception may be the apex of the heart if close to the surface).	Heaves are felt with an enlarged right or left ventricular aneurysm.
		Thrills indicate aortic, mitral, or pulmonic stenosis and regurgitation that may originate from rheumatic fever.
		Pulsations suggest an aortic or ventricular aneurysm, right ventricular enlargement, or mitral regurgitation.
Auscultate heart sounds. The accumulation of lipofuscin, amyloid, collagen, and fats in the pacemaker cells of the heart and loss of pacemaker cells in the sinus node predispose the older adult to dysrhythmias, even in the absence of heart disease.	A soft systolic murmur heard best at the base of the heart may result from calcification, stiffening, and dilation of the aortic and mitral valve.	Abnormal heart sounds are generally considered to be disease related only if there is additional evidence of compromised cardiovascular function. However, any previously undetected extra heart sound warrants further investigation.

ASSESSMENT PROCEDURE	NORMAL FINDINGS/VARIATIONS	ABNORMAL FINDINGS
		S_3 and S_4 sounds may reflect the cardiac and fluid overloads of heart failure, aortic stenosis, cardiomyopathy, or myocardial infarction.
		Note: Falls, dyspnea, fatigue, and palpitations are common symptoms seen with dysrhythmias in older adults.

BREASTS

Inspect and palpate breast and axillae. When viewing axillae and contour of breasts, assist a client with arthritis to raise the arms over the head. Do this gently and without force and only if it is not painful for the client.	The breasts of older women are often described as pendulous due to the atrophy of breast tissue and supporting tissues and the forward thrust of the client brought about by kyphosis.	Pain upon palpation may indicate an infectious process or cancer. Or breast tenderness, pain, or swelling may be side effects of hormone replacement therapy and an indication that a lower dosage is needed.
	Decreases in fat composition and increase in fibrotic tissue may make the terminal ducts feel more fibrotic and palpable as linear, spoke-like strands.	Male breast enlargement (gynecomastia) may result from a decrease in testosterone.
If the breasts are pendulous, assist the client to lean slightly so the breasts hang away from the chest wall, enabling you to best observe symmetry and form.	Nipples may retract due to loss in musculature. Unlike nipple retraction due to a mass, nipples retracted because of aging can be everted with gentle pressure (Stephan, 2010).	*Note: A greater percentage of older women have had radical mastectomies. If so, inquiring about pain and swelling from lymphedema is important.*

Continued on following page

BREASTS (Continued)

ASSESSMENT PROCEDURE	NORMAL FINDINGS/VARIATIONS	ABNORMAL FINDINGS
Inspect skin under breasts.	Skin intact without lesions or rashes.	Macerated skin under the breasts may result from perspiration or fungal infection (usually seen in an immunocompromised client).

ABDOMEN

ASSESSMENT PROCEDURE	NORMAL FINDINGS/VARIATIONS	ABNORMAL FINDINGS
Motility		
Assess GI motility and auscultate bowel sounds. Review fiber intake and laxative use.	Five to 30 sounds/minute are heard. A decrease in gastric emptying time occurs with aging and may cause early satiety. Intestinal motility is generally reduced from a general loss of muscle tone. Risk of constipation is increased by diminished physical activity, fluid intake, fiber in diet, and certain medications such as iron or narcotics.	Absence of bowel sounds and vomiting of undigested food are abnormal. Decreased motility is exacerbated by common pathologies such as Parkinson, stroke, and diabetes mellitus. Results in propensity for chronic constipation and diverticula. Hiatal hernia may manifest by postprandial chest fullness, heartburn, or nausea.

ASSESSMENT PROCEDURE	NORMAL FINDINGS/VARIATIONS	ABNORMAL FINDINGS
Determine absorption or retention problems in older adult clients receiving enteral feedings. *Note: An abdominal radiograph, flat plate, should be taken to check for correct placement of newly inserted nasogastric tubes.*	Less than 100 mL residual is a normal finding for intermittent feedings.	More than 100 mL residual measured before a scheduled feeding is a sign of insufficient absorption and excessive retention. Abdominal distention, diarrhea, fluid overload, aspiration pneumonia, or fluid/electrolyte imbalances may indicate excessive retention although mental status changes may be the first or only sign.
Inspect and percuss abdomen. Use the same manner as you would for younger adults. *Note: The loss of abdominal musculature that occurs with aging may make it easier to palpate abdominal organs. Atrophy of intestinal villi is a common aging change.*	Liver, pancreas, and kidneys normally decrease in size, but the decrease is not generally appreciable upon physical examination.	Anorexia, abdominal pain and distention, impaired protein digestion, and vitamin B_{12} malabsorption suggest inflammatory gastritis or a peptic ulcer. Abdominal distention, cramping, diarrhea, and increased flatus are signs of lactose intolerance, which may occur for the first time in old age. Bruits over aorta suggest an aneurysm. If present, do not palpate because this could rupture the aneurysm.

Continued on following page

ABDOMEN (Continued)

ASSESSMENT PROCEDURE	NORMAL FINDINGS/VARIATIONS	ABNORMAL FINDINGS
Palpate the bladder. Ask the client to empty bladder before the examination. If the bladder is palpable, percuss from symphysis pubis to umbilicus. If the client is incontinent, postvoid residual content may also need to be measured.	Empty bladder is not palpable or percussible.	Full bladder sounds dull. More than 100 mL drained from bladder is considered abnormal for a postvoid residual. A distended bladder with an associated small-volume urine loss may indicate overflow incontinence (see Box 26-3, p. 660). Guarding upon palpation, rebound tenderness, or a friction rub (sounds like pieces of sandpaper rubbing together) often suggests peritonitis, which could be secondary to ruptured diverticula, tumor, or infarct.

GENITALIA

ASSESSMENT PROCEDURE	NORMAL FINDINGS/VARIATIONS	ABNORMAL FINDINGS
Female		
Inspect external genitalia. Assist the client into the lithotomy position. Inspect the urethral meatus and vaginal opening.	Many atrophic changes begin in women at menopause. Pubic hair is usually sparse, and labia are flattened. Clitoris is decreased in size. The size of ovaries, uterus, and cervix also decreases.	White, glistening particles attached to pubic hair may be a sign of lice. Redness or swelling from the urethral meatus indicates a possible urinary tract infection.

ASSESSMENT PROCEDURE	NORMAL FINDINGS/VARIATIONS	ABNORMAL FINDINGS
Note: Arthritis may make the lithotomy position particularly uncomfortable for the elderly woman, necessitating a change in position.		
Ask the client to cough while in the lithotomy position. *Note: Incontinence is not a normal part of aging. If embarrassment or acceptance is preventing the client from acknowledging the problem, the genital examination may be a more acceptable time to introduce the topic.*	No leakage of urine occurs.	Leakage of urine that occurs with coughing is a sign of stress incontinence and may be due to lax pelvic muscles from childbirth, surgery, obesity, cystocele, rectocele, or a prolapsed uterus. *Note: In noncommunicative patients, an excoriated perineum may be the result of incontinence.*
Test for prolapse. Ask the client to bear down while you observe the vaginal opening.	No prolapse is evident.	A protrusion into the vaginal opening may be a cystocele, rectocele, or uterine prolapse, which is a common sequela of relaxed pelvic musculature in older women.

Continued on following page

GENITALIA (Continued)

ASSESSMENT PROCEDURE	NORMAL FINDINGS/VARIATIONS	ABNORMAL FINDINGS
Perform a pelvic examination. Put on disposable gloves and use a small speculum if the vaginal opening has narrowed with age. Use lubrication on speculum and hand because natural lubrication is decreased.	Vagina narrows and shortens. A loss of elastic tissue and vascularity in vagina results in a thin, pale epithelium. Atrophic changes are intensified by infrequent intercourse. Loss of elasticity and reduced vaginal lubrication due to lower levels of estrogen can cause dyspareunia (painful intercourse). Sexual desire, pleasure are not necessarily diminished by these structural changes, nor do women lose capacity for orgasm with age.	Atrophic vaginitis symptoms can mimic malignancy, vulvar dystrophies, urinary tract infections, and other infections, such as *Candida albicans*, bacterial vaginosis, gonorrhea, or chlamydia (Better Medicine, 2011).
	Because the ovaries, uterus, and cervix shrink with age, the ovaries may not be palpable.	
	The vaginal wall should constrict around the examiner's finger, and the perineum should feel smooth.	If the client has a cystocele, the examiner's finger in the vagina will feel pressure from the anterior surface of the vagina.
Test pelvic muscle tone. Ask the woman to squeeze muscles while the examiner's finger is in the vagina. Assess perineal strength by turning fingers posterior to the perineum while the woman squeezes muscles in the vaginal area.		In clients with uterine prolapse, protrusion of the cervix is felt down through the vagina.
		A bulging of the posterior vaginal wall and part of the rectum may be felt with a rectocele.

ASSESSMENT PROCEDURE	NORMAL FINDINGS/VARIATIONS	ABNORMAL FINDINGS
Male		
Inspect the male genital area with the client in standing position if possible.	Decreased testosterone leads to atrophic changes. Pubic hair is thinner. Scrotal skin slightly darker than surrounding skin, smooth and flaccid in the older man. Penis and testicular size decreases, scrotum hangs lower. In addition, there is a decrease in amount and viscosity of seminal fluid. Sperm count may decrease by 50%. Orgasm may be briefer; time to obtain an erection may increase. These changes alone do not usually result in any loss of libido or satisfaction.	Scrotal edema may be present with portal vein obstruction or heart failure. Lesions on the penis may be a sign of infection. Associated symptoms frequently include discharge, scrotal pain, and difficulty with urination.
Observe and palpate for inguinal swelling or bulges suggestive of hernia in the same manner as for a younger male.	No swelling or bulges are present.	Masses or bulges are abnormal, and pain may be a sign of testicular torsion. A mass may be due to a hydrocele, spermatocele, or cancer.
Auscultate the scrotum if a mass is detected; otherwise palpate the right and left testicles using the thumb and first two fingers.	No detectable sounds or masses are present.	Bowel sounds heard over the scrotum may suggest an indirect inguinal hernia. Masses are abnormal, and the client should be referred to a specialist for follow-up examination.

Continued on following page

ANUS, RECTUM, AND PROSTATE

ASSESSMENT PROCEDURE	NORMAL FINDINGS/VARIATIONS	ABNORMAL FINDINGS
Inspect the anus and rectum.	The anus is darker than the surrounding skin.	Lesions, swelling, inflammation, and bleeding are abnormalities.
	Bluish, grape-like lumps at the anus are indicators of hemorrhoids.	If hemorrhoids account for discomfort, the degree to which bleeding, swelling, or inflammation interferes with bowel activity generally determines if treatment is warranted.
Put on gloves to palpate the anus and rectum. Also palpate the prostate in the male client.	Normal findings include no internal masses, polyps, hemorrhoids, rectal prolapse, or fecal impaction.	Palpation of internal masses could indicate polyps, internal hemorrhoids, rectal prolapse, cancer, or fecal impaction.
Note: The left side-lying position with knees tucked up toward the chest is the preferred one for comfort. Pillows may be needed for positioning and client comfort.	The prostate is normally soft or rubbery-firm and smooth, and the median sulcus is palpable. Some degree of benign prostatic hypertrophy almost always occurs by age 85.	Obliteration of the median sulcus is seen with prostatic hyperplasia. A hard, asymmetrically enlarged, and nodular prostate is suggestive of malignancy (Barry, 2009). Tender and softer prostate is more common with prostatitis. Fever and dysuria are common with acute prostatitis. Obstructive symptoms seen with both prostate malignancy and infection.

MUSCULOSKELETAL SYSTEM

ASSESSMENT PROCEDURE	NORMAL FINDINGS/VARIATIONS	ABNORMAL FINDINGS
Observe the client's posture and balance when standing, especially the first 3–5 seconds. *Note: The ability to reach for everyday items without losing balance can be assessed by asking the client to remove an object from a shelf that is high enough to require stretching or standing on the toes and to bend down to pick up a small object, such as a pen, from the floor.*	Client stands reasonably straight with feet positioned fairly widely apart to form a firm base of support. This stance compensates for diminished sense of proprioception in lower extremities. Body usually bends forward as well.	A "humpback" curvature of the spine, called kyphosis, usually results from osteoporosis. The combination of osteoporosis, calcification of tendons and joints, and muscle atrophy makes it difficult for the frail elderly person to extend the hips and knees fully when walking. This impairs the ability to maintain balance early enough to prevent a fall. Client cannot maintain balance without holding onto something. Postural instability increases the risk of falling and immobility from the fear of falling.
Observe the client's gait by performing the timed "Get Up and Go" test (Fig. 26-3). 1. Have the client rise from a straight-backed armchair, stand momentarily, and walk about 3 m toward a wall.	Widening of pelvis and narrowing of shoulders. Client walks steadily without swaying, stumbling, or hesitating during the walk. The client does not appear to be at risk of falling. Older adult clients without impairments in gait or balance can complete the test within 10 seconds.	Shuffling gait, characterized by smaller steps and minimal lifting of the feet, increases the risk of tripping when walking on uneven or unsteady surfaces.

Continued on following page

MUSCULOSKELETAL SYSTEM (Continued)

ASSESSMENT PROCEDURE	NORMAL FINDINGS/VARIATIONS	ABNORMAL FINDINGS

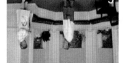
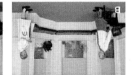
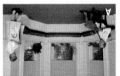
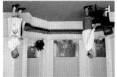
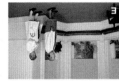
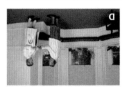
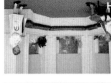
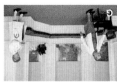

FIGURE 26-3 "Get Up and Go" test. (Photo by B. Proud.)

ASSESSMENT PROCEDURE	NORMAL FINDINGS/VARIATIONS	ABNORMAL FINDINGS
2. Ask client to turn without touching the wall and walk back to chair; then turn around and sit down. 3. Using watch with second hand, determine how long it takes the client to complete test.	**Score performance (1–5):** 1. Normal. 2. Very slightly abnormal. 3. Mildly abnormal. 4. Moderately abnormal. 5. Severely abnormal.	Abnormal findings from the timed "Get Up and Go" test include hesitancy, staggering, stumbling, and abnormal movements of the trunk and arms. People who take >30 seconds to complete the test tend to be dependent in some activities of daily living such as bathing, getting in and out of bed, or climbing stairs.
Inspect the general contour of limbs, trunk, and joints. Palpate wrist and hand joints. 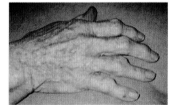 **FIGURE 26-4** Degenerative joint disease.	Enlargement of the distal, interphalangeal joints of the fingers, called Heberden nodes, is an indicator of degenerative joint disease (DJD), a common age-related condition involving joints in the hips, knees, and spine as well as the fingers (Fig. 26-4).	With accumulated damage and loss of cartilage, bony overgrowths protrude from the bone into the joint capsule, causing deformities, limited mobility, and pain. Hand deformities such as ulnar deviation, swan-neck deformity, and boutonnière deformity are of concern because of pain and limitations they impose on activities of daily living.

Continued on following page

MUSCULOSKELETAL SYSTEM (Continued)

ASSESSMENT PROCEDURE	NORMAL FINDINGS/VARIATIONS	ABNORMAL FINDINGS
Test ROM. Ask client to touch each finger with the thumb of the same hand, to turn wrists up toward the ceiling and down toward the floor, to push each finger against yours while you apply resistance, and to make a fist and release it.	There is full ROM of each joint and equal bilateral resistance.	Limitations in ROM or strength may be due to DJD, rheumatoid arthritis, or a neurologic disorder, which, if unilateral, suggests stroke (CVA). Signs of pain such as grimacing, pulling back, or verbal messages are indicators of the need to do a pain assessment (see Box 26-1, p. 624). Grating, popping, crepitus, and palpation of fluid are abnormalities. Crepitus and joint pain that is worse with activity and relieved by rest in the absence of systemic symptoms is often associated with DJD.
Similarly assess ROM and strength of shoulders (left) and elbows (right).	There is full ROM of each joint and equal strength in each joint.	Tenderness, stiffness, and pain in the shoulders and elbows (and hips), which is aggravated by movement, are common signs associated with polymyalgia rheumatica.

ASSESSMENT PROCEDURE	NORMAL FINDINGS/VARIATIONS	ABNORMAL FINDINGS
Assess hip joint for strength and ROM. Use the same technique as you would for a younger adult.	Intact flexion, extension, and internal and external rotation.	Hip pain that is worse with weightbearing and relieved with rest may indicate *DJD*. Often an association exists between crepitation and a decrease in ROM.
		Complaints of hip, thigh, or groin pain, external rotation and adduction of the affected leg, and an inability to bear weight are the most common signs of a hip fracture. If the fracture is complete, there will also be minimal shortening of the leg (AAOS, 2009).
Inspect and palpate knees, ankles, and feet. Also assess comfort level, particularly with movement (flexion, extension, rotation).	The common problems associated with the aged foot, such as soreness and aching, are most frequently due to improperly fitting footwear.	A great toe overriding or underlying the second toe may be hallux valgus (bunion).
		Enlargement of the medial portion of the first metatarsal head and inflammation of the bursae over the medial aspect of the joint are noticed.
		Bunions are associated with pain and difficulty walking.

Continued on following page

MUSCULOSKELETAL SYSTEM (Continued)

ASSESSMENT PROCEDURE	NORMAL FINDINGS/VARIATIONS	ABNORMAL FINDINGS
Inspect client's muscle bulk and tone.	Atrophy of the hand muscles may occur with normal aging.	Muscle atrophy from rheumatoid arthritis, muscle disuse, malnutrition, motor neuron disease, or diseases of the peripheral nervous system. Increased resistance to passive ROM is a classic sign of Parkinson disease, especially in clients with bradykinesia. Decreased resistance may also suggest peripheral nervous system disease, cerebellar disease, or acute spinal cord injury.

NEUROLOGIC SYSTEM

ASSESSMENT PROCEDURE	NORMAL FINDINGS/VARIATIONS	ABNORMAL FINDINGS
Observe for tremors and involuntary movements.	Resting tremors increase in the aged. In the absence of an identifiable disease process, they are not considered pathologic.	The tremors of Parkinson may occur when the client is at rest. They usually diminish with voluntary movement, begin in the hand and affect one side of the body early in the disease and/or are accompanied by muscle rigidity.

SENSORY SYSTEM

ASSESSMENT PROCEDURE	NORMAL FINDINGS/VARIATIONS	ABNORMAL FINDINGS
Test sensation to pain, temperature, touch position, and vibration. Use the same assessment techniques as you would use for a younger adult.	Touch and vibratory sensations may diminish normally with aging.	Unilateral sensory loss suggests a lesion in the spinal cord or higher pathways; a symmetric sensory loss suggests a neuropathy that may be associated with a condition such as diabetes.
Assess positional sense by using the Romberg test as presented in Chapter 21. The exceptions to the test are clients who must use assistive devices such as a walker.	There is minimal swaying without loss of balance.	Significant swaying with appearance of a potential fall.

BOX 26-3 UNDERSTANDING URINARY INCONTINENCE: ASSESSMENT AND INTERVENTION

TYPES OF INCONTINENCE

The signs and symptoms associated with the involuntary loss of urine have been clustered into three categories: urge, stress, and overflow incontinence. Any one or a combination of all three types may be present in an individual. Voiding diaries are useful for determining the type of incontinence that is occurring based on the amount, timing, and associated symptoms of incontinent episodes.

Urge Incontinence

Urge incontinence is the involuntary loss of urine associated with an abrupt and strong desire to void. It is frequently caused by a neurologic disorder such as a stroke (CVA) or multiple sclerosis (MS), which impairs the ability of the bladder or urinary sphincter to contract and relax.

Stress Incontinence

Stress incontinence is the involuntary loss of urine during coughing, sneezing, laughing, or other physical activities that increase abdominal pressure. In women, stress incontinence may result from weakened and relaxed muscles from the combined effects of aging superimposed on the effects of childbirth.

Overflow Incontinence

Overflow incontinence is the involuntary loss of urine associated with overdistention of the bladder. Prostatic hypertrophy is a common cause in men, and diabetic neuropathy is a common cause in both sexes.

Functional Incontinence

Functional incontinence is the inability to get to the bathroom in time or to understand the cues to void due to problems with mobility or cognition.

STEPS OF ASSESSMENT

The nursing assessment varies somewhat depending on the client's general health status and whether the problem is an acute or chronic one. In general, however, a comprehensive nursing assessment can be described as a five-step process that includes screening for an infection with a urinalysis, obtaining a voiding diary, evaluating

Note: Atrophic vaginitis from estrogen deficiency usually results in symptoms of urge incontinence as well as stress incontinence (mixed incontinence).

functional status, compiling a health history, and performing a physical examination. Key features within the five steps follow.

- Record all incontinent and continent episodes for 3 days in a voiding diary.
- Review medication for any newly prescribed drugs that may be triggering incontinence. Follow-up with physician regarding the need to discontinue therapy or change medication.
- Rule out constipation or fecal impaction as a source of urinary incontinence. If client has had no bowel movement within the last 3 days or is oozing stool continuously, check for impaction by digital examination or abdominal palpation. Problem should be treated if identified.
- Assess functional status along with signs and symptoms as they relate to incontinence. Contributors to incontinence may include immobility, insufficient fluid intake, and confusion. Accompanying signs and symptoms include polyuria, nocturia, dysuria, hesitancy, poor or interrupted urine stream, straining, suprapubic or perineal pain, urgency and characteristics of incontinent episodes (precipitated by walking, coughing, getting in and out of bed and so forth).

- Consult physician regarding physical examination and need to measure postvoid residual volume by straight catheterization (particularly if client dribbles, reports urgency, has difficulty starting stream). Components of the physical examination include direct observation of urine loss using a cough stress test; abdominal, rectal, genital, and pelvic examination; and identification of neurologic abnormalities. Abdominal and vaginal examinations are performed to detect prolapse or a palpable bladder after micturition.

INTERVENTIONS

The physician is responsible for identifying and treating the conditions causing reversible or chronic incontinence. A physical therapist may play a role in identifying specific activities that are associated with incontinent episodes. Either a nurse or physical therapist may be involved in teaching Kegel exercises to help relieve stress incontinence. When functional incontinence and urgency have been identified, the expertise of an occupational therapist in appropriate dressing and undressing and for choosing incontinence aids may be beneficial.

Appendices

APPENDIX 1

Nursing Assessment Form Based on Functional Health Patterns

Client Profile

Name	Birthdate	Sex

Ethnic origin ——————————— Religion ———————————

Medical diagnoses ————————————————————————

Present treatment ————————————————————————

Past treatments ————————————————————————

Past hospitalizations ————————————————————————

Allergies ————————————————————————

Current Medications	Name	Dose	Purpose	Problems
	_____	_____	_____	_____
	_____	_____	_____	_____
	_____	_____	_____	_____

Subjective

Health Perception–Health Management Pattern

Reason for seeking health care _____

_____

Health rating	1	2	3
	Poor	Fair	Excellent

Perception of illness _____
Effect of illness on ADLs _____
Use of alcohol _____
   tobacco _____
   drugs _____
Special health habits _____
Last immunizations _____
Compliance with treatments _____

_____

Objective

Appearance _____
Grooming _____
Posture _____
Expressions _____
Ht _____ Wt _____
P _____ R _____ T _____
(oral, axillary, rectal)
BP sitting   R _____ L _____
   standing   R _____ L _____

Nutritional–Metabolic Pattern

Daily Food and Fluid Intake

Breakfast ——————————————
Lunch ——————————————
Supper ——————————————
Snacks ——————————————
Food intolerances ——————————————
Difficulty chewing ——————————————
Dysphagia ——————————————
Sore gums ——————————————
Sore tongue ——————————————
N and V ——————————————
Abdominal pains ——————————————
Antacids ——————————————
Laxatives ——————————————
Skin condition ——————————————
Hair condition ——————————————
Nail condition ——————————————
Difficulty gaining   Ideal wt. ———— Difficulty gaining ————
losing ——————————————
Cold/heat intolerances ——————————————
Voice changes ——————————————
Difficulty with nervousness ——————————————

Skin: Color ———— Texture ————
Lesions ————
Temp ———— Moisture ————
Turgor ————

Hair: Color ————
Amt ———— Texture ————
Scalp lesions ———— Dry ————

Nails: Color ————
Shape ———— Condition ————
Texture ———— Tenderness ————

Oral Mucosa: Number of teeth ————
Condition ————
Lesions ————
Gums ———— Tongue ————

Elimination Pattern

Bowel habits

Frequency _____ Color _____ Pain _____

Consistency _____ Laxatives _____

Enemas _____ Suppositories _____

Ileostomy _____ Colostomy _____

Bladder habits

Frequency _____ Amt _____ Color _____

Pain _____ Hematuria _____

Incontinence _____ Nocturia _____

Retention _____ Infections _____

Catheter _____ Type _____

Abdomen

Contour _____

Lesions _____ Umbilicus _____

Striae _____ Veins _____

Bowel sounds char. _____

Frequency _____

Size of liver dullness _____

Masses palpated _____

Liver palpated _____

Spleen palpated _____

Rectum

Rashes _____

Lesions _____ Tenderness _____

Activity–Exercise Pattern

Daily Activities

Hygiene _____

Cooking _____

Shopping _____

Housework _____

Yard work _____

Eating times _____

Dyspnea _____ Palpitations _____

Chest pain _____ Stiffness _____

Weakness _____ Aching _____

Leisure activities _____

Exercise routine _____

Occupation _____

Effect of illness on activities _____

_____

Musculoskeletal

Gait _____ Posture _____

Extremity swelling _____

Symmetry _____ ROM _____

Crepitus _____ Tone _____

Strength _____

Respiratory

Thorax shape _____

Symmetry _____ Retractions _____

Tenderness _____

Diaphragmatic level _____

Breath sounds _____

Adventitious sounds _____

Cardiovascular

Jugular venous pressure _____

Pulsations _____ Heaves _____

Lifts _____

PMI _____ S_1 _____ S_2 _____

S_3 _____ S_4 _____ Murmurs _____

Peripheral Vascular Pulses

Carotid R ____ L ____	Radial	R ____ L ____
Ulnar R ____ L ____	Brachial	R ____ L ____
Popliteal R ____ L ____	Femoral	R ____ L ____
Pedal R ____ L ____	Posterior tibial	R ____ L ____
Bruits R ____ L ____		

Sleep–Rest Pattern

Sleep time _____ Quality _____
Difficulty falling asleep _____
Difficulty remaining asleep _____
Sleep aids _____
Sleep medications _____

Appearance _____
Yawning _____ Irritability _____
Short attention span _____

Sexuality–Reproduction Pattern

Female Menstruation
Age of onset _____ Last menstrual period _____
Length _____
Problems _____
_____
_____

Gravida _____ Para _____ Abortions _____
Current pregnancy _____
Infertility _____

Breasts
BSE _____ When _____
  Shape _____ Symmetry _____
  Nipples _____ Discharge _____
  Masses _____ Lymph nodes _____

Male Genitalia
Testicular exam When _____
  Masses _____ Swelling _____
  Texture _____

Male-Female

Contraception used _____

_____

Undesirable side effects _____

Problems with sexual activities _____

_____

_____

Effect of illness on sexuality _____

_____

_____

Sexually transmitted diseases _____

_____

Pain _____ Burning _____

Discomfort during intercourse _____

Penile exam _____

Masses _____ Growths _____

Lesions _____ Discharge _____

Foreskin retraction _____

Urethral opening _____

Lymph nodes _____

Inguinal masses _____

Female Genitalia

Labia _____ Color _____

Swelling _____ Symmetry _____

Urethral opening _____

Discharge _____

Vaginal opening _____

Lesions _____ Discharge _____

Hymen _____ Inflammation _____

Sensory–Perceptual Pattern

Perceptions of: Vision _____

Hearing _____ Taste _____

Smell _____ Sensation _____

Pain _____

Vision aids _____

Hearing aids _____

Visual Acuity: OD _____ OS _____

OU _____ Visual fields _____

EOMs _____

PERRLA _____

Funduscopic Exam: Red reflex

Optic disc _____ Macula _____

Arterioles/venules _____

Hearing: Weber _____ Rinne _____
External canal _____
Tympanic membrane _____
Sensations: Superficial _____ Deep pressure _____
2-point discrimination _____
Cranial Nerves
I. Olfactory _____
II. Optic _____
V. Trigeminal _____
III, IV, VI. Oculomotor, trochlear, abducens _____
VII. Facial _____ Acoustic _____

Cognitive Pattern

Understanding of illness _____
Understanding of treatments _____
Ability to express self _____
Ability to recall:
Remote _____
Recent _____
Ability to make decisions _____
Expression of feelings _____

Behavior _____
Speech _____ Vocabulary _____
Mood _____
Thought processes _____
Orientation: Person _____
Time _____ Place _____
Attention _____ Information _____
Vocabulary _____
Abstract reasoning _____
Similarities _____ Judgment _____
Sensory perception and coordination _____

Role–Relationship Pattern

Role in family _____

Responsibility _____

Work role _____

Social role _____

Level of satisfaction _____

Effect of illness on roles _____

_____

Communication between family members _____

Family visits _____ Length _____

Draw family genogram:

Self-Perception–Self-Concept Pattern

Identity _____

Perception of abilities _____

Body image _____

Coping–Stress Tolerance Pattern

Stressors _____

Coping methods _____

Support systems _____

Value–Belief Pattern

Values _____

Goals _____

Source of hope/strength _____

Significant religious person _____

Religious practices _____

Relationship with God _____

Presence of religious articles _____

Religious activities _____

_____

Visits from clergy _____

Information adapted from: Gordon, M. (2010). *Manual of nursing diagnosis* (12th ed.). Sudbury, MA: Jones & Bartlett.

Physical Assessment Guide: Pulling It All Together

Following is an outline guide for performing a head-to-toe physical assessment. This guide will help you pull together all your assessment skills to complete an integrated and comprehensive physical examination efficiently.

Equipment for a Head-To-Toe Assessment

- Assessment documentation forms
- Coin or key
- Cotton ball
- Cover card (for eye assessment)
- Gloves
- Goniometer
- Gown for client
- Lubricating jelly
- Magnifying glass
- Marking pencil

- Newspaper print or Rosenbaum pocket screener
- Notepad and pencil
- Ophthalmoscope
- Otoscope
- Paper clip
- Penlight
- Pillows (two small pillows)
- Platform scale with height attachment
- Reflex hammer
- Ruler with centimeter markings
- Skinfold calibers, flexible tape measure
- Small cup of water for client to drink
- Snellen chart
- Stethoscope and sphygmomanometer
- Substances for testing smell (eg, soap, coffee)
- Substances for testing taste (eg, salt, lemon, sugar, pickle juice)
- Supplies for collecting vaginal specimen (slides, spatula, cotton-tip applicator)
- Thermometer (electronic, tympanic)
- Tongue depressor
- Tuning fork
- Vaginal speculum
- Watch

Preparing the Client

Discuss the purpose of the physical assessment with your client and acquire his or her permission to perform the various examinations. Ensure privacy and confidentiality. Respect the client's right to refuse any part of the assessment. Ask him or her to change into a gown for the examination.

General Survey

- **Observe appearance including:**
  - Overall physical and sexual development
  - Apparent age (compare with stated age)
  - Overall skin coloring
  - Dress, grooming, and hygiene
  - Body build, as well as muscle mass and fat distribution
  - Behavior (compare with developmental stage)
- **Assess the client's vital signs:**
  - Temperature
  - Pulse
  - Respiration
  - Blood pressure
  - Pain (as the fifth vital sign)

Mental Status Examination

- **In addition to data collected about the client's appearance during the general survey, observe:**
  - Level of consciousness
  - Posture and body movements
  - Facial expressions
  - Speech
  - Mood, feelings, and expressions
  - Thought processes and perceptions
- **Assess the client's cognitive abilities:**
  - Orientation to person, time, and place
  - Concentration, ability to focus and follow directions
  - Recent memory of happenings today
  - Remote memory of the past
  - Recall of unrelated information in 5-, 10-, and 30-minute periods
  - Abstract reasoning (Explain a "Stitch in time saves nine.")
  - Judgment ("What one would do in case of . . . ?")
  - Visual perceptual and constructional ability (draw a clock or shapes of square, etc.)

Ask the client to empty the bladder (give the client a specimen cup if a urine sample is needed) and change into a gown. Ask him or her to sit on the examination table.

Skin, Hair, and Nails

- As you perform each part of the head-to-toe assessment, assess skin for color variations, texture, temperature, turgor, edema, and lesions.
- Assess hair for distribution, color, and texture.
- Assess nails for condition, texture, and shape.
- Teach the client skin self-examination.

- **Take body measurements:**
  - Height
  - Weight
  - Waist and hip circumference; mid-arm circumference
  - Triceps skinfold thickness (TSF)
- Calculate ideal body weight, body mass index, waist-to-hip ratio, and mid-arm muscle area and circumference.
- Test vision using the Snellen chart.

Head and Face

- Inspect and palpate the head for size, shape, and configuration.
- Note consistency, distribution, and color of hair.
- Observe face for symmetry, facial features, expressions, and skin condition.
- Check function of cranial nerve (CN) VII: Have the client smile, frown, show teeth, blow out cheeks, raise eyebrows, and tightly close eyes.
- Evaluate function of CN V: Using the sharp and dull sides of a paper clip, test sensations of forehead, cheeks, and chin.
- Palpate the temporal arteries for elasticity and tenderness.
- As the client opens and closes the mouth, palpate the temporomandibular joint for tenderness, swelling, and crepitation.

Eyes

- Determine function:
  - Test visual fields.
  - Assess corneal light reflex.
  - Perform cover and position tests.
- Inspect external eye:
  - Position and alignment of the eyeball in eye socket

- Bulbar conjunctiva and sclera
  - Palpebral conjunctiva
  - Lacrimal apparatus
  - Cornea, lens, iris, and pupil
- Test pupillary reaction to light.
- Test accommodation of pupils.
- Assess corneal reflex (CN VII—facial).
- Use the ophthalmoscope to inspect:
  - Optic disc for shape, color, size, and physiologic cup
  - Retinal vessels for color and diameter and arteriovenous (AV) crossings
  - Retinal background for color and lesions
  - Fovea centralis (sharpest area of vision) and macula
  - Anterior chamber for clarity

Ears and Nose

- Inspect the auricle, tragus, and lobule for shape, position, lesions, discolorations, and discharge.
- Palpate the auricle and mastoid process for tenderness.
- Use the otoscope to inspect:
  - External auditory canal for color and cerumen (ear wax)

- Tympanic membrane for color, shape, consistency, and landmarks
- Test hearing:
  - Whisper test
  - Weber's test for diminished hearing in one ear
  - Rinne test to compare bone and air conduction (tuning fork on mastoid, then in front of ear)
- Inspect the external nose for color, shape, and consistency.
- Palpate the external nose for tenderness.
- Check patency of airflow through nostrils (occlude one nostril at a time and ask client to sniff).
- Test CN I: Ask the client to close his or her eyes and smell for soap, coffee, or vanilla. (Occlude each nostril.)
- Use an otoscope with a short wide tip to inspect internal nose for color and integrity of nasal mucosa, nasal septum, and inferior and middle turbinates.
- Transilluminate maxillary sinuses with a penlight to check for fluid or pus.

Mouth and Throat

Put on gloves. Use a tongue depressor and penlight as needed.

- Inspect lips for consistency, color, and lesions.
- Inspect the teeth for number and condition.
- Check the gums and buccal mucosa for color, consistency, or lesions.
- Inspect the hard (anterior) and soft (posterior) palates for color and integrity.
- Ask the client to say "aah" and observe the rise of the uvula.
- Test CN X: Touch the soft palate to assess for gag reflex.
- Inspect the tonsils for color, size, lesions, and exudates.
- Inspect the tongue for color, moisture, size, and texture.
- Inspect the ventral surface of the tongue for frenulum, color, lesions, and Wharton ducts.
- Palpate the tongue for lesions.
- Test CN IX and CN X: Assess tongue strength by asking the client to press the tongue against the tongue blade.
- Assess CN VII and CN IX: Have the client close his or her eyes. Check taste by placing salt, sugar, and lemon on the tongue.

Neck

- Inspect the neck for appearance of lesions, masses, swelling, and symmetry.
- Test range of motion (ROM).

- Palpate the preauricular, postauricular, occipital, tonsillar, submandibular, and submental nodes.
- Palpate the trachea.
- Palpate the thyroid gland for size, irregularity, or masses.
- Auscultate an enlarged thyroid for bruits.
- Palpate carotid arteries and auscultate for bruits.

Arms, Hands, and Fingers

- Inspect the upper extremities for overall skin color, texture, moisture, masses, and lesions.
- Test function of CN XI (spinal) by shoulder shrug and turning head against resistance.
- Palpate arms for tenderness, swelling, and temperature.
- Assess epitrochlear lymph nodes.
- Test ROM of the elbows.
- Palpate the brachial pulse.
- Palpate ulnar and radial pulses.
- Test ROM of the wrist.
- Inspect palms of hands and palpate for temperature.
- Test ROM of the fingers.
- Use a reflex hammer to test biceps, triceps, and brachioradialis reflexes.

- Test rapid alternating movements of hands.
- Ask the client to close the eyes; test sensation:
  - Assess light touch, pain, and temperature sensation in scattered locations over hands and arms.
  - Evaluate sensitivity of position of fingers.
  - Place a quarter or key in the client's hand to test stereognosis.
  - Assess graphesthesia by writing a number in the palm of the client's hand.
  - Assess two-point discrimination in the fingertips, forearm, and dorsal hands.

Ask client to continue sitting with arms at sides and stand behind client. Untie gown to expose posterior chest.

Posterior and Lateral Chest

- Inspect configuration and shape of scapulae and chest wall.
- Note use of accessory muscles when breathing and posture.
- Palpate for tenderness, sensation, crepitus, masses, lesions, and fremitus.
- Evaluate chest expansion at level T9 or T10.
- Percuss for tone at posterior intercostal spaces (comparing bilaterally).

Anterior Chest

- Inspect anteroposterior diameter of chest, slope of ribs, and color of chest.
- Note quality and pattern of respirations (rate, rhythm, and depth).
- Observe intercostal spaces for bulging or retractions and use of accessory muscles.
- Palpate for tenderness, sensation, masses, lesions, fremitus, and anterior chest expansion.
- Percuss for tone at apices above clavicles, then at intercostal spaces (comparing bilaterally).

Move to front of client and expose anterior chest. Allow client to maintain modesty.

- Ask client to lean forward and exhale; use bell of stethoscope to listen over the apex and left sternal border of the heart.
- Test for two-point discrimination on the client's back.
- Auscultate for breath sounds, adventitious sounds, and voice sounds (bronchophony, egophony, and whispered pectoriloquy).
- Determine diaphragmatic excursion.

Breasts

Ask client to fold gown to waist and sit with arms hanging freely.

- Pinch skin over sternum to assess mobility (ease to pinch) and turgor (return to original shape).
- Auscultate for anterior breath sounds, adventitious sounds, and voice sounds.

FEMALE BREASTS

- Inspect size, symmetry, color, texture, superficial venous pattern, areolae, and nipples of both breasts.
- Inspect for retractions and dimpling of nipples: Have the client raise her arms overhead, press her hands on her hips, press her hands together in front of her, and lean forward.
- Palpate axillae for rashes, infection, and anterior, central, and posterior lymph nodes.

MALE BREASTS

- Inspect for swelling, nodules, and ulcerations.
- Palpate the breast tissue and axillae.

Assist client to supine position with the head elevated to 30° to 45°.

Stand on client's right side.

Neck

Observe and evaluate jugular venous pressure.

Assist client to supine position (lower examination table).

Complete examination of female breasts:
- Palpate breasts for masses and the nipples for discharge.
- Teach breast self-examination.

Heart

- Inspect and palpate for apical impulse.
- Palpate the apex, left sternal border, and base of the heart for any abnormal pulsations.
- Auscultate over aortic area, pulmonic area, Erb's point, tricuspid area, and mitral area (apex) for:
  - Heart rate and rhythm (with diaphragm of stethoscope). If irregular, auscultate for a pulse rate deficit.
  - S_1 and S_2 (with diaphragm of stethoscope)
  - Extra heart sounds, S_3 and S_4 (with diaphragm and bell of stethoscope)
  - Murmurs (using bell and diaphragm of the stethoscope)

- *Ask the client to lie on left side;* use bell of stethoscope to listen to apex of the heart.

Cover chest with gown and arrange draping to expose abdomen.

Abdomen

- Inspect for:
  - Overall skin color
  - Vascularity, striae, lesions, and rashes
  - Location, contour, and color of umbilicus
  - Symmetry and contour of abdomen
  - Aortic pulsations or peristaltic waves
- Auscultate for:
  - Bowel sounds (intensity, pitch, and frequency)
  - Vascular sounds and friction rubs (over spleen, liver, aorta, iliac artery, umbilicus, and femoral artery)
- Percuss for:
  - Tone over four quadrants
  - Liver location, size, and span
  - Spleen location and size
- Lightly palpate:
  - Abdominal reflex

– Four quadrants to identify tenderness and muscular resistance
- Deeply palpate:
  – Four quadrants for masses
  – Aorta
  – Liver, spleen, and kidneys for enlargement or irregularities

Replace gown and position draping so lower extremities are exposed.

Legs, Feet, and Toes

- Inspect the lower extremities for overall skin coloration, texture, moisture, masses, lesions, and varicosities.
- Observe muscles of the legs and feet.
- Note hair distribution.
- Palpate joints of hips and test ROM. Palpate the femoral pulse.
- Palpate for:
  – Edema, skin temperature
  – Muscle size and tone of legs and feet
- Palpate knees including popliteal pulse.
- Palpate the ankles; assess dorsalis pedis and posterior tibial pulses. Test ROM.

- Assess capillary refill.
- Test
  – Sensation to dull and sharp sensations
  – Two-point discrimination (on thighs)
  – Patellar reflex, Achilles reflex, and plantar reflex
  – Position sense
  – Vibratory sensation on bony surface of big toe
- Perform heel-to-shin test.
- As warranted, perform special tests:
  – Position change for arterial insufficiency
  – Manual compression test
  – Trendelenburg test
  – Bulge knee test
  – Ballottement test
  – McMurray's test

Secure gown and assist client to standing position.

Musculoskeletal and Neurologic Examination

Note: Parts of these systems have already been assessed throughout the physical examination.

- Check for spinal curvatures and scoliosis.
- Observe gait including base of support, weight-bearing stability, foot position, stride, arm swing, and posture.
- Observe as the client:
  - Walks heel to toe (tandem walk)
  - Hops on one leg, then the other
  - Performs Romberg's test
  - Performs finger-to-nose test

Perform the female and male genitalia examination last, moving from the less private to more private examination for client comfort.

Genitalia

FEMALE GENITALIA

Have female client assume the lithotomy position. Apply gloves. Apply lubricant as appropriate.

- Inspect:
  - Distribution of pubic hair
  - Mons pubis, labia majora, and perineum for lesions, swelling, and excoriations
  - Labia minora, clitoris, urethral meatus, and vaginal opening for lesions, swelling, or discharge

- Palpate:
  - Bartholin glands, urethra, and Skene glands
  - Size of vaginal opening and vaginal musculature
- Insert speculum and inspect:
  - Cervix for lesions and discharge
  - Vagina for color, consistency, and discharge
- Obtain cytologic smears and cultures.
- Perform bimanual examination; palpate:
  - Cervix for contour, consistency, mobility, and tenderness
  - Uterus for size, position, shape, and consistency
  - Ovaries for size and shape

Discard gloves and apply clean gloves and lubricant.

- Perform the rectovaginal examination; palpate rectovaginal septum for tenderness, consistency, and mobility.

MALE GENITALIA AND RECTUM

Sit on a stool. Have client stand and face you with gown raised. Apply gloves.

- Inspect the penis, including:
  - Base of penis and pubic hair for excoriation, erythema, and infestation
  - Skin and shaft of penis for rashes, lesions, lumps, or hardened or tender areas

- Color, location, and integrity of foreskin in uncircumcised men
  - Glans for size, shape, lesions, or redness and location of urinary meatus
- Palpate for urethral discharge by gently squeezing glans.
- Inspect scrotum, including:
  - Size, shape, and position
  - Scrotal skin for color, integrity, lesions, or rashes
  - Posterior skin (by lifting scrotal sac)
- Palpate both testis and epididymis between thumb and first two fingers for size, shape, nodules, and tenderness. Palpate spermatic cord and vas deferens.
- Transilluminate scrotal contents for red glow, swelling, or masses. If a mass is found during inspection and palpation, have the client lie down and inspect and palpate for scrotal hernia.
- As client bears down, inspect for bulges in inguinal and femoral areas and palpate for femoral hernias.
- While client shifts weight to each corresponding side, palpate for inguinal hernia.
- Teach testicular self-examination.

Ask the client to remain standing and to bend over the exam table. Change gloves.

- Inspect:
  - Perianal area for lumps, lesions, ulcers, rashes, redness, fissures, or thickening of epithelium
  - Sacrococcygeal area for swelling, redness, dimpling, or hair
- While client bears down or performs Valsalva maneuver, inspect for bulges or lesions.
- Apply lubrication and use finger to palpate:
  - Anus
  - External sphincter for tenderness, nodules, and hardness
  - Rectum for tenderness, irregularities, nodules, and hardness
  - Peritoneal cavity
  - Prostate for size, shape, tenderness, and consistency
- Inspect stool for color and test feces for occult blood.

Abbreviated Physical Assessment Format

The following is a brief "Head-to-Toe Physical Assessment Guide" that may be used to establish the client's physical status. This type of assessment is frequently used by nurses at the beginning of a hospital shift when the nurse has multiple clients to whom she will provide nursing care. Often a total physical examination is done upon admission to the hospital by the physician or nurse practitioner. Therefore this shorter format is more practical for ongoing client assessments.

PROCEDURE	NORMAL FINDINGS	ABNORMAL FINDINGS
General Survey		
Assess level of consciousness (LOC)	Awake, alert, and oriented to person, place, and time.	If altered LOC, consider the Glasgow Coma Scale
Assess speech	Speech clear. Makes and maintains conversation appropriately.	
Assess comfort level	Denies c/o pain/discomfort.	If the patient reports or c/o pain: rate the pain using the 0–10 pain scale, intervene to provide comfort measures and evaluate the effectiveness of such interventions.
Skin color, temperature, moisture, turgor	Skin: pink, warm, and dry. Immediate recoil noted at the clavicle.	Pale, pallor ← anemia Erythema ← infection Warmth ← infection Increased tenting ← dehydration

Continued on following page

Abbreviated Physical Assessment Format (Continued)

PROCEDURE	NORMAL FINDINGS	ABNORMAL FINDINGS
Eyes		
Assess pupils	Pupils equal, round, react to light and accommodation (PERRLA).	Pupils unequal or nonreactive to light.
Chest		
Assess breath sounds	Lungs: clear to auscultation (CTA) anterior and posterior (A & P), bilaterally. Respiratory rate 18, no reports of dyspnea	Note any wheezes or crackles and identify their location (anterior or posterior, upper or lower lobes, right or left).
Assess heart sounds	Heart: S_1 and S_2 present, regular rate (82) and rhythm. No S_3 or S_4 appreciated. No murmur, rub, or gallop (MRG).	Heart sounds irregular or irregularly irregular.
Note if rhythm is irregular.		Murmurs, rub, or gallop—if present.
Abdomen		
Assess contour and firmness	Nondistended, soft, and nontender.	Distended and firm, visible palpations
Assess bowel sounds	Active bowel sounds noted in all four quadrants. ($+ABS \times 4Q$)	Absence of bowel sounds in one or more quadrants. One must listen for 5 minutes to document absent bowel sounds. Normal bowel sounds 5–35/min.
Extremities		
Assess mobility of extremities, strength of extremities, and peripheral pulses	Able to actively move all extremities. Equal strength. 5/5. Radial, dorsalis pedis, and posterior tibia pulses 2+. No peripheral edema.	Unable to actively or passively move one or more extremities.

PROCEDURE	NORMAL FINDINGS
Other	
Note any wounds or lesions	Describe: size, shape, location, color, characteristics of any drainage, type of dressing.
Note any drains: Jackson-Pratt, Foley catheter, Hemovac, nasogastric tube.	Describe insertion site: color, consistency, and/or odor of any drainage.
Note any venous access devices	Describe the location, appearance, type and size of device, type of intravenous fluids and rate of infusion, and infusion device(s).
Note any other therapies: external ice/heat devices, continuous passive motion devices, TENS unit, etc.	Describe the presence of correct functioning of any of these devices.

APPENDIX 3

Sample Adult Nursing Health History and Physical Assessment

Health History

A. CLIENT PROFILE

S.L. is a 72-year-old white female, born on a small farm in south-ern Missouri. Appears younger than stated age. English speaking, with a German ethnic origin. High school graduate and presently retired from restaurant work. Lives in a one-bedroom apartment on first floor. Drives own car. Seeks health care in local community hospital 4 miles from home. Major reason for seeking health care is for routine checkup—has not had one for 8 years. Understands that she has adult-onset diabetes mellitus (type 2), which is controlled with 1800-calorie diet and moderate amount of exercise. Also has "mild rheumatoid arthritic" pains in right hip and finger joints in early mornings; relieved with exercise, warm baths, and ASA.

Treatments/Medications

1. Prescribed: none
2. OTC
   a. ASA gr at H.S. for "arthritis aches." Takes about 2× per month. Denies nausea, abdominal pains or evidence of bleeding while taking.
   b. Mylanta at H.S. for "gas pains."
   c. Dulcolax suppository 3×/week for past 4 years.
   d. Multivitamin 1 qd, for past 4 years.

Past Illnesses/Hospitalizations

1. Appendectomy age 18.
2. Left arm fracture age 20.
3. Cholecystectomy age 56, performed for complaint of gas pains after eating fatty foods. Satisfied with care received at local hospital.

Allergies

Denies food, drug, and environmental allergies.

B. DEVELOPMENTAL HISTORY

Developmental Level: Integrity vs Despair

Describes childhood as a very happy time for her. Becomes excited and smiles as she relates stories of her childhood on the farm. States she was an average child and ran and played like all the others. Companions were brothers and sisters. Has been married for 55 years. Describes relationship with husband as close and sharing. Owned and operated a restaurant for 30 years with husband and was a waitress at another restaurant after they retired from their own. Lived in a large house until 1988. Currently lives in a one-bedroom apartment. Active in church and society. Volunteers at community functions. She and her husband are active in their church. States she enjoys being retired and lives a "comfortable" life. Does not voice financial concerns. Has begun to write will and distribute personal heirlooms to son and grandchildren. States she is not afraid of death and wishes to have the "business part taken care of" in order to enjoy the rest of her life together with her husband.

C. HEALTH PERCEPTION–HEALTH MANAGEMENT PATTERN

1. Client's rating of health:
   Scale: 10-best; 1-worst
   5 years ago: 10

Now: 8
5 years from now: 6

Sees health deterioration as normal aging process and states,
"I feel really good when I look at a lot of people my age with
all their problems and the medicine they take."

2. Health does not interfere with self-care or other desired
activities of daily living. Unaware of signs, symptoms, and Tx
of hyperglycemia and hypoglycemia. Denies use of alcohol,
tobacco, and drugs.

3. Client seeks health care only in emergencies. Last medical
exam September 1996. Keeps active and feels well. Feels lifestyle and faith "keep her going." Does not check own blood
sugar or do breast self-exams.

D. NUTRITIONAL–METABOLIC PATTERN

States she is on a "no concentrated sweet" meal pattern as follows: Eats breakfast of whole wheat toast, one boiled egg, orange
juice, and decaf. coffee at 7 AM. Eats lunch at noon. Today had
tuna, lettuce salad, apple, and milk. Eats light supper around
6 PM. Typical dinner includes small serving broiled meat, green
vegetables, piece of fruit, and glass of milk. Tries not to snack
but will have fruit if she feels the urge. Drinks two 8-oz glasses
of water a day. Drinks decaf. coffee—no tea or colas. Voices no
dislikes or food intolerances.

Wears dentures. Last dental exam October 1996. Denies problems with proper fit, eating, chewing, swallowing, sore throat,
sore tongue, or colds. Complains of "canker sore" if she eats
strawberries. Denies n/v, abdominal pain, or excessive gas. Complains of dyspepsia approx. 2×/month, relieved by Mylanta.
Does not associate this with the time she takes ASA.

Describes skin and scalp as dry. Uses lotions frequently. Denies
easy bruising, pruritus, or nonhealing sores. Nails are hard and
brittle. Hair is fine and soft.
Current weight: 120 lb; height: 5'4"
Previous weight: 150 lb 10 years ago. Desires to maintain current weight.
Weight fluctuates ± 5 lb/month. Client states, "I've always had
to watch what I eat because I gain so easily." Denies intolerance
to heat or cold, or voice changes.

E. ELIMINATION PATTERN

Bowel habits: Soft, formed, med. brown bowel movement (BM)
every third day after Dulcolax suppository. States she becomes
constipated without use of laxative. Denies mucous, bloody, or

tarry stools. States discomfort with BMs starting in September 1996. When having to strain with BMs felt "some kind of mass" prolapsing from rectum. Consulted her doctor, who explained to her "it was a piece of my colon slipping out." No surgical treatment or exercises prescribed. Gently reinserts tissue when this happens. Denies rectal bleeding, change in color, consistency, or habits.

Bladder habits: Voids 4–5×/day, clear yellow urine. Denies current problems with dysuria, hematuria, polyuria, hesitancy, incontinence, or nocturia. Complaint of urgency during the colder months with no increase in frequency. Had polyuria and polydipsia prior to diagnosis of diabetes type 2. Developed UTI at age 60, at which time she sought medical advice and was diagnosed with type 2 diabetes mellitus.

F. ACTIVITY–EXERCISE PATTERN

1. ADLs on an average day: Arises at 6 AM. Eats breakfast and does housekeeping. In early afternoon goes to the community center to eat lunch, quilt, and visit. Goes home around 2 PM. Walks about four blocks with a friend every day. Cleans own house daily for one 2-hour period (includes dusting, vacuuming, washing). Denies palpitations, chest pain, SOB, fatigue, wheezing, claudication, cramps, stiffness, or joint pain or swelling with activity. Walking relieves ache in hips and makes her feel good. After walking, returns home and relaxes with crafts and visiting with husband. During evenings attends church-related activities. Expresses satisfaction with activity and believes she functions above the level of the average person her age.
2. Hygiene: Showers and washes hair every day.
3. Occupational activities: Retired from being a cook and waitress. Volunteers to cook for church group. Occasionally has lower back pains when carrying large amounts of food or when carrying large trays.

G. SEXUALITY–REPRODUCTION PATTERN

Menstrual history: Age of menarche: approx. 12 years; age of menopause: 50 years. States, "going through my change of life wasn't difficult for me physically or emotionally." Described menstrual period as regular, lasting 4 days with moderate flow. Denies postmenopausal spotting at this time.

Obstetric history: Gravida 1, Para 1. No complications with pregnancy or childbirth.

Contraception: Never used any form.

Sexual activities: Sexually active. States, "My husband and I have good relations." Denies pain, discomfort, or postcoital bleeding.

Special problems: Denies history of any sexually transmitted diseases. Denies problem with vaginal itching. Last Pap smear negative in 1988.

H. SLEEP–REST PATTERN

Goes to bed at 10 PM. Denies difficulty falling asleep or sleeping. Feels well rested when she arises at 6 AM. Never used sleep medications. Denies orthopnea and nocturnal dyspnea. Enjoys reading 1 to 2 pages of Bible history each evening.

I. SENSORY–PERCEPTUAL PATTERN

1. *Vision:* Has worn glasses "all of my life." Cannot recall age at which they were prescribed. Prescription change from bifocals to trifocals August 1996. Complains of blurred vision without glasses. Denies diplopia, itching, excessive tearing, discharge, redness, or trauma to eyes.

2. *Hearing:* Believes she is "a little slow to grasp, and I think it may be because of my hearing." Does not wear hearing aid. Cannot recall last hearing test. Denies tinnitus, pain, discharge, or trauma to ears. Does not ask for questions to be repeated when asked at normal voice tone and level.

3. *Smell:* Denies difficulty with smell, pain, postnasal drip, sneezing, or frequent nosebleeds.

4. *Touch:* States "occasionally my feet feel numb"; subsides on own.

5. *Taste:* No difficulty tasting foods.

J. COGNITIVE PATTERN

Speech clear without slur or stutter. Follows verbal cues. Expresses ideas and feelings clearly and concisely. States she has had a gradual loss of memory over past 5 to 6 years. Believes long-term memory is better than short term. She can recall past weekly events but has trouble recalling dates, times, and places of events. Learns best by writing information down and then reviewing it. Makes major decisions jointly with husband after prayer.

K. ROLE–RELATIONSHIP PATTERN

Client has been married 55 years. Describes relationship as the best part of her life right now. Only son lives in Minnesota, and they visit one to two times a year. Is very fond of three grandchildren. Expresses desire to visit more often but states, "He has his own life and family now." Communicates once a month by phone. Explains her relationship with other members of the church and community groups as friendly and "familylike." Lives

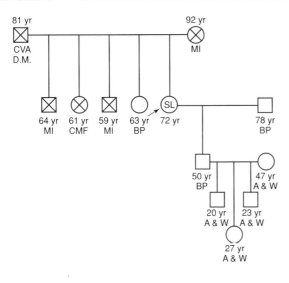

with husband in first-floor apartment. Has casual relationship with apartment neighbors—friendly but distant. Was the oldest of five children. See family genogram.

L. SELF-PERCEPTION–SELF-CONCEPT PATTERN

Describes self as a normal person. Talkative, outgoing, and likes to be around people but hates noisy environments. Happy with the person she has become and states, "I can definitely live with myself." States a weakness is that she worries about "little things" more now than she used to and tends to be irritated more easily. Cannot place specific onset of these feelings. Feels good about self-control of diabetes.

M. COPING–STRESS TOLERANCE PATTERN

States husband's high blood pressure has never been a source of stress to her. Shares confidences with husband and with a few close friends. Most stressful time in life was losing two brothers and a sister, all in 1994. States with the support of husband and church she handled it "better than most people would have." States she prays and eats when under stress. Cannot identify any major stresses that have occurred in the last year.

N. VALUE-BELIEF PATTERN

Religious preference is Lutheran. Values relationship with husband, family, and God. Enjoys helping others in the church and community. Believes God is loving, supportive, and forgiving. Places God as first priority in life. States prayer is extremely important to her and practices it daily. States this personalizes her relationship with God. Has been Lutheran all her life and states she and her husband share in church activities together.

Physical Assessment

A. GENERAL PHYSICAL SURVEY

Ht: 5'4", Wt: 120 lb, Radial pulse: 71, Resp: 16, BP: R arm—120/72, L arm—120/70, Temp: 98.6°F. Client alert and cooperative. Sitting comfortably on table with arms crossed and shoulders slightly slouched forward. Smiling with mild anxiety. Dress is neat and clean. Walks steadily with posture slightly stooped.

B. SKIN, HAIR, AND NAIL ASSESSMENT

1. *Skin:* Pale pink, warm and dry to touch. Skinfold returns to place after 1 second when lifted over clavicle. Tan "age spots" on posterior hands bilaterally in clusters of four to five and evenly distributed over lower extremities. A 3-cm nodule with 2-mm macule in center noted in right axilla; indurated, nontender, and nonmobile. No evidence of vascular or purpuric lesions. No edema.

2. *Hair:* Chin length, gray, straight, clean, styled, medium-textured, evenly distributed on head. No scalp lesions or flaking. Fine blond hair evenly distributed over arms bilaterally and sparsely on legs bilaterally. No hair noted on axilla or on chest, back, or face.

3. *Nails:* Fingernails medium length, and thickness, clear. Splinter hemorrhages noted on right thumb near fingertip in midline. No clubbing or Beau lines.

C. HEAD AND NECK ASSESSMENT

Head symmetrically rounded, neck nontender with full ROM. Neck symmetrical without masses, scars, pulsations. Lymph nodes nonpalpable. Trachea in midline. Thyroid nonpalpable. Carotid arteries equally strong without bruits. Identifies light and deep touch to various parts of face.

CN V: Identifies light touch and sharp touch to forehead, check, and chin. Bilateral corneal reflex intact. Masseter muscles contract equally and bilaterally. Jaw jerk + 1.

CN VII: Identifies sugar and salt on anterior two thirds of tongue. Smiles, frowns, shows teeth, blows cheeks, and raises eyebrows as instructed.

D. EYE ASSESSMENT

Eyes 2 cm apart without protrusion. Eyebrows sparse with equal distribution. No scaliness noted. Lids pink without ptosis, edema, or lesions, and freely closeable bilaterally. Lacrimal apparatus nonedematous. Sclera white without increased vascularity or lesions noted. Palpebral and bulbar conjunctiva slightly reddened without lesions noted. Irises uniformly blue. PERRLA, EOMs intact bilaterally. Peripheral vision equal to examiner's.

Visual acuity: With glasses off vision is blurred at 14″ away, but can identify number of fingers held up. With glasses on reads newspaper print at 14″.

Funduscopic exam: Red reflex present bilaterally. Optic disc round with well-defined margins. Physiologic cup occupies disc. Arterioles smaller than venules. No A-V nicking, no hemorrhages, or exudates noted. Macula not seen. (CNs II, III, IV, and VI intact.)

E. EAR ASSESSMENT

Auricle without deformity, lumps, or lesions. Right auricle with tag at top of pinna. Auricles and mastoid processes nontender. Bilateral auditory canals contain moderate amount dark-brown cerumen. Tympanic membrane difficult to view due to wax.

Whisper test: Client identifies one out of two words in four attempts. Weber test: No lateralization of sound to either ear. Rinne test: AC is greater than BC both ears (CN VIII).

F. NOSE AND SINUSES ASSESSMENT

External structure without deformity, asymmetry, or inflammation. Nares patent. Turbinates and middle meatus pale pink, without swelling, exudate, lesions, or bleeding. Nasal septum midline without bleeding, perforation, or deviation. Frontal and maxillary sinuses nontender. Identifies smells of coffee and soap (CN I).

G. MOUTH AND PHARYNX ASSESSMENT

Lips moist with peach lipstick. No lesions or ulcerations. Buccal mucosa pink and moist without discoloration or increased pigmentation. No ulcers or nodules. Upper and lower dentures secure. Gums pink and moist without inflammation, bleeding, or discoloration. Hard and soft palates smooth without lesions or masses. Tongue midline when protruded without fasciculations (CN XII intact), lesions, or masses. No lesions, discolorations, or ulcerations on floor of mouth, oral mucosa, or gums. Gag reflex intact, and client identifies sugar and salt on posterior tongue. Uvula in midline and elevates on phonation. (CNS IX and X intact.) Tonsils present without exudate, edema, ulcers, or enlargement.

H. CARDIAC ASSESSMENT

No pulsations visible. No heaves, lifts, or vibrations. PMI: 5th ICS to LMCL. Clear, brief heart sounds throughout. Physiologic S_2. No gallops, murmurs, or rubs. AP = 72/min and regular.

I. PERIPHERAL VASCULAR SYSTEM ASSESSMENT

Arms: Equal in size and symmetry bilaterally; pale pink; warm and dry to touch without edema, bruising, or lesions noted. Radial pulses equal in rate and amplitude, and strong. Allen test: Right equal 2-second refill, left equal 2-second refill. Brachial pulses strong, equal, and even. Epitrochlear nodes nonpalpable.

Legs: Large in size and bilaterally symmetrical. Skin intact, pale pink; warm and dry to touch without edema, bruising, lesions, or increased vascularity. Superficial inguinal, horizontal, and vertical lymph nodes nonpalpable. Femoral pulses strong and equal without bruits. Popliteal pulse nonpalpable with client supine or prone. Dorsalis pedis and posterior tibial pulses strong and equal. No edema palpable. Homans negative bilaterally. No

retrograde filling noted when client stands. Toenails thick and yellowed. Special maneuver for arterial insufficiency: feet regain color after 4 seconds and veins refilled in 5 seconds.

J. THORAX AND LUNG ASSESSMENT

Skin pale pink without scars, pulsations, or lesions. No hair noted. Thorax expands evenly bilaterally without retractions or bulging. Slope of ribs = 40°. No use of auxiliary respiratory muscles and no nasal flaring. Respirations even, unlabored, and regular (16/min). No cough noted. No tenderness, crepitus, or masses. Tactile fremitus decreases below T5 bilaterally posteriorly, and 4th ICS anteriorly bilaterally. Thorax resonance throughout. Diaphragmatic excursion: Left—on inspiration diaphragm descends to T11, and on expiration diaphragm ascends to T9. Right—on inspiration diaphragm descends to T12, and on expiration diaphragm ascends to T9. Vesicular breath sounds heard in all lung fields. No rales, rhonchi, friction rubs, or abnormal whispered pectoriloquy, bronchophony, or egophony noted.

K. BREAST ASSESSMENT

Breasts moderate in size, round, and symmetrical bilaterally. Skin pale pink with light-brown areola. No dimpling or retraction. Free movement in all positions. Engorged vein noted running across UOQ to areola in right breast. Nipples inverted bilaterally. No discharge expressed. No thickening or tenderness noted. A 2-cm, hard, immobile round mass noted in left breast in LUOQ. Client denies ever noticing this. Nontender to palpation. Lymph nodes nonpalpable. Client does not know how to do breast self-exam.

L. ABDOMINAL ASSESSMENT

Abdomen rounded, symmetrical without masses, lesions, pulsations, or peristalsis noted. Abdomen free of hair, bruising, and increased vasculature. Healed with appendectomy scar. Umbilicus in midline, without herniation, swelling, or discoloration. Bowel sounds low pitched and gurgling at 22/minute × four quads. Aortic, renal, and iliac arteries auscultated without bruit. No venous hums or friction rubs auscultated over liver or spleen. Tympany percussed over all four quads. An 8-cm liver span percussed in RMCL. Area of dullness percussed at 9th ICS in left postaxillary line. No tenderness or masses noted with light and deep palpation in all four quadrants. Liver and spleen nonpalpable.

M. GENITOURINARY–REPRODUCTIVE ASSESSMENT

No bulging or masses in inguinal area. A 1-cm nodule palpated in right groin. Labia pink with decreased elasticity and vaginal secretions. No bulging of vaginal wall, purulent foul drainage, or lesions. Skene's gland not visible. Anal area pink with small amount of hair. Rectal mucosa bulges with straining.

N. MUSCULOSKELETAL ASSESSMENT

Posture slightly stooped with mild kyphosis. Gait steady, smooth, and coordinated with even base. Limited ROM of lateral flexion and extension of spine. Paravertebrals equal in size and strength. Shrugs shoulders and moves head to right and left against resistance (CN XI intact); upper extremities and lower extremities have full ROM. Muscles moderately firm bilaterally. No deviations, inflammations, or bony deformities. Small callus on left heel. Moves upper and lower extremities freely against gravity and against resistance. Rheumatoid nodule noted on dorsal surface of left hand.

O. NEUROLOGIC ASSESSMENT

Mental status: Pleasant and friendly. Appropriately dressed for weather with matching colors and patterns. Clothes neat and clean. Facial expressions symmetrical and correlate with mood and topic discussed. Speech clear and appropriate. Follows through with train of thought. Carefully chooses words to convey feelings and ideas. Oriented to person, place, time, and events. Remains attentive and able to focus on exam during entire interaction. Short-term memory intact, long-term memory before 1992 unclear—especially cannot recall dates and sequencing of events. General information questions answered correctly 100% of the time. Vocabulary suitable to educational level. Explains proverb accurately. Gives semiabstract answers and enjoys joking. Is able to identify similarities 5 seconds after asked. Answers to judgment questions in realistic manner.

Cranial nerves: I–XII intact (integrated throughout exam).

Cerebellar and motor function: Alternates finger to nose with eyes closed; occasionally tends to hit opposite side of nose. Rapidly opposes fingers to thumb bilaterally without difficulty. Alternates pronation and supination of hands rapidly without difficulty. Heel to shin intact bilaterally. Romberg: minimal swaying. Tandem walk: steady. No involuntary movements noted.

Sensory status: Superficial light- and deep-touch sensation intact on arms, legs, neck, chest, and back. Position sense of toes and fingers intact bilaterally. Identifies point localization correctly. Identifies coin placed in hand and number written on palm of hand correctly.

Two-Point Discrimination (in mm)	Right	Left
Fingertips	6	6
Dorsal hand	15	15
Chest	45	49
Forearm	39	35
Back	45	45
Upper arm	40	45

Reflexes	Right	Left
Biceps	2+	2+
Triceps	2+	2+
Patellar	3+	3+
Achilles	2+	2+
Abdominal	1+	1+
Babinski	neg	neg

Motor status: Muscle tone firm at rest, abdominal muscles slightly relaxed. Muscle size adequate for age. No fasciculations or involuntary movements noted. Muscle strength moderately strong and equal bilaterally.

CLIENT'S STRENGTHS

- Positive attitude and outlook in life
- Motivation to comply with prescribed diet
- Strong support systems: husband and spiritual beliefs
- No physical limitations

NURSING DIAGNOSES

- Risk for Ineffective Health Maintenance related to lack of knowledge concerning importance of regular medical checkups, re: lesion in UOQ of left breast not seen by physician, no Pap smear, and no follow-up with diabetes
- Acute right hip pain
- Constipation related to lack of bowel routine and laxative overuse
- Knowledge Deficit: Signs, symptoms, and treatment of hyperglycemia/hypoglycemia
- Knowledge Deficit: Management and causes of constipation
- Knowledge Deficit: self breast exam technique
- Knowledge Deficit: Importance of self-blood glucose monitoring

COLLABORATIVE PROBLEMS

- Risk for complication: Hyperglycemia, hypoglycemia
- Risk for complication: Hypertension

Assessment of Family Functional Health Patterns

The nurse obtains data about the family's functional health patterns by interviewing the family as a group or by interviewing one or two family members who are reliable historians and seem knowledgeable about their family's health patterns. If data reveal a particular problem identified with an individual family member, the nurse can then focus attention on obtaining more data from that individual.

I. Family Profile

The purpose of the family profile is to obtain biographical family data (age, sex, and current health status of each family member). A genogram may be used to illustrate this information.

II. Health Perception–Health Management Pattern

SUBJECTIVE DATA

- Describe your family's general health during the past few years.
- Has your family been able to participate in its usual activities (work, school, sports)?
- Describe what your family does to try to stay healthy (diet, exercise, etc.).
- From whom does your family seek health care? When?
- Describe how your family members check their health status (eg, eye exams, dental exams, breast exams, testicular exams, medical checkups).
- Describe any behaviors in your family that are considered unhealthy.
- Who cares for family members who are or who become ill?
- How would you know if a family member were ill?

OBJECTIVE DATA

1. Observe the appearance of family members.
2. Observe the home (hazards and safety devices, storage facilities, cooking facilities).

III. Nutritional–Metabolic Pattern

SUBJECTIVE DATA

- Describe typical breakfast, lunch, supper, and snacks that you eat as a family.
- What type of drinks do you usually have during the day and at night?
- How would you describe your family's appetite in general?
- How often does your family seek dental care? Are there any dental problems in your family?
- Does anyone in your family have skin rashes or problems with sores healing? Explain.
- Who usually prepares the family meals? Who shops for groceries?

OBJECTIVE DATA

1. Observe kitchen appliances, availability of food, and types of foods kept in the home, if possible.
2. Observe preparation of a family meal, if possible.
3. Observe family members for obvious signs of malnutrition or obesity.

IV. Elimination Pattern

SUBJECTIVE DATA

• How often do family members have bowel movements? Urinate?
• Are laxatives used in your family? Explain.
• Are there problems with disposing of waste or garbage?
• Describe any recycling you do.
• Does your family have pets (indoor or outdoor)? How are their wastes disposed?
• Do you have problems with insects in your home? Explain.

OBJECTIVE DATA

1. Observe bathroom facilities.
2. Inspect home for insects.
3. Observe garbage and waste disposal.

V. Activity–Exercise Pattern

SUBJECTIVE DATA

• Describe how your family exercises. Frequency?
• How does your family relax?
• What does your family do for enjoyment?
• Describe a typical day of activities in your family (work, school, play, games, meals, hobbies, house cleaning, yard work, cooking, exercise).

OBJECTIVE DATA

1. Observe the pace of family activities.
2. Observe any exercise equipment kept in home.

VI. Sleep–Rest Pattern

SUBJECTIVE DATA

• When does your family generally go to bed and awaken? Do family members go to bed and arise at different times? Explain.
• Does your family seem to get enough time to sleep? To rest and relax?
• Do any family members work at night? How does this affect other family members?

OBJECTIVE DATA

1. Observe sleeping areas.
2. Observe temperament and energy level of family members.

VII. Sensory–Perceptual Pattern

SUBJECTIVE DATA

- Are there any hearing or visual problems that affect your family members?
- Are there any deficits in a family member's ability to taste and smell that affect how food is prepared for the family?
- Does pain seem to be a family problem? Explain. How is this managed?
- What is the usual form of pain relief used by family members?

OBJECTIVE DATA

1. Observe any visual or hearing aids used by family members.
2. Observe medications kept on hand to relieve pain.

VIII. Cognitive Pattern

SUBJECTIVE DATA

- Who makes the major family decisions? How?
- Describe the highest educational level of all family members.
- Does your family understand any illnesses and treatments that affect any of your family members?
- How does your family enjoy learning (eg, reading, watching television, attending classes)?
- Are there any problems with memory in the family? Explain.

OBJECTIVE DATA

1. Observe language spoken by all family members.
2. Observe use of words (vocabulary level), and ability to grasp ideas and express self.
3. Are family decisions present or future oriented? Observe family decision-making strategies.
4. Observe school attended by children.

IX. Self-Perception–Self-Concept Pattern

SUBJECTIVE DATA

- Describe the general mood of your family (eg, sad, happy, eager, depressed, anxious, relaxed).
- Do you consider yourselves to be a close family? How do you spend time together? Is this time satisfying?
- Do family members share any common goals? Explain.
- What does the family enjoy doing most together?
- How does your family deal with disagreements?

X. Role–Relationship Pattern

SUBJECTIVE DATA

- Describe how your family members support each other, show affection, and express concerns.
- Describe any problems with relationships between family members.
- Describe your family resources (financial, community support systems, family support systems).
- How do your family members express their affection, feelings, and/or concerns? Are they allowed to do so freely? Explain.
- Does your family seem to discuss problems that affect individual members?
- How does your family deal with change?

OBJECTIVE DATA

1. Observe family discussions.
2. Observe mood and temperament of family.
3. Observe how family members deal with conflict.
4. How do family members show concern and consideration for each other's needs and desires?

- How active is your family in your neighborhood and/or community?
- Explain family responsibilities for various household chores (washing, cooking, driving, lawn maintenance, etc.).
- Explain how discipline is used in your family. How are family members rewarded? Describe any aggression and/or violence that occurs in your family.

OBJECTIVE DATA

1. Observe family interaction patterns (verbal and nonverbal).
2. Explore which family members take responsibility for managing and leading family activities.
3. Observe living space and ownership of rooms by family members.

XI. Sexuality–Reproductive Pattern

SUBJECTIVE DATA

If appropriate: Are sexual partners within home satisfied with sexual relationship and activities? Describe any problems.

- Are contraceptives used?
- Is family planning used? How?

- Are parents comfortable answering questions and explaining topics related to sexuality to their children?

XII. Coping–Stress Tolerance Pattern

SUBJECTIVE DATA

- What major changes have occurred in your family during the past year (eg, divorce, marriage, family members leaving home, new members coming into home, death, illness, births, accidents, change in finances and/or occupation)?
- How does your family *cope* with major stressors (eg, exercise, discussion, prayer, drugs, alcohol, violence)?
- Who in the family copes best with stressors?
- Who has the most difficult time coping with stress?
- Who outside the family (eg, friends, church, support groups) seems to help your family most during difficult times?

OBJECTIVE DATA

1. Observe effect and pace of family interactions.

XIII. Value–Belief Pattern

SUBJECTIVE DATA

- What does your family consider to be most important in life?
- What does your family want from life?
- What rules does your family hold most important?
- Is religion important in the family? What religion are family members? What religious practices are important to the family? Is a relationship with God important to the family?
- What does your family look forward to in the future?
- From where do the family's hope and strength come?

OBJECTIVE DATA

1. Observe family rituals and/or traditions.
2. Observe pictures and other articles (religious or other) in home.
3. Listen to general topics discussed in home by family members.
4. Observe the type of television programs viewed by family members and the type of music to which family members listen.

Developmental Information—Age 1 Month to 18 Years

Age	Physical Development	Language (Cognitive) Development (Based on PIAGET)	Psychosocial Development (Based on ERIKSON)	Nurse's Approach To Assessment
Overview of birth to 1 year		*Sensorimotor stage of development.*	*Developmental task: trust vs mistrust.* Learns to trust and to anticipate satisfaction. Sends cues to	Involve caretaker in assessment (eg, allow him or her to hold

Age	Physical Development	Language (Cognitive) Development (Based on PIAGET)	Psychosocial Development (Based on ERIKSON)	Nurse's Approach To Assessment
			mother/caretaker. Begins understanding self as separate from others (body image).	child in lap for parts of examination).
1–2 months	Lifts chin and chest off bed. Holds extremities in flexion and moves at random; weak neck muscles. Activity varies from quiet sleep to drowsiness to alert activity.	Can discriminate between various sensations and prefers certain ones. Follows moving objects with eyes.	Begins to bond with mother during alert periods.	Conserve infant's body heat. Assess while asleep or quiet. Place infant on table or in caretaker's arms. Give bottle if awake.
3–4 months	Head and back control developing. Holds rattle. Looks at own hands. Infant reflexes begin to disappear. Able to sit propped. Props self on forearm in prone position. Rolls	Responds to parent. Social smile. Begins to vocalize; coos, babbles. Locates sounds by turning head, looking.	Learns to signal displeasure. Shows excitement with whole body. Begins to discriminate strangers. Squeals.	Speak softly to infant. Use brightly colored toys, bells, rattles to elicit necessary responses and to distract. Assess ears, mouth, nose last. Assess lungs and heart when quiet.

Continued on following page

Age	Physical Development	Language (Cognitive) Development (Based on PIAGET)	Psychosocial Development (Based on ERIKSON)	Nurse's Approach To Assessment
5–8 months	from side to back and vice versa and from back to abdomen. Takes objects to mouth. Drools with eruption of lower teeth. Begins to develop teeth. Birth weight doubled. Grasps objects. Sits unsupported.	Begins to imitate sounds, two-syllable words ("dada," "mama,").	Increased fear of strangers. Definite likes/dislikes. Responds to "no."	Place on caretaker's lap (same as above).
9–12 months	Birth weight tripled. Anterior fontanelle nearly closed. Learns to pull in order to stand, creep, and crawl.	Responds to own name. Says two-syllable words besides "dada," "mama." Understands simple commands, imitates animal sounds. Looks for hidden objects.	Unceasing determination to move about. Clings to mother. Shows emotion. Plays peek-a-boo and pat-a-cake.	

Age	Physical Development	Language (Cognitive) Development (Based on PIAGET)	Psychosocial Development (Based on ERIKSON)	Nurse's Approach To Assessment
1–3 years	Begins to walk and run well. Drinks from cup, feeds self. Develops fine motor control. Climbs. Begins self-toileting. Kneels without support. Steady growth in height/ weight. Adult height will be approximately double the height at age 2. Dresses self by age 3.	*Preoperational stage of development.* Has poor time sense. Increasing verbal ability. Formulates sentences of 4 to 5 words by age 3. Talks to self and others. Has misconceptions about cause and effect. Interested in pictures. *Fears:* • Loss/separation from parents—peak • Dark • Machines/equipment • Intrusive procedures • Bedtime Speaks to dolls and animals. Increasing attention span. Knows own sex by age 3.	*Developmental task: autonomy vs shame and doubt.* Establishes self-control, decision making, independence (autonomy). Extremely curious and prefers to do things by self. Demonstrates independence through negativism. Very egocentric; believes he or she controls the world. Attempts to please parents. Participates in parallel play; able to share some toys by age 3.	Be flexible. Begin assessment with play period to establish rapport. Be honest. Praise for cooperation. Begin slowly; speak to child. Involve caretaker/ parent in holding on exam table. Let child hold security object. Allow child to play with stethoscope, tongue blade, flashlight before using on child if possible. Assess face, mouth, eyes, ears last. May need to restrain when lying prone. If resistant, save that part of the assessment for later.

Continued on following page

Age	Physical Development	Language (Cognitive) Development (Based on PIAGET)	Psychosocial Development (Based on ERIKSON)	Nurse's Approach To Assessment
4–6 years	Growth slows. Locomotion skills increase and coordination improves. Tricycle/bicycle riding. Throws ball but has difficulty catching. Constantly active, increasing dexterity. Eruption of permanent teeth. Skips, hops, jumps rope.	Preoperational stage of development continues. Language skills flourish. Generates many questions (eg, How, Why, What?) Simple problem solving. Uses fantasy to understand and problem solve. *Fears:* • Mutilation • Castration • Dark • Unknown • Unfamiliar objects • Inanimate • Unknown Causality related to proximity of events. Enjoys mimicking and imitating adults.	*Developmental tasks: initiative vs guilt.* Attempts to establish self like his or her parents, but independent. Explores environment on own initiative. Boasts, brags, has feelings of indestructibility. Family is primary social group. Peers increasingly important. Assumes sex roles. Aggressive, very curious. Enjoys activities such as sports, cooking, shopping. Cooperative play. Likes rules. May stretch the truth and tell large stories.	Establish rapport through talking and play. Introduce self to child. Have parent present but direct conversation to child. Games such as "follow the leader" and "Simon says" can be used to elicit necessary behaviors. Explain each assessment in simple language. Ask for child's help and use flattery. Use pictures, models, or items he or she can see or touch. Reserve genital examination for last; drape accordingly.

Age	Physical Development	Language (Cognitive) Development (Based on PIAGET)	Psychosocial Development (Based on ERIKSON)	Nurse's Approach To Assessment
6–11 years	Moves constantly. Physical play prevalent; sports, swimming, skating, etc. Increased smoothness of movement. Grows at rate of 2 in/7 lb a year. Eyes/hands well coordinated.	*Concrete operations stage of development.* Organized thought; memory concepts more complicated. Reads, reasons better. Focuses on concrete understanding. *Fears:* • Mutilation • Death • Immobility • Rejection • Failure	*Developmental task: industry vs inferiority.* Learns to include values and skills of school, neighborhood, peers. Peer relationships important. Focuses more on reality, less on fantasy. Family is main base of security and identity. Sensitive to reactions of others. Seeks approval and recognition. Enthusiastic, noisy, imaginative, desires to explore. Likes to complete a task. Enjoys helping others.	Explain all procedures and impact on body. Encourage questioning and active participation in care. Be direct about explanation of procedures, based on what child will hear, see, smell, and feel. (In addition, explain body part involved, and use anatomical names and pictures to explain step by step.) Be honest. Reassure child that he or she is

Continued on following page

Age	Physical Development	Language (Cognitive) Development (Based on PIAGET)	Psychosocial Development (Based on ERIKSON)	Nurse's Approach To Assessment
				liked. Provide privacy. Involve parents, but give child choice as to whether parent will stay during exam. Reason and explain. Allow child some choice as to direction of assessment. May be able to proceed as if assessing adult. Praise cooperation.
12–18 years	Well developed. Rapid physical growth (early adolescence: maximum growth). Secondary sex characteristics. (See Chapter 17, Genitourinary Assessment.)	*Formal operations stage of development.* Abstract reasoning, problem solving. Understanding of multiple cause-and-effect relationships. May plan for future career.	*Developmental task: identity vs role confusion.* Predominant values are those of peer group. Early adolescence: outgoing and enthusiastic. Emotions are extreme, with mood swings. Seeking self-identity, sexual identity. Wants privacy and	Respect privacy. Accept expression of feelings. Direct discussions of care and condition to child. Ask for child's opinions and encourage questions. Allow input into decisions.

Age	Physical Development	Language (Cognitive) Development (Based on PIAGET)	Psychosocial Development (Based on ERIKSON)	Nurse's Approach To Assessment
		Fears: • Mutilation • Disruption of body image • Rejection by peers	independence. Develops interests not shared with family. Concern with physical self. Explores adult roles.	Be flexible with routines. Explain all procedures/treatments. Encourage continuance of peer relationships. Listen actively. Identify impact of illness on body image, future, and level of functioning. Correct misconceptions. Involve parent in assessment only if child requests presence.

Information adapted from: Erikson, E. H. (1991). *Erikson's stages of personality development. Childhood and society.* New York: W. W. Norton & Company
Piaget, J. (1981). *The psychology of intelligence* (M. Piercy & D. E. Berlyne, Trans.). Totowa, NJ: Littlefield & Adams.

APPENDIX 9

Recommended Childhood and Adolescent Immunization Schedule

TABLE 1   Recommended Immunization Schedule for Persons Aged 0–6 Years—United States—2012

Vaccine ▼ Age ►	Birth	1 month	2 months	4 months	6 months	9 months	12 months	15 months	18 months	19–23 months	2–3 years	4–6 years	
Hepatitis B[1]	Hep B	HepB			HepB								Range of recommended ages for all children
Rotavirus[2]			RV	RV	RV[2]								
Diphtheria, tetanus, pertussis[3]			DTaP	DTaP	DTaP		see footnote[3]	DTaP				DTaP	Range of recommended ages for certain high-risk groups
Haemophilus influenzae type b[4]			Hib	Hib	Hib[4]		Hib						
Pneumococcal[5]			PCV	PCV	PCV		PCV				PPSV		
Inactivated poliovirus[6]			IPV	IPV		IPV						IPV	Range of recommended ages for all children and certain high-risk groups
Influenza[7]					Influenza (Yearly)								
Measles, mumps, rubella[8]							MMR		see footnote[8]			MMR	
Varicella[9]							Varicella		see footnote[9]			Varicella	
Hepatitis A[10]							Dose 1[10]				HepA Series		
Meningococcal[11]							MCV4 — see footnote[11]						

This schedule includes recommendations in effect as of December 23, 2011. Any dose not administered at the recommended age should be administered at a subsequent visit, when indicated and feasible. The use of a combination vaccine generally is preferred over separate injections of its equivalent component vaccines. Vaccination providers should consult the relevant Advisory Committee on Immunization Practices (ACIP) statement for detailed recommendations, available online at http://www.cdc.gov/vaccines/pubs/acip-list.htm. Clinically significant adverse events that follow vaccination should be reported to the Vaccine Adverse Event Reporting System (VAERS) online (http://www.vaers.hhs.gov) or by telephone (800-822-7967).

Continued on following page

TABLE 1 Recommended Immunization Schedule for Persons Aged 0–6 Years—United States—2012 (Continued)

1. **Hepatitis B (HepB) vaccine.** (Minimum age: birth)

At birth:
- Administer monovalent HepB vaccine to all newborns before hospital discharge.
- For infants born to hepatitis B surface antigen (HBsAg)–positive mothers, administer HepB vaccine and 0.5 mL of hepatitis B immune globulin (HBIG) within 12 hours of birth. These infants should be tested for HBsAg and antibody to HBsAg (anti-HBs) 1 to 2 months after receiving the last dose of the series.
- If mother's HBsAg status is unknown, within 12 hours of birth administer HepB vaccine for infants weighing 22,000 grams, and HepB vaccine plus HBIG for infants weighing <2,000 grams. Determine mother's HBsAg status as soon as possible and, if she is HBsAg-positive, administer HBIG for infants weighing 22,000 grams (no later than age 1 week).

Doses after the birth dose:
- The second dose should be administered at age 1 to 2 months. Monovalent HepB vaccine should be used for doses administered before age 6 weeks.
- Administration of a total of 4 doses of HepB vaccine is permissible when a combination vaccine containing HepB is administered after the birth dose.
- Infants who did not receive a birth dose should receive 3 doses of a HepB-containing vaccine starting as soon as feasible (Figure 3).
- The minimum interval between dose 2 is 4 weeks, and between dose 2 and 3 is 8 weeks. The final (third or fourth) dose in the HepB vaccine series should be administered no earlier than age 24 weeks and at least 16 weeks after the first dose.

2. **Rotavirus (RV) vaccines.** (Minimum age: 6 weeks for both RV-1 [Rotarix] and RV-5 [Rota Teq])
- If RV-1 (Rotarix) is administered at ages 2 and 4 months, a dose at 6 months is not indicated.
- The maximum age for the first dose in the series is 14 weeks, 6 days; and 8 months, 0 days for the final dose in the series. Vaccination should not be initiated for infants aged 15 weeks, 0 days or older.

3. **Diphtheria and tetanus toxoids and acellular pertussis (DTaP) vaccine.** (Minimum age: 6 weeks)
- The fourth dose may be administered as early as age 12 months, provided at least 6 months have elapsed since the third dose.

4. **Haemophilus influenzae type b (Hib) conjugate vaccine.** (Minimum age: 6 weeks)
- If PRP-OMP (PedvaxHIB or Comvax [HepB-Hib]) is administered at ages 2 and 4 months, a dose at age 6 months is not indicated.
- Hiberix should only be used for the booster (final) dose in children aged 12 months through 4 years.

5. **Pneumococcal vaccines.** (Minimum age: 6 weeks for pneumococcal conjugate vaccine [PCV]; 2 years for pneumococcal polysaccharide vaccine [PPSV])
- Administer 1 dose of PCV to all healthy children aged 24 through 59 months who are not completely vaccinated for their age.
- For children who have received an age-appropriate series of 7-valent PCV (PCV7), a single supplemental dose of 13-valent PCV (PCV13) is recommended for:
  — All children aged 14 through 59 months
  — Children aged 60 through 71 months with underlying medical conditions.

TABLE 1   **Recommended Immunization Schedule for Persons Aged 0–6 Years—United States—2012** (Continued)

- Administer PPSV at least 8 weeks after last dose of PCV to children aged 2 years or older with certain underlying medical conditions, including a cochlear implant. See *MMWR* 2010:59(No. RR-11), available at http://www.cdc.gov/mmwr/pdf/rr/rr5911.pdf.
6. **Inactivated poliovirus vaccine (IPV).** (Minimum age: 6 weeks)
   - If 4 or more doses are administered before age 4 years, an additional dose should be administered at age 4 through 6 years.
   - The final dose in the series should be administered on or after the fourth birthday and at least 6 months after the previous dose.
7. **Influenza vaccines.** (Minimum age: 6 months for trivalent inactivated influenza vaccine [TIV]; 2 years for live, attenuated influenza vaccine [LAIV])
   - For most healthy children aged 2 years and older, either LAIV or TIV may be used. However, LAIV should not be administered to some children, including 1) children with asthma, 2) children 2 through 4 years who had wheezing in the past 12 months, or 3) children who have any other underlying medical conditions that predispose them to influenza complications. For all other contraindications to use of LAIV, see *MMWR* 2010;59(No. RR-8), available at http://www.cdc.gov/mmwr/pdf/rr/rr5908.pdf.
   - For children aged 6 months through 8 years:
     — For the 2011–12 season, administer 2 doses (separated by at least 4 weeks) to those who did not receive at least 1 dose of the 2010–11 vaccine. Those who received at least 1 dose of the 2010–11 vaccine require 1 dose for the 2011–12 season.

     — For the 2012–13 season, follow dosing guidelines in the 2012 ACIP influenza vaccine recommendations.
8. **Measles, mumps, and rubella (MMR) vaccine.** (Minimum age: 12 months)
   - The second dose may be administered before age 4 years, provided at least 4 weeks have elapsed since the first dose.
   - Administer MMR vaccine to infants aged 6 through 11 months who are traveling internationally. These children should be revaccinated with 2 doses of MMR vaccine, the first at ages 12 through 15 months and at least 4 weeks after the previous dose, and the second at ages 4 through 6 years.
9. **Varicella (VAR) vaccine.** (Minimum age: 12 months)
   - The second dose may be administered before age 4 years, provided at least 3 months have elapsed since the first dose.
   - For children aged 12 months through 12 years, the recommended minimum interval between doses is 3 months. However, if the second dose was administered at least 4 weeks after the first dose, it can be accepted as valid.
10. **Hepatitis A (HepA) vaccine.** (Minimum age: 12 months)
    - Administer the second (final) dose 6 to 18 months after the first.
    - Unvaccinated children 24 months and older at high risk should be vaccinated. See *MMWR* 2006;55(No. RR-7), available at http://www.cdc.gov/mmwr/pdf/rr/rr5507.pdf.
    - A 2-dose HepA vaccine series is recommended for anyone aged 24 months and older, previously unvaccinated, for whom immunity against hepatitis A virus infection is desired.

Continued on following page

TABLE 1 Recommended Immunization Schedule for Persons Aged 0–6 Years—United States—2012 (Continued)

11. Meningococcal conjugate vaccines, quadrivalent (MCV4). (Minimum age: 9 months for Menactra [MCV4-D], 2 years for Menveo [MCV4-CRM])

- For children aged 9 through 23 months 1) with persistent complement component deficiency; 2) who are residents of or travelers to countries with hyperendemic or epidemic disease; or 3) who are present during outbreaks caused by a vaccine serogroup, administer 2 primary doses of MCV4-D, ideally at ages 9 months or 12 months or at least 8 weeks apart.
- For children aged 24 months and older with 1) persistent complement component deficiency who have not been previously vaccinated; or 2) anatomic/functional asplenia, administer 2 primary doses of either MCV4 at least 8 weeks apart.

- For children with anatomic/functional asplenia, if MCV4-D (Menactra) is used, administer at a minimum age of 2 years and at least 4 weeks after completion of all PCV doses.
- See *MMWR* 2011;60:72–6, available at http://www.cdc.gov/mmwr/pdf/wk/mm6003. pdf, and Vaccines for Children Program resolution No. 6/11–1, available at http://www.cdc.gov/vaccines/programs/vfc/downloads/resolutions/06–11mening-mcv.pdf, and *MMWR* 2011;60:1391–2, available at http://www.cdc.gov/mmwr/pdf/wk/mm6040. pdf, for further guidance, including revaccination guidelines.

This schedule is approved by the Advisory Committee on Immunization Practices (http://www.cdc.gov/vaccines/recs/acip), the American Academy of Pediatrics (http://www.aap.org), and the American Academy of Family Physicians (http://www.aafp.org).

Department of Health and Human Services • Centers of Disease Control and Prevention

TABLE 2 Recommended Immunization Schedule for Persons Aged 7–18 Years—United States—2012

Vaccine ▼ Age ▶	7–10 years	11–12 years	13–18 years	
Tetanus, diphtheria, pertussis[1]	1 dose (if indicated)	1 dose	1 dose (if indicated)	Range of recommended ages for all children
Human papillomavirus[2]	*see footnote[2]*	3 doses	Complete 3-dose series	
Meningococcal[3]	See footnote[3]	Dose 1	Booster at 16 years old	
Influenza[4]	Influenza (yearly)			Range of recommended ages for catch-up immunization
Pneumococcal[5]	See footnote[5]			
Hepatitis A[6]	Complete 2-dose series			
Hepatitis B[7]	Complete 3-dose series			Range of recommended ages for certain high-risk groups
Inactivated poliovirus[8]	Complete 3-dose series			
Measles, mumps, rubella[9]	Complete 2-dose series			
Varicella[10]	Complete 2-dose series			

This schedule includes recommendations in effect as of December 23, 2011. Any dose not administered at the recommended age should be administered at a subsequent visit, when indicated and feasible. The use of a combination vaccine generally is preferred over separate injections of its equivalent component vaccines. Vaccination providers should consult the relevant Advisory Committee on Immunization Practices (ACIP) statement for detailed recommendations, available online at http://www.cdc.gov/vaccines/pubs/acip-list.htm. Clinically significant adverse events that follow vaccination should be reported to the Vaccine Adverse Event Reporting System (VAERS) online (http://www.vaers.hhs.gov) or by telephone (800-822-7967).

Continued on following page

TABLE 2 Recommended Immunization Schedule for Persons Aged 7–18 Years—United States—2012 (Continued)

1. **Tetanus and diphtheria toxoids and acellular pertussis (Tdap) vaccine.** (Minimum age: 10 years for Boostrix and 11 years for Adacel)
- Persons aged 11 through 18 years who have not received Tdap vaccine should receive a dose followed by tetanus and diphtheria toxoids (Td) booster doses every 10 years thereafter.
- Tdap vaccine should be substituted for a single dose of Td in the catchup series for children aged 7 through 10 years. Refer to the catch-up schedule if additional doses of tetanus and diphtheria toxoid–containing vaccine are needed.
- Tdap vaccine can be administered regardless of the interval since the last tetanus and diphtheria toxoid–containing vaccine.

2. **Human papillomavirus (HPV) vaccines (HPV4 [Gardasil] and HPV2 [Cervarix]).** (Minimum age: 9 years)
- Either HPV4 or HPV2 is recommended in a 3-dose series for females aged 11 or 12 years. HPV4 is recommended in a 3-dose series for males aged 11 or 12 years.
- The vaccine series can be started beginning at age 9 years.
- Administer the third dose 6 months after the first dose and the second dose 1 to 2 months after the first dose (at least 24 weeks after the first dose).
- See *MMWR* 2010;59:626–32, available at http://www.cdc.gov/mmwr/pdf/wk/mm5920.pdf.

3. **Meningococcal conjugate vaccines, quadrivalent (MCV4).**
- Administer MCV4 at age 11 through 12 years with a booster dose at age 16 years.
- Administer MCV4 at age 13 through 18 years if patient is not previously vaccinated.
- If the first dose is administered at age 13 through 15 years, a booster dose should be administered at age 16 through 18 years with a minimum interval of at least 8 weeks after the preceding dose.
- If the first dose is administered at age 16 years or older, a booster dose is not needed.
- Administer 2 primary doses at least 8 weeks apart to previously unvaccinated persons with persistent complement component deficiency or anatomic/functional asplenia, and 1 dose every 5 years thereafter.
- Adolescents aged 11 through 18 years with human immunodeficiency virus (HIV) infection should receive a 2-dose primary series of MCV4, at least 8 weeks apart.
- See *MMWR* 2011;60:72–76, available at http://www.cdc.gov/mmwr/pdf/wk/mm6003.pdf, and Vaccines for Children Program resolution No. 6/11–1, available at http://www.cdc.gov/vaccines/programs/vfc/downloads/resolutions/06–11mening-mcv.pdf, for further guidelines.

4. **Influenza vaccines (trivalent inactivated influenza vaccine [TIV] and live, attenuated influenza vaccine [LAIV]).**
- For most healthy, nonpregnant persons, either TIV or LAIV may be used, except LAIV should not be used for some persons, including those with asthma or any other underlying medical conditions that predispose them to influenza complications. For all other contraindications to use of LAIV, see *MMWR* 2010;59(No.RR-8), available at http://www.cdc.gov/mmwr/pdf/rr/rr5908.pdf.

TABLE 2   **Recommended Immunization Schedule for Persons Aged 7–18 Years—United States—2012** (Continued)

- Administer 1 dose to persons aged 9 years and older.
- For children aged 6 months through 8 years:
  — For the 2011–12 season, administer 2 doses (separated by at least 4 weeks) to those who did not receive at least 1 dose of the 2010–11 vaccine. Those who received at least 1 dose of the 2010–11 vaccine require 1 dose for the 2011–12 season.
  — For the 2012–13 season, follow dosing guidelines in the 2012 ACIP influenza vaccine recommendations.

5. **Pneumococcal vaccines (pneumococcal conjugate vaccine [PCV] and pneumococcal polysaccharide vaccine [PPSV]).**
   - A single dose of PCV may be administered to children aged 6 through 18 years who have anatomic/functional asplenia, HIV infection or other immunocompromising condition, cochlear implant, or cerebral spinal fluid leak. See *MMWR* 2010:59(No. RR-11), available at http://www.cdc.gov/mmwr/pdf/rr/rr5911.pdf.
   - Administer PPSV at least 8 weeks after the last dose of PCV to children aged 2 years or older with certain underlying medical conditions, including a cochlear implant. A single revaccination should be administered after 5 years to children with anatomic/functional asplenia or an immunocompromising condition.

6. **Hepatitis A (HepA) vaccine.**
   - HepA vaccine is recommended for children older than 23 months who live in areas where vaccination programs target older children, who are at increased risk for infection, or for whom immunity against hepatitis A virus infection is desired. See *MMWR* 2006;55(No. RR-7), available at http://www.cdc.gov/mmwr/pdf/rr/rr5507.pdf.
   - Administer 2 doses at least 6 months apart to unvaccinated persons.

7. **Hepatitis B (HepB) vaccine.**
   - Administer the 3-dose series to those not previously vaccinated.
   - For those with incomplete vaccination, follow the catch-up recommendations (Figure 3).
   - A 2-dose series (doses separated by at least 4 months) of adult formulation Recombivax HB is licensed for use in children aged 11 through 15 years.

8. **Inactivated poliovirus vaccine (IPV).**
   - The final dose in the series should be administered at least 6 months after the previous dose.
   - If both OPV and IPV were administered as part of a series, a total of 4 doses should be administered, regardless of the child's current age.
   - IPV is not routinely recommended for U.S. residents aged 18 years or older.

9. **Measles, mumps, and rubella (MMR) vaccine.**
   - The minimum interval between the 2 doses of MMR vaccine is 4 weeks.

Continued on following page

TABLE 2   Recommended Immunization Schedule for Persons Aged 7–18 Years—United States—2012 (Continued)

10. Varicella (VAR) vaccine.
- For persons without evidence of immunity (see *MMWR* 2007;56[No. RR-4], available at http://www.cdc.gov/mmwr/pdf/rr/rr5604.pdf), administer 2 doses if not previously vaccinated or the second dose if only 1 dose has been administered.
- For persons aged 7 through 12 years, the recommended minimum interval between doses is 3 months. However, if the second dose was administered at least 4 weeks after the first dose, it can be accepted as valid.
- For persons aged 13 years and older, the minimum interval between doses is 4 weeks.

This schedule is approved by the Advisory Committee on Immunization Practices (http://www.cdc.gov/vaccines/recs/acip), the American Academy of Pediatrics (http://www.aap.org), and the American Academy of Family Physicians (http://www.aafp.org). Department of Health and Human Services • Centers of Disease Control and Prevention

TABLE 3 Catch-up Immunizations Schedule for Persons Aged 4 Months–18 Years Who Start Late or Who are More Than 1 Month Behind—United States—2012

	Persons aged 4 months through 6 years				
	Minimum Age for Dose 1	Minimum Interval Between Doses			
Vaccine		Dose 1 to dose 2	Dose 2 to dose 3	Dose 3 to dose 4	Dose 4 to dose 5
Hepatitis B	Birth	4 weeks	8 weeks and at least 16 weeks after first dose; minimum age for the final dose is 24 weeks		
Rotavirus[1]	6 weeks	4 weeks	4 weeks[1]		
Diphtheria, tetanus, pertussis[2]	6 weeks	4 weeks	4 weeks	6 months	6 months[2]
Haemophilus influenzae type b[3]	6 weeks	4 weeks if first dose administered at younger than age 12 months 8 weeks (as final dose) if first dose administered at age 12–14 months No further doses needed if first dose administered at age 15 months or older	4 weeks[3] if current age is younger than 12 months 8 weeks (as final dose)[3] if current age is 12 months or older and first dose administered at younger than 12 months and second dose administered at younger than 15 months No further doses needed if previous dose administered at age 15 months or older	8 weeks (as final dose) This dose only necessary for children aged 12 months through 59 months who received 3 doses before age 12 months	

Continued on following page

TABLE 3   Catch-up Immunizations Schedule for Persons Aged 4 Months–18 Years Who Start Late or Who are More Than 1 Month Behind—United States—2012 (Continued)

Vaccine	Minimum Age for Dose 1	Minimum Interval Between Doses			
		Dose 1 to dose 2	Dose 2 to dose 3	Dose 3 to dose 4	Dose 4 to dose 5
			Persons aged 4 months through 6 years		
Pneumococcal[1]	6 weeks	4 weeks if first dose administered at younger than age 12 months 8 weeks (as final dose for healthy children) if first dose administered at age 12 months or older or current age 24 through 59 months No further doses needed for healthy children if first dose administered at age 24 months or older	4 weeks if current age is younger than 12 months 8 weeks (as final dose for healthy children) if current age is 12 months or older No further doses needed for healthy children if previous dose administered at age 24 months or older	This dose only necessary for children aged 12 months through 59 months who received 3 doses before age 12 months or for children at high risk who received 3 doses at any age	8 weeks (as final dose) This dose only necessary for children aged 12 months through 59 months who received 3 doses before age 12 months or for children at high risk who received 3 doses at any age
Inactivated poliovirus[5]	6 weeks	4 weeks	4 weeks	6 months[5] minimum age 4 years for final dose	
Meningococcal[5]	9 months	8 weeks[5]			
Measles, mumps, rubella[2]	12 months	4 weeks			
Varicella[8]	12 months	3 months			
Hepatitis A	12 months	6 months			

TABLE 3 Catch-up Immunizations Schedule for Persons Aged 4 Months–18 Years Who Start Late or Who are More Than 1 Month Behind—United States—2012 (Continued)

		Persons aged 7 through 18 years			
	Minimum Age for Dose 1	**Minimum Interval Between Doses**			
Vaccine		**Dose 1 to dose 2**	**Dose 2 to dose 3**	**Dose 3 to dose 4**	**Dose 4 to dose 5**
Tetanus, diphtheria/ tetanus, diphtheria, pertussis[9]	7 years[9]	4 weeks	4 weeks if first dose administered at younger than age 12 months 6 months if first dose administered at 12 months or older	6 months if first dose administered at younger than age 12 months	
Human papilloma-virus[10]	9 years		Routine dosing intervals are recommended[10]		
Hepatitis A	12 months	6 months			
Hepatitis B	Birth	4 weeks	8 weeks (and at least 16 weeks after first dose)		
Inactivated poliovirus[5]	6 weeks	4 weeks	4 weeks[5]	6 months[5]	
Meningococcal[6]	9 months	8 weeks[6]			
Measles, mumps, rubella[7]	12 months	4 weeks			
Varicella[8]	12 months	3 months if person is younger than age 13 years 4 weeks if person is aged 13 years or older			

Continued on following page

TABLE 3 Catch-up Immunizations Schedule for Persons Aged 4 Months–18 Years Who Start Late or Who are More Than 1 Month Behind—United States—2012 (Continued)

1. **Rotavirus (RV) vaccines (RV-1 [Rotarix] and RV-5 [Rota Teq]).**
   - The maximum age for the first dose in the series is 14 weeks, 6 days; and 8 months, 0 days for the final dose in the series. Vaccination should not be initiated for infants aged 15 weeks, 0 days or older.
   - If RV-1 was administered for the first and second doses, a third dose is not indicated.

2. **Diphtheria and tetanus toxoids and acellular pertussis (DTaP) vaccine.**
   - The fifth dose is not necessary if the fourth dose was administered at age 4 years or older.

3. **Haemophilus influenzae type b (Hib) conjugate vaccine.**
   - Hib vaccine should be considered for unvaccinated persons aged 5 years or older who have sickle cell disease, leukemia, human immunodeficiency virus (HIV) infection, or anatomic/functional asplenia.
   - If the first 2 doses were PRP-OMP (PedvaxHIB or Comvax) and were administered at age 11 months or younger, the third (and final) dose should be administered at age 12 through 15 months and at least 8 weeks after the second dose.
   - If the first dose was administered at age 7 through 11 months, administer the second dose at least 4 weeks later and a final dose at age 12 through 15 months.

4. **Pneumococcal vaccines.** (Minimum age: 6 weeks for pneumococcal conjugate vaccine [PCV]; 2 years for pneumococcal polysaccharide vaccine [PPSV])
   - For children aged 24 through 71 months with underlying medical conditions, administer 1 dose of PCV if 3 doses of PCV were received previously, or administer 2 doses of PCV at least 8 weeks apart if fewer than 3 doses of PCV were received previously.
   - A single dose of PCV may be administered to certain children aged 6 through 18 years with underlying medical conditions. See age-specific schedules for details.
   - Administer PPSV to children aged 2 years or older with certain underlying medical conditions. See MMWR 2010;59(No. RR-11), available at http://www.cdc.gov/mmwr/pdf/rr/rr5911.pdf.

5. **Inactivated poliovirus vaccine (IPV).**
   - In the first 6 months of life, minimum age and minimum intervals are only recommended if the person is at risk for imminent exposure to circulating poliovirus (i.e., travel to a polio-endemic region or during an outbreak).
   - IPV is not routinely recommended for U.S. residents aged 18 years or older.
   - A fourth dose is not necessary if the third dose was administered at age 4 years or older and at least 6 months after the previous dose.

6. **Meningococcal conjugate vaccines, quadrivalent (MCV4).** (Minimum age: 9 months for Menactra [MCV4-D]; 2 years for Menveo [MCV4-CRM])
   - See Figure 1 ("Recommended immunization schedule for persons aged 0 through 6 years") and Figure 2 ("Recommended immunization schedule for persons aged 7 through 18 years") for further detail.

7. **Measles, mumps, and rubella (MMR) vaccine.**
   - Administer the second dose routinely at age 4 through 6 years.

8. **Varicella (VAR) vaccine.**
   - Administer the second dose routinely at age 4 through 6 years. If the second dose was administered at least 4 weeks after the first dose, it can be accepted as valid.

9. **Tetanus and diphtheria toxoids (Td) and tetanus and diphtheria toxoids and acellular pertussis (Tdap) vaccines.**
   - For children aged 7 through 10 years who are not fully immunized with the childhood DTaP vaccine series, Tdap vaccine should be substituted for a single dose of Td vaccine in the catch-up series; if additional doses are needed, use Td vaccine. For these children, an adolescent Tdap vaccine dose should not be given.
   - An inadvertent dose of DTaP vaccine administered to children aged 7 through 10 years can count as part of the catch-up series. This dose can count as the adolescent Tdap dose, or the child can later receive a Tdap booster dose at age 11–12 years.

10. **Human papillomavirus (HPV) vaccines (HPV4 [Gardasil] and HPV2 [Cervarix]).**
    - Administer the vaccine series to females (either HPV2 or HPV4) and males (HPV4) at age 13 through 18 years if patient is not previously vaccinated.
    - Use recommended routine dosing intervals for vaccine series catch-up; see Figure 2 ("Recommended immunization schedule for persons aged 7 through 18 years").

Clinically significant adverse events that follow vaccination should be reported to the Vaccine Adverse Event Reporting System (VAERS) online (http://www.vaers.hhs.gov) or by telephone (800-822-7967). Suspected cases of vaccine-preventable diseases should be reported to the state or local health department. Additional information, including precautions and contraindications for vaccination, is available from CDC online (http://www.cdc.gov/vaccines) or by telephone (800-CDC-INFO [800-232-4636]).

Recommended Adult
Immunization Schedules

Recommended Adult Immunization Schedule—United States - 2012

Note: These recommendations must be read with the footnotes on
http://www.cdc.gov containing number of doses, intervals between doses,
and other important information.

Figure 1. Recommended adult immunization schedule, by vaccine and age group[1]

VACCINE ▼ AGE GROUP ►	19-21 years	22-26 years	27-49 years	50-59 years	60-64 years	≥ 65 years
Influenza[2]	1 dose annually					
Tetanus, diphtheria, pertussis (Td/Tdap)[3,*]	Substitute 1-time dose of Tdap for Td booster; then boost with Td every 10 yrs					Td/Tdap[3]
Varicella[4,*]	2 Doses					
Human papillomavirus (HPV) Female[5,*]	3 doses					
Human papillomavirus (HPV) Male[5,*]	3 doses					
Zoster[6]					1 dose	
Measles, mumps, rubella (MMR)[7,*]	1 or 2 doses				1 dose	
Pneumococcal (polysaccharide)[8,9]	1 or 2 doses					1 dose
Meningococcal[10,*]	1 or more doses					

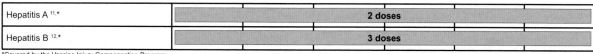

Hepatitis A [11,*]	2 doses	
Hepatitis B [12,*]	3 doses	

*Covered by the Vaccine Injury Compensation Program

[1-12]See footnotes on http://www.cdc.gov/mmwr/preview/mmwrhtml/mm6104a9.htm

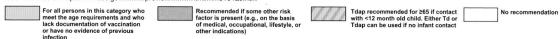

For all persons in this category who meet the age requirements and who lack documentation of vaccination or have no evidence of previous infection	Recommended if some other risk factor is present (e.g., on the basis of medical, occupational, lifestyle, or other indications)	Tdap recommended for ≥65 if contact with <12 month old child. Either Td or Tdap can be used if no infant contact	No recommendation

Report all clinically significant postvaccination reactions to the Vaccine Adverse Event Reporting System (VAERS). Reporting forms and instructions on filing a VAERS report are available at www.vaers.hhs.gov or by telephone, 800-822-7967.

Information on how to file a Vaccine Injury Compensation Program claim is available at www.hrsa.gov/vaccinecompensation or by telephone, 800-338-2382. To file a claim for vaccine injury, contact the U.S. Court of Federal Claims, 717 Madison Place, N.W., Washington, D.C. 20005; telephone, 202-357-6400.

Additional information about the vaccines in this schedule, extent of available data, and contraindications for vaccination is also available at www.cdc.gov/vaccines or from the CDC-INFO Contact Center at 800-CDC-INFO (800-232-4636) in English and Spanish, 8:00 a.m. - 8:00 p.m. Eastern Time, Monday - Friday, excluding holidays.

Use of trade names and commercial sources is for identification only and does not imply endorsement by the U.S. Department of Health and Human Services.

APPENDIX 8

Height–Weight–Head Circumference Charts for Children

2 to 20 Years: Stature-for-age and Weight-for-age percentiles: Girls (and Boys)
"Published May 30, 2000 (modified 11/21/00)."

Weight-for-stature percentiles: Girls (and Boys)
"Published May 30, 2000 (modified 10/16/00)."

SOURCE: Developed by the National Center for Health Statistics in collaboration with the National Center for Chronic Disease Prevention and Health Promotion (2013). http://www.cdc.gov/growthcharts.

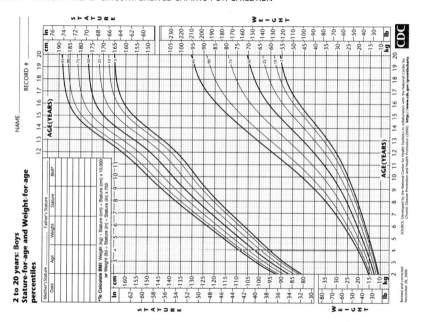

2 to 20 years: Boys
Stature-for-age and Weight-for-age percentiles

NAME

RECORD #

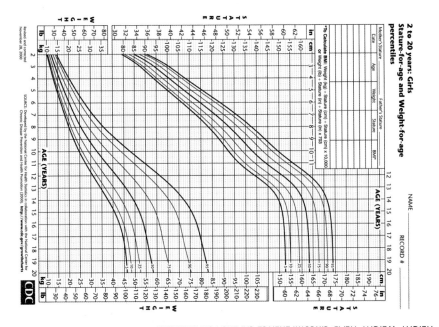

2 to 20 years: Girls
Stature-for-age and Weight-for-age
percentiles

NAME

RECORD #

SOURCE: Developed by the National Center for Health Statistics in collaboration with the National Center for Chronic Disease Prevention and Health Promotion (2000). http://www.cdc.gov/growthcharts

Revised and corrected November 28, 2000

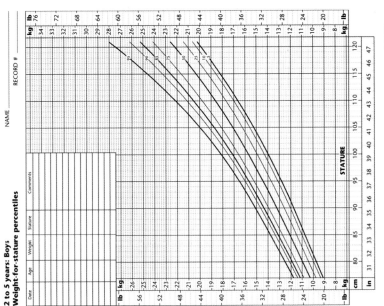

2 to 5 years: Boys
Weight-for-stature percentiles

NAME _____ RECORD # _____

SOURCE: Developed by the National Center for Health Statistics in collaboration with the National Center for Chronic Disease Prevention and Health Promotion (2000). http://www.cdc.gov/growthcharts.

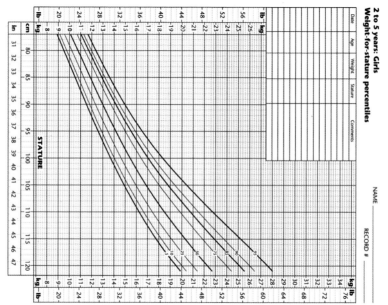

2 to 5 years: Girls
Weight-for-stature percentiles

NAME

RECORD #

Date	Age	Weight	Stature	Comments

STATURE

SOURCE: Developed by the National Center for Health Statistics in collaboration with the National Center for Chronic Disease Prevention and Health Promotion (2000). http://www.cdc.gov/growthcharts

NANDA Approved Nursing Diagnoses 2012–2014

Newly Approved Nursing Diagnoses

Risk for Ineffective Activity Planning
Risk for Adverse Reaction to Iodinated Contrast Media
Risk for Allergy Response
Insufficient Breast Milk
Ineffective Childbearing Process
Risk for Ineffective Childbearing Process
Risk for Dry Eye

Deficient Community Health
Ineffective Impulse Control
Risk for Neonatal Jaundice
Risk for Disturbed Personal Identity
Ineffective Relationship
Risk for Ineffective Relationship
Risk for Chronic Low Self-Esteem
Risk for Thermal Injury
Risk for Ineffective Peripheral Tissue Perfusion

Domain 1: Health Promotion

Deficient Diversional Activity
Sedentary Lifestyle
Deficient Community Health
Risk-Prone Health Behavior
Ineffective Health Maintenance
Readiness for Enhanced Immunization Status
Ineffective Protection
Ineffective Self-Health Management
Readiness for Enhanced Self-Health Management
Ineffective Family Therapeutic Regimen Management

Domain 2: Nutrition

Insufficient Breast Milk
Ineffective Infant Feeding Pattern
Imbalanced Nutrition: Less Than Body Requirements
Imbalanced Nutrition: More Than Body Requirements
Risk for Imbalanced Nutrition: More Than Body Requirements
Readiness for Enhanced Nutrition
Impaired Swallowing

Risk for Unstable Blood Glucose Level
Neonatal Jaundice
Risk for Neonatal Jaundice
Risk for Impaired Liver Function
Risk for Electrolyte Imbalance
Readiness for Enhanced Fluid Balance
Deficient Fluid Volume
Excess Fluid Volume
Risk for Deficient Fluid Volume
Risk for Imbalanced Fluid Volume

Domain 3: Elimination and Exchange

Functional Urinary Incontinence
Overflow Urinary Incontinence
Reflex Urinary Incontinence
Stress Urinary Incontinence
Urge Urinary Incontinence
Risk for Urge Urinary Incontinence
Impaired Urinary Elimination
Readiness for Enhanced Urinary Elimination
Urinary Retention

Constipation
Perceived Constipation
Risk for Constipation
Diarrhea
Dysfunctional Gastrointestinal Motility
Risk for Dysfunctional Gastrointestinal Motility
Bowel Incontinence
Impaired Gas Exchange

Domain 4: Activity/Rest

Insomnia
Sleep Deprivation
Readiness for Enhanced Sleep
Disturbed Sleep Pattern
Risk for Disuse Syndrome
Impaired Bed Mobility
Impaired Physical Mobility
Impaired Wheelchair Mobility
Impaired Transfer Ability
Impaired Walking

Disturbed Energy Field
Fatigue
Wandering
Activity Intolerance
Risk for Activity Intolerance
Ineffective Breathing Pattern
Decreased Cardiac Output
Risk for Ineffective Gastrointestinal Perfusion
Risk for Ineffective Renal Perfusion
Impaired Spontaneous Ventilation
Ineffective Peripheral Tissue Perfusion
Risk for Decreased Cardiac Tissue Perfusion
Risk for Ineffective Cerebral Tissue Perfusion
Risk for Ineffective Peripheral Tissue Perfusion
Dysfunctional Ventilatory Weaning Response
Impaired Home Maintenance
Readiness for Enhanced Self-Care
Bathing Self-Care Deficit
Dressing Self-Care Deficit
Feeding Self-Care Deficit
Toileting Self-Care Deficit
Self-Neglect

Domain 5: Perception/Cognition

Unilateral Neglect
Impaired Environmental Interpretation Syndrome
Acute Confusion
Chronic Confusion
Risk for Acute Confusion
Ineffective Impulse Control
Deficient Knowledge
Readiness for Enhanced Knowledge
Impaired Memory
Readiness for Enhanced Communication
Impaired Verbal Communication

Domain 6: Self-Perception

Hopelessness
Risk for Compromised Human Dignity
Risk for Loneliness
Disturbed Personal Identity
Risk for Disturbed Personal Identity
Readiness for Enhanced Self-Control

Domain 7: Role Relationships

Ineffective Breastfeeding
Interrupted Breastfeeding
Readiness for Enhanced Breastfeeding
Caregiver Role Strain
Risk for Caregiver Role Strain
Impaired Parenting
Readiness for Enhanced Parenting

Chronic Low Self-Esteem
Risk for Chronic Low Self-Esteem
Risk for Situational Low Self-Esteem
Situational Low Self-Esteem
Disturbed Body Image
Stress Overload
Risk for Disorganized Infant Behavior
Autonomic Dysreflexia
Risk for Autonomic Dysreflexia
Disorganized Infant Behavior
Readiness for Enhanced Organized Infant Behavior
Decreased Intracranial Adaptive Capacity

Risk for Impaired Parenting
Risk for Impaired Attachment
Dysfunctional Family Processes
Interrupted Family Processes
Readiness for Enhanced Family Processes
Ineffective Relationship
Readiness for Enhanced Relationship
Risk for Ineffective Relationship
Parental Role Conflict
Ineffective Role Performance
Impaired Social Interaction

Domain 8: Sexuality

Sexual Dysfunction
Ineffective Sexuality Pattern
Ineffective Childbearing Process
Readiness for Enhanced Childbearing Process
Risk for Ineffective Childbearing Process
Risk For Disturbed Maternal–Fetal Dyad

Domain 9: Coping/Stress Tolerance

Post-Trauma Syndrome
Risk for Post-Trauma Syndrome
Rape-Trauma Syndrome
Relocation Stress Syndrome
Risk for Relocation Stress Syndrome
Ineffective Activity Planning
Risk for Ineffective Activity Planning
Anxiety
Compromised Family Coping
Defensive Coping
Disabled Family Coping
Ineffective Coping
Ineffective Community Coping
Readiness for Enhanced Coping
Readiness for Enhanced Family Coping
Death Anxiety
Ineffective Denial
Adult Failure To Thrive
Fear

Grieving
Complicated Grieving
Risk for Complicated Grieving
Readiness for Enhanced Power
Powerlessness
Risk for Powerlessness
Impaired Individual Resilience
Readiness for Enhanced Resilience
Risk for Compromised Resilience
Chronic Sorrow
Stress Overload
Risk for Disorganized Infant Behavior
Autonomic Dysreflexia
Risk for Autonomic Dysreflexia
Disorganized Infant Behavior
Readiness for Enhanced Organized Infant Behavior
Decreased Intracranial Adaptive Capacity

Domain 10: Life Principles

Readiness for Enhanced Hope
Readiness for Enhanced Spiritual Well-Being

Readiness for Enhanced Decision Making
Decisional Conflict
Moral Distress
Noncompliance
Impaired Religiosity
Readiness for Enhanced Religiosity
Risk for Impaired Religiosity
Spiritual Distress
Risk for Spiritual Distress

Domain 11: Safety/Protection

Risk for Infection
Ineffective Airway Clearance
Risk for Aspiration
Risk for Bleeding
Impaired Dentition
Risk for Dry Eye
Risk for Falls
Risk for Injury
Impaired Oral Mucous Membrane
Risk for Perioperative Positioning Injury

Risk for Peripheral Neurovascular Dysfunction
Risk for Shock
Impaired Skin Integrity
Risk for Impaired Skin Integrity
Risk for Sudden Infant Death Syndrome
Risk for Suffocation
Delayed Surgical Recovery
Risk for Thermal Injury
Impaired Tissue Integrity
Risk for Trauma
Risk for Vascular Trauma
Risk for Other-Directed Violence
Risk for Self-Directed Violence
Self-Mutilation
Risk for Self-Mutilation
Risk for Suicide
Contamination
Risk for Contamination
Risk for Poisoning

Risk for Adverse Reaction to Iodinated Contrast Media
Risk for Allergy Response
Latex Allergy Response
Risk for Latex Allergy Response
Risk for Imbalanced Body Temperature
Hyperthermia
Hypothermia
Ineffective Thermoregulation

Domain 12: Comfort

Impaired Comfort
Readiness for Enhanced Comfort
Nausea
Acute Pain
Chronic Pain
Impaired Comfort
Readiness for Enhanced Comfort
Social Isolation

Selected Collaborative Problems*

Risk for Complication: Cardiac/Vascular

RC: Decreased Cardiac Output
RC: Dysrhythmias
RC: Pulmonary Edema
RC: Deep Vein Thrombosis
RC: Hypovolemia
RC: Compartmental Syndrome
RC: Pulmonary Embolism

Risk for Complication: Respiratory

RC: Hypoxemia
RC: Atelectasis, Pneumonia
RC: Tracheobronchial Constriction
RC: Pneumothorax

(Carpenito-Moyet, L. J. (2012). *Nursing diagnosis: Application to clinical practice* [14th ed.]. Philadelphia, PA: Lippincott Williams & Wilkins.)
*Frequently used collaborative problems are represented on this list. Other situations not listed here could qualify as collaborative problems.

Risk for Complication: Metabolic/Immune/Hematopoietic

RC: Hypo/Hyperglycemia
RC: Negative Nitrogen Balance
RC: Electrolyte Imbalances
RC: Sepsis
RC: Acidosis (Metabolic, Respiratory)
RC: Alkalosis (Metabolic, Respiratory)
RC: Allergic Reaction
RC: Thrombocytopenia
RC: Opportunistic Infections
RC: Sickling Crisis

Risk for Complication: Renal/Urinary

RC: Acute Urinary Retention
RC: Renal Insufficiency
RC: Renal Calculi

Risk for Complication: Neurologic/Sensory

RC: Increased Intracranial Pressure
RC: Seizures
RC: Increased Intraocular Pressure
RC: Neuroleptic Malignant Syndrome
RC: Alcohol Withdrawal

Risk for Complication: Gastrointestinal/Hepatic/Biliary

RC: Paralytic Ileus
RC: GI Bleeding
RC: Hepatic Dysfunction
RC: Hyperbilirubinemia

Risk for Complication: Muscular/Skeletal

RC: Pathologic Fractures
RC: Joint Dislocation

Risk for Complication: Reproductive

RC: Prenatal Bleeding
RC: Preterm Labor
RC: Pregnancy-Associated Hypertension
RC: Fetal Distress
RC: Postpartum Hemorrhage

Risk for Complication: Medication Therapy Adverse Effects

RC: Anticoagulant Therapy Adverse Effects
RC: Antianxiety Therapy Adverse Effects

RC: Adrenocorticosteroid Therapy Adverse Effects
RC: Antineoplastic Therapy Adverse Effects
RC: Anticonvulsant Therapy Adverse Effects
RC: Antidepressant Therapy Adverse Effects
RC: Antiarrhythmic Therapy Adverse Effects
RC: Antipsychotic Therapy Adverse Effects
RC: Antihypertensive Therapy Adverse Effects
RC: β-Adrenergic Blocker Therapy Adverse Effects
RC: Calcium Channel Blocker Therapy Adverse Effects
RC: Angiotensin-Converting Enzyme Inhibitor Therapy Adverse Effects

Spanish Translation for Nursing Health History and Physical Examination

Biographical Data

English	Spanish
What is your name?	¿Cómo se llama Ud.?
	¿Cómo te llamas? (For child)
How old are you?	¿Cuántos años tiene?
Where do you live?	¿Dónde vive Ud.?
Are you allergic to anything?	¿Tiene Ud. alérgias a algún medicamento?
Do you have any handicaps?	¿Tiene minusvalía?
	¿Incapacidad física?
Do you have any illnesses that you know of?	¿Padece Ud. de una enfermedad?
	¿Más de una?
Have you had any past surgeries?	¿Ha sido operado?

Functional Health Pattern History

HEALTH PERCEPTION/HEALTH MANAGEMENT PATTERN

English	Spanish
Rate your health on a scale of 1 to 10 (1 being poor, 10 being good).	Estime su salud en una escala de uno a diez (cuando uno significa malo y diez bueno).
Describe your current health.	Describa cómo está su salud.
When was your last tetanus shot?	¿Ha tenido inyección de tétano? ¿Cuándo fue la última?
Do you use drugs? If yes, explain.	¿Toma Ud. medicamentos? ¿drogas? Si 'si,' ¿cuales son?
Do you use alcohol? If yes, explain.	¿Toma alcohol? Si 'si,' ¿de qué clase y cuánto toma?
Do you use caffeine? If yes, explain.	¿Toma cafeína? ¿En qué forma y cuánto por dia?

NUTRITIONAL/METABOLIC PATTERN

English	Spanish
What do you eat for breakfast? For lunch? For supper? For snacks?	¿Qué come por el desayuno? ¿por el almuerzo? ¿por la cena? ¿bocaditos? ¿tapas?
Describe the condition of your: • Skin • Hair • Nails	Por favor, describa la condición • de la piel • del pelo • de las uñas
Have you recently gained or lost weight? How much?	¿Ha experimentado un bajo o aumento de peso?

ELIMINATION PATTERN

English	Spanish
Describe your bowel pattern. How often? Color and consistency?	¿Cuándo hizo la deposición/defecación/evacuación la última vez? (¿Cuándo fue al baño la última vez?) ¿Puede describir el patrón de la defecación? ¿Cuántas veces a la semana? ¿Color? ¿Textura?
Describe your urinary pattern. How often? Color?	¿Puede describir el color de la orina? ¿Cuántas veces al día orina? (hace pi pi)
Do you need to urinate at night?	¿Hay que orinar de noche?
Is there a sense of urgency?	¿Hay un sentido de urgencia?

ACTIVITY/EXERCISE PATTERN

English	Spanish
What activities do you in do a normal day?	Describa un día normal. ¿Cuáles actividades hace?
What do you do to relax?	¿Qué hace para descansar?
Do you physically exercise? Explain.	¿Hace ejercicio? Descríbalo, por favor.

SEXUAL/REPRODUCTION PATTERN

English	Spanish
How old were you when you started menstruating? Or when you stopped menstruating?	¿Cuántos años tenía cuando comenzó la menstruación? (a menstruar) ¿Cuándo paró la menstruación?
How many times have you been pregnant?	¿Cuántos embarazos ha tenido?
How many children do you have?	¿Cuántos ninos/hijos tiene?
Do you do anything to prevent pregnancy?	¿Hace algo por evitar el embarazo?
Do you have any sexually transmitted diseases?	¿Padece de enfermedades transmitidos por el sexo?

SLEEP/REST PATTERN

English	Spanish
What time do you go to bed at night?	¿A qué hora se aqueste?
How long do you sleep each night?	¿Cuántas horas se duerme de noche?
Does anything wake you?	¿Hay algo que lo despierte?
What helps you fall asleep?	¿Qué le ayuda dormir?
Do you take naps? How often?	¿Toma siestas? ¿Con frecuencia?

SENSORY/PERCEPTUAL PATTERN

English	Spanish
When was your last eye exam?	¿Cuándo fue el último examen de los ojos?
Do you have any problems:	¿Padece de problemas de
• Seeing?	• la vista?
• Hearing?	• oír? escuchar?
• Smelling?	• oler?
• Tasting?	• saber?
• Feeling?	• sentir sensaciones?
Do you have any pain now? Show me on this picture	¿Tiene dolor ahora? ¿En dónde le duele? Muéstramelo en este dibujo.
• What causes it?	• ¿Qué cree que causa el dolor?
• What relieves it?	• ¿Qué reduce o quita el dolor?
• When does it occur?	• ¿Cuándo ocurre el dolor?
• How often?	• ¿y la frecuencia del dolor?
• How long does it last?	• ¿Cuánto tiempo dura el dolor?
• Show me on this scale how bad it hurts (use facial scale).	• Muéstreme lo malo que es el dolor en esta escala.

COGNITIVE PATTERN

English	Spanish
What did your doctor tell you?	¿Qué es lo que le dijo el medico?
Do you have questions about your illness? Or treatments?	¿Quiere preguntar algo sobre la enfermedad? ¿sobre los tratamientos?

ROLE/RELATIONSHIP PATTERN

English	Spanish
Who do you live with?	¿Con quién vive Ud.?
Are you married?	¿Está Ud. casado? casada (fem.)
Does your family get along well?	¿La familia se acuerdan/se portan bien?
What is your role in your family?	¿Qué es el papel que hace en la familia?

SELF-PERCEPTION/SELF-CONCEPT PATTERN

English	Spanish
What are your strengths?	¿Cuáles son las fuerzas que tiene en cuanto a la salud?
What are your weaknesses?	¿Cuáles son las debilidades?

COPING/STRESS TOLERANCE PATTERN

English	Spanish
What is stressful in your life?	¿Cuáles son los estreses de su vida?
What or who helps you most when you have a problem?	Cuándo hay un problema, ¿quién lo ayuda mas?

VALUE/BELIEF PATTERN

English	Spanish
What is very important to you in life?	¿Qué mas le importa en la vida?
What religion are you?	¿A qué religion corresponde?
Are there certain foods you cannot have?	¿Hay comidas o ingredients que no puede comer?
Do you want a priest or hospital chaplain to visit you?	¿Quiere que el padre el capillán del hospital le hace una visita?

Phrases to Use to Help the Client Through the Physical Assessment

English	Spanish
Please	Por favor
Take off all your clothes and put on this gown.	Saque toda la ropa y ponga esta bata.
Urinate in this cup.	Orina (hace pi pi) en esta taza.
Lie down.	Acuéstese, por favor.
Stand up.	Póngase en pie, por favor.
Sit up.	Siéntese.
Get up and sit again.	Levántese y siéntese de nuevo.
Roll over to your right.	Gírese a la derecha.
Roll over to your left.	Gírese a la izquierda.
Take a deep breath.	Respira profundo.
Hold it.	Manténgalo.
Breathe out.	Respira de nuevo.
Cough.	Tosa.
Bend your leg	Doble la pierna.
Bend your arm.	Doble el brazo.
Look up.	Mire para arriba.
Look down.	Mire para abajo.
Look to your right.	Mire al lado derecho.
Look to your left.	Mire al lado izquierdo.

Canada's Food Guide

APPENDIX 12

Advice for different ages and stages...

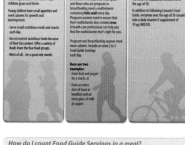

Children

Following *Canada's Food Guide* helps children grow and thrive.

Young children have small appetites and need calories for growth and development.

- Serve small nutritious meals and snacks each day.
- Do not restrict nutritious foods because of their fat content. Offer a variety of foods from the four food groups.
- Most of all... be a good role model.

Women of childbearing age

All women who could become pregnant and those who are pregnant or breastfeeding need a multivitamin containing **folic acid** every day. Pregnant women need to ensure that their multivitamin also contains **iron**. A health care professional can help you find the multivitamin that's right for you.

Pregnant and breastfeeding women need more calories. Include an extra 2 to 3 Food Guide Servings each day.

Here are two examples:
- Have fruit and yogurt for a snack, or
- Have an extra slice of toast at breakfast and an extra glass of milk at supper.

Men and women over 50

The need for **vitamin D** increases after the age of 50.

In addition to following *Canada's Food Guide*, everyone over the age of 50 should take a daily vitamin D supplement of 10 μg (400 IU).

How do I count Food Guide Servings in a meal?

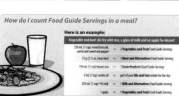

Here is an example:

Vegetable and beef stir-fry with rice, a glass of milk and an apple for dessert		
250 mL (1 cup) mixed broccoli, carrot and sweet red pepper	=	2 **Vegetables and Fruit** Food Guide Servings
75 g (2½ oz.) lean beef	=	1 **Meat and Alternatives** Food Guide Serving
250 mL (1 cup) brown rice	=	2 **Grain Products** Food Guide Servings
5 mL (1 tsp) canola oil	=	part of your **Oils and Fats** intake for the day
250 mL (1 cup) 1% milk	=	1 **Milk and Alternatives** Food Guide Serving
1 apple	=	1 **Vegetables and Fruit** Food Guide Serving

Eat well and be active today and every day!

The benefits of eating well and being active include:
- Better overall health.
- Lower risk of disease.
- A healthy body weight.
- Feeling and looking better.
- More energy.
- Stronger muscles and bones.

Be active

To be active every day is a step towards better health and a healthy body weight.

It is recommended that adults accumulate at least 2½ hours of moderate to vigorous physical activity each week and that children and youth accumulate at least 60 minutes per day. You don't have to do it all at once. Choose a variety of activities spread throughout the week.

Start slowly and build up.

Eat well

Another important step towards better health and a healthy body weight is to follow *Canada's Food Guide* by:

- Eating the recommended amount and type of food each day.
- Limiting foods and beverages high in calories, fat, sugar or salt (sodium) such as cakes and pastries, chocolate and candies, cookies and granola bars, doughnuts and muffins, ice cream and frozen desserts, french fries, potato chips, nachos and other salty snacks, alcohol, fruit flavoured drinks, soft drinks, sports and energy drinks, and sweetened hot or cold drinks.

Read the label

- Compare the Nutrition Facts table on food labels to choose products that contain less fat, saturated fat, trans fat, sugar and sodium.
- Keep in mind that the calories and nutrients listed are for the amount of food found at the top of the Nutrition Facts table.

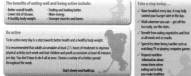

Nutrition Facts
Per 1 mL (0 g)

Amount	% Daily Value
Calories 0	
Fat 0 g	0 %
Saturated 0 g	0 %
+ Trans 0 g	
Cholesterol 0 mg	
Sodium 0 mg	0 %
Carbohydrate 0 g	0 %
Fibre 0 g	0 %
Sugars 0 g	
Protein 0 g	
Vitamin A 0 %	Vitamin C 0 %
Calcium 0 %	Iron 0 %

Limit trans fat

When a Nutrition Facts table is not available, ask for nutrition information to choose foods lower in trans and saturated fats.

Take a step today...

✓ Have breakfast every day. It may help control your hunger later in the day.
✓ Walk wherever you can – get off the bus early, use the stairs.
✓ Benefit from eating vegetables and fruit at all meals and as snacks.
✓ Spend less time being inactive such as watching TV or playing computer games.
✓ Request nutrition information about menu items when eating out to help you make healthier choices.
✓ Enjoy eating with family and friends!
✓ Take time to eat and savour every bite!

For more information, interactive tools, or additional copies visit Canada's Food Guide on-line at:
www.healthcanada.gc.ca/foodguide

or contact:
Publications
Health Canada
Ottawa, Ontario K1A 0K9
E-Mail: publications@hc-sc.gc.ca
Tel.: 1-866-225-0709
Fax: (613) 941-5366
TTY: 1-800-267-1245

Également disponible en français sous le titre :
Bien manger avec le Guide alimentaire canadien

This publication can be made available on request on diskette, large print, audio-cassette and braille.

© Her Majesty the Queen in Right of Canada, represented by the Minister of Health Canada, 2011. This publication may be reproduced without permission.
No changes permitted. HC Pub.: 4651 Cat.: H164-38/1-2011E-PDF ISBN 978-1-100-19255-0

Health Canada / Santé Canada
Your health and safety... our priority.
Votre santé et votre sécurité... notre priorité.

Eating Well with Canada's Food Guide

Canada

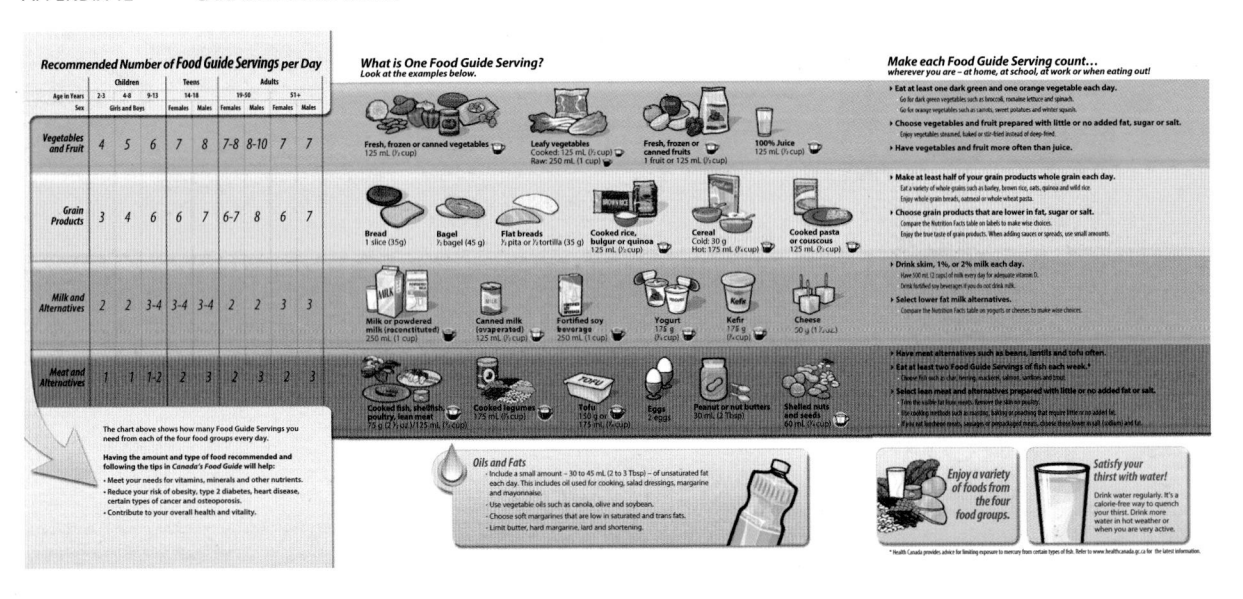

Recommended Number of Food Guide Servings per Day

Age in Years	Children 2-3	Children 4-8	Children 9-13	Teens 14-18 Females	Teens 14-18 Males	Adults 19-50 Females	Adults 19-50 Males	Adults 51+ Females	Adults 51+ Males
Sex	Girls and Boys			Females	Males	Females	Males	Females	Males
Vegetables and Fruit	4	5	6	7	8	7-8	8-10	7	7
Grain Products	3	4	6	6	7	6-7	8	6	7
Milk and Alternatives	2	2	3-4	3-4	3-4	2	2	3	3
Meat and Alternatives	1	1	1-2	2	3	2	3	2	3

The chart above shows how many Food Guide Servings you need from each of the four food groups every day.

Having the amount and type of food recommended and following the tips in *Canada's Food Guide* will help:
- Meet your needs for vitamins, minerals and other nutrients.
- Reduce your risk of obesity, type 2 diabetes, heart disease, certain types of cancer and osteoporosis.
- Contribute to your overall health and vitality.

What is One Food Guide Serving?
Look at the examples below.

Fresh, frozen or canned vegetables
125 mL (½ cup)

Leafy vegetables
Cooked: 125 mL (½ cup)
Raw: 250 mL (1 cup)

Fresh, frozen or canned fruits
1 fruit or 125 mL (½ cup)

100% Juice
125 mL (½ cup)

Bread
1 slice (35g)

Bagel
½ bagel (45 g)

Flat breads
½ pita or ½ tortilla (35 g)

Cooked rice, bulgur or quinoa
125 mL (½ cup)

Cereal
Cold: 30 g
Hot: 175 mL (¾ cup)

Cooked pasta or couscous
125 mL (½ cup)

Milk or powdered milk (reconstituted)
250 mL (1 cup)

Canned milk (evaporated)
125 mL (½ cup)

Fortified soy beverage
250 mL (1 cup)

Yogurt
175 g (¾ cup)

Kefir
175 g (¾ cup)

Cheese
50 g (1½ oz.)

Cooked fish, shellfish, poultry, lean meat
75 g (2 ½ oz.)/125 mL (½ cup)

Cooked legumes
175 mL (¾ cup)

Tofu
150 g or
175 mL (¾ cup)

Eggs
2 eggs

Peanut or nut butters
30 mL (2 Tbsp)

Shelled nuts and seeds
60 mL (¼ cup)

Oils and Fats
- Include a small amount – 30 to 45 mL (2 to 3 Tbsp) – of unsaturated fat each day. This includes oil used for cooking, salad dressings, margarine and mayonnaise.
- Use vegetable oils such as canola, olive and soybean.
- Choose soft margarines that are low in saturated and trans fats.
- Limit butter, hard margarine, lard and shortening.

Make each Food Guide Serving count...
wherever you are – at home, at school, at work or when eating out!

▸ Eat at least one dark green and one orange vegetable each day.
Go for dark green vegetables such as broccoli, romaine lettuce and spinach.
Go for orange vegetables such as carrots, sweet potatoes and winter squash.

▸ Choose vegetables and fruit prepared with little or no added fat, sugar or salt.
Enjoy vegetables steamed, baked or stir-fried instead of deep-fried.

▸ Have vegetables and fruit more often than juice.

▸ Make at least half of your grain products whole grain each day.
Eat a variety of whole grains such as barley, brown rice, oats, quinoa and wild rice.
Enjoy whole grain breads, oatmeal or whole wheat pasta.

▸ Choose grain products that are lower in fat, sugar or salt.
Compare the Nutrition Facts table on labels to make wise choices.
Enjoy the true taste of grain products. When adding sauces or spreads, use small amounts.

▸ Drink skim, 1%, or 2% milk each day.
Have 500 mL (2 cups) of milk every day for adequate vitamin D.
Drink fortified soy beverages if you do not drink milk.

▸ Select lower fat milk alternatives.
Compare the Nutrition Facts table on yogurts or cheeses to make wise choices.

▸ Have meat alternatives such as beans, lentils and tofu often.

▸ Eat at least two Food Guide Servings of fish each week.*
Choose fish such as char, herring, mackerel, salmon, sardines and trout.

▸ Select lean meat and alternatives prepared with little or no added fat or salt.
Trim the visible fat from meats. Remove the skin on poultry.
Use cooking methods such as roasting, baking or poaching that require little or no added fat.
If you eat luncheon meats, sausage or prepackaged meats, choose those lower in salt (sodium) and fat.

Enjoy a variety of foods from the four food groups.

Satisfy your thirst with water!
Drink water regularly. It's a calorie-free way to quench your thirst. Drink more water in hot weather or when you are very active.

* Health Canada provides advice for limiting exposure to mercury from certain types of fish. Refer to www.health.canada.gc.ca for the latest information.

References and Bibliography

Abrams, S. (2011). Dietary guidelines for calcium and vitamin D: A new era. *Pediatrics, 127*(3), 566–568. Available at http://pediatrics.aappublications.org/content/127/3/566.full

Alfaro-Lefevre, R. (2009). *Applying nursing process: A tool for critical thinking* (7th ed.). Philadelphia, PA: Lippincott-Raven.

Alzheimer's Association. (2001–2011). Alzheimer's and other dementias: Understanding the differences. Available at http://www.helpguide.org/elder/alzheimers_dementias_types.htm

Alzheimer's Association. (2011). 10 early signs and symptoms of Alzheimer's association. Available at http://www.alz.org/alzheimers_disease_10_signs_of_alzheimers.asp

American Academy of Dermatology. (2010). Squamous cell carcinoma. Available at http://www.aad.org/dermatology-a-to-z/diseases-and-treatments/q—t/squamous-cell-carcinoma

American Academy of Dermatology. (2012). Atopic dermatitis. Available at http://www.aad.org/skin-conditions/dermatology-a-to-z/atopic-dermatitis

American Academy of Neurology. (2010). Clinical dementia rating. Available at http://www.aan.com/Guidelines/Home/GetGuidelineContent/425

American Academy of Ophthalmology (AAO). (2007). Eye examination in infants, children, and young adults by pediatricians—2003; Reaffirmed May 2007. Available at http://one.aao.org/CE/PracticeGuidelines/ClinicalStatements_Content.aspx?cid=e57de45b-2c03-4fbd-9c83-02374a6c09e0

American Academy of Pediatrics. (2012). SIDS and other sleep-related infant deaths: Expansion of recommendations for a safe infant sleeping environment. Available at http://pediatrics.aappublications.org/content/128/5/e1341.full

American Cancer Society (ACS). (2012). Smokeless tobacco. Available at http://www.cancer.org/cancer/cancercauses/tobaccocancer/smokeless-tobacco

American Cancer Society (ACS). (2012/2013). Screening guidelines for the early detection of cancer. Available at http://www.cancer.org/Healthy/FindCancerEarly/CancerScreeningGuidelines/american-cancer-society-guidelines-for-the-early-detection-of-cancer

American Cancer Society (ACS). (2013a). Cancer facts & figures. Available at http://www.cancer.org/acs/groups/content/@epidemiologysurveilance/documents/document/acspc-036845.pdf

American Cancer Society (ACS). (2013b). Skin cancer prevention and early detection: How do I protect myself from UV rays? Available at http://www.cancer.org/cancer/cancercauses/sunanduvexposure/skincancerpreventionandearlydetection/skin-cancer-prevention-and-early-detection-u-v-protection

American College of Obstetricians and Gynecologists (ACOG). (2010). The initial reproductive health visit. Available at http://www.acog.org/Resources%20And%20Publications/Committee%20Opinions/Committee%20on%20Adolescent%20Health%20Care/The%20Initial%20Reproductive%20Health%20Visit.aspx

American College of Obstetricians and Gynecologists (ACOG). (2012). Intimate partner violence. Available at http://www.acog.org/Resources_And_Publications/Committee_Opinions/Committee_on_Health_Care_for_Underserved_Women/Intimate_Partner_Violence

American College of Obstetricians and Gynecologists (ACOG). (2013). Changes in the 2010 STD treatment guidelines what adolescent health care providers should know. Available at http://www.acog.org/About%20ACOG/ACOG%20Departments/Adolescent%20Health%20Care/Changes%20in%20the%202010%20STD%20Treatment%20Guidelines%20%20What%20Adolescent%20Health%20Care%20Providers%20Should%20Know.aspx

American Dental Association. (2012). Oral health topics: Cleaning your teeth & gums. Available at http://www.ada.org/2624.aspx

American Diabetes Association. (2010). Position statement: Standards of medical care in diabetes—2010. *Diabetes Care, 33*(Suppl. 1), S11–S61.

American Heart Association. (2008). Seventh Report of the Joint National Committee on Prevention, Detection, Evaluation of Hypertension. Available at www.nhlbi.nih.gov/guidelines/hypertension

American Heart Association. (2011). Exercise guidelines. Available at http://www.livestrong.com/article/224429-american-heart-association-exercise-guidelines/

American Heart Association. (2012a). Diet and lifestyle recommendations. Available at http://www.heart.org/HEARTORG/GettingHealthy/Diet-and-Lifestyle-Recommendations_UCM_305855_Article.jsp

American Heart Association. (2012b). Heart attack risk assessment. Available at http://www.heart.org/HEARTORG/Conditions/HeartAttack/HeartAttackToolsResources/Heart-Attack-Risk-Assessment_UCM_303944_Article.jsp#.Tx6isG_2ZrA

American Medical Association (AMA) National Advisory Council on Violence and Abuse Policy Compendium. (2008, April). Policy statement on family and intimate partner violence: H-515.965. Available at http://www.ama-assn.org/ama1/pub/upload/mm/386/vio_policy_comp.pdf

American Optometric Association (AOA). (2012). Comprehensive eye and vision examination. Available at http://www.aoa.org/x4725.xml

American Stroke Association. (2012). About stroke. Available at http://www.strokeassociation.org/STROKEORG/AboutStroke/About-Stroke_UCM_308529_SubHomePage.jsp

Andrews, M., & Boyle, J. (2011). *Transcultural concepts in nursing care* (6th ed.). Philadelphia, PA: Lippincott Williams & Wilkins.

Andrews, M., & Boyle, J. (2013). *Transcultural concepts in nursing care* (6th ed.). Philadelphia, PA: Lippincott Williams & Wilkins.

Apgar, V. (1953, July, August). A proposal for a new method of evaluation of the newborn infant. *Current Researchers in Anesthesia and Analgesia.* Available at http://profiles.nlm.nih.gov/ps/access/CPBBKG.pdf

Ashburn, S. S. (1992). Selected theories of development. In C. S. Schuster & S. S. Ashburn (Eds.), *The process of human development: A holistic life-span approach* (3rd ed.; p. 884). Philadelphia, PA: J. B. Lippincott.

Asher, C., & Northington, L. (2008). Society of Pediatric Nurses. Position statement for measurement of temperature/fever in children. Available at http://www.pedsnurses.org/pdfs/downloads/gid,126/index.pdf

Assessing confusion. (2011). Exams for nursing. Available at http://www.examsfornursing.com/elderly/71-confusion

Ayello, E. A. (2012). Predicting pressure ulcer risk. *The Hartford Institute for Geriatric Nursing, 1*(5). Available at http://consultgerirn.org/uploads/File/trythis/try_this_5.pdf

Baker, C. M., & Wong, D. L. (1987). Q.U.E.S.T.: A process of pain assessment. *Orthopaedic Nursing, 6*(1), 1–21.

Ballard, J. L., Khoury, J. C., Wedig, K., Want, L., Eilers-Walsman, B. L., & Lipp, R. (1991). New Ballard score: Expanded to include extremely premature infants. *Journal of Pediatrics, 19*(3), 417–423.

Banicek, J. (2010). How to ensure acute pain in older people is appropriately assessed and managed. Available at http://www.nursingtimes.net/how-to-ensure-acute-pain-in-older-people-is-appropriately-assessed-and-managed/5017667.article

Barry, M. (2009). *Primary care medicine: Office evaluation and management of the adult patient* (6th ed.). Philadelphia, PA: Lippincott Williams & Wilkins.

Berry, P.H., & Dahl, J. (2000). The new JCAHO pain standards: implications for pain management nurses. *Pain Management Nursing, 1*(1), 3–12.

Better Medicine (2011). Atrophic vaginitis. Available at http://www.bettermedicine.com/article/atrophic-vaginitis 527. Available at http://www.localhealth.com/article/atrophic-vaginitis

Bickley, L. S., & Szilagyi, P. G. (2012). *Bates guide to physical examination and history taking* (11th ed.). Philadelphia, PA: Lippincott Williams & Wilkins.

Braden, B., & Bergstrom, N. (1988). Braden Scale for predicting pressure sore risk. Available at http://www.healthcare.uiowa.edu/igec/tools/pressureulcers/bradenScale.pdf

Braden Scale for Predicting Pressure Sore Risk. (1988). Copyright Barbara Braden and Nancy Bergstrom. Available at www.med-pass.com

Braes, T., Milisen, K., & Foreman, M. (201). Assessing cognitive function. Available at http://consultgerirn.org/topics/assessing_cognitive_function/want_to_know_more/

Brown, M. (2012). AAFP, USPSTF recommend screening all adults for obesity, offering some patients lifestyle intervention. Available at http://www.aafp.org/news-now/health-of-the-public/20120704obesityrecs.html

Burn Survivors Throughout the World. (n.d.). Visual Analog Scale (VAS). Available at www.burnsurvivorsttw.org/articles/painass3.html

Byers A. L., Covinsky, K. E., Barnes, D. E., & Yaffe, K. (2012). Dysthymia and depression increase risk of dementia and mortality among older veterans. *American Journal of Geriatric Psychiatry, 20*(8):664–672. Available at www.ncbi.nlm.nih.gov/pubmed/21597358

Campbell, J. C. (1981). Misogyny and homicide of women. *Advances in Nursing Science, 3*, 67–85.

Campbell, J. C. (1986). Nursing assessment for risk of homicide with battered women. *Advances in Nursing Science 8*, 36–51.

Campbell, J. C. (1992). "If I can't have you, no one can": Power and control in homicide of female partners. In J. Radford & D. E. H. Russell (Eds.), *Femicide: The politics of woman killing* (pp. 99–113). New York, NY: Twayne.

Campbell, J. C. (1995). *Assessing dangerousness*. Newbury Park, CA: Sage.

Campbell, W. (2004). Revised 'SAD PERSONS' helps assess suicide risk. *The Journal of Family Practice, 3*(3) [Online].

Campbell, J. C., Webster, D., & Glass, N. (2009). The danger assessment: Validation of a lethality risk assessment instrument for intimate partner femicide. *Journal of Interpersonal Violence, 24*(4), 653–674. Available at http://www.dangerassessment.net/uploads/DA_Validation_of_a_Lethality_Risk_Assessment_Instrument-Campbell.pdf

Campinha-Bacote, J. (2012). *The process of cultural competence in the delivery of healthcare services*. Available at www.transculturalcare.net

Canada's food guide. (2012). Available at http://www.hc-sc.gc.ca/fn-an/food-guide-aliment/order-commander/index-eng.php

Carpenito-Moyet, L. J. (2012). *Nursing diagnosis: Application to clinical practice* (14th ed.). Philadelphia, PA: Lippincott Williams & Wilkins.

Center for Nutrition Policy and Promotion. (2012). Ethnic/cultural food guide pyramid. Available at http://fnic.nal.usda.gov/dietary-guidance/myplatefood-pyramid-resources/ethnicultural-food-pyramids

Centers for Disease Control and Prevention (CDC). (2012a). FASTSTATS: Suicide and self-inflicted injury. Available at http://www.cdc.gov/nchs/fastats/suicide.htm

Centers for Disease Control and Prevention (CDC). (2012b). HPV vaccine—Questions & answers. Available at http://www.cdc.gov/vaccines/vpd-vac/hpv/vac-faqs.htm

Centers for Disease Control and Prevention (CDC). (2012c). Injury prevention & control: Traumatic brain injury. Available at http://www.cdc.gov/traumaticbraininjury/prevention.html

Centers for Disease Control and Prevention (CDC). (2012d). Prevalence of stroke—United States 2006–2010. Available at http://www.cdc.gov/mmwr/preview/mmwrhtml/mm6120a5.htm

Centers for Disease Control and Prevention (CDC). (2013a). Adolescent and school health: Childhood obesity facts. Available at http://www.cdc.gov/healthyyouth/obesity/facts.htm

Centers for Disease Control and Prevention (CDC). (2013b). HIV incidence. Available at http://www.cdc.gov/hiv/statistics/surveillance/incidence/index.html

Centers for Disease Control and Prevention (CDC). (2013c). Prostate cancer screening. Available at http://www.cdc.gov/cancer/prostate/basic_info/screening.htm

Centers for Disease Control and Prevention (CDC). (2013d). Sexually transmitted diseases (STDs). Available at http://www.cdc.gov/std/

Centers for Disease Control and Prevention (CDC). (2013e). Stroke facts. Available at http://www.cdc.gov/stroke/facts.htm

Chan, P. (2011). Clarifying the confusion about confusion: Current practices in managing geriatric delirium. *British Columbia Medical Journal (BCMJ)*, *53*(8), 409–415. Available at http://www.bcmj.org/articles/clarifying-confusion-about-confusion-current-practices-managing-geriatric-delirium

Child abuse and neglect stats. (2012). Available at http://www.firststar.org/library/child-welfare-resources.aspx

Cleeland, C. (1992). Brief pain inventory short form [BPI SF]. In C. Cleeland, D. Turk, & R. Melzack, *Handbook of pain assessment* (pp. 367–370, 383–384). New York, NY: Guildford Press.

Colarossi, L., Breitbart, V., & Betancourt, G. (2010). Barriers to screening for intimate partner violence: A mixed-methods study of providers in family planning clinics. *Perspectives on Sexual and Reproductive Health*, *42*(4), 236–243.

Colby, A., Kohlberg, L., Gibbs, J. C., & Lieberman, M. (1983). A longitudinal study of moral judgment. *Monographs of the Society for Research in Child Development*, *48*(1–2, serial No. 200).

Committee on Health Care for Underserved Women of American Congress of Obstetricians and Gynecologists (ACOG). (2012). Committee opinion: Intimate partner violence. Available at http://www.acog.org/

Denver II Developmental Screening Test. (1992). Available at www.denverii.com

Devi, S. (2012). US guidelines for domestic violence screening spark debate. *The Lancet*, *379*(9815), 506. Available at http://www.thelancet.com/journals/lancet/article/PIIS0140-6736%2812%2960215-3/fulltext

Devrim, I., Kara, A., Ceyhan, M., Tezer, H., Uludag, A. K., Cengiz, A. B., … Secmeer, G. (2007). Measurement accuracy of fever by tympanic and axillary thermometry. *Pediatric Emergency Care*, *23*(1), 16–19.

Dietary guidelines for Americans, 2010. (2011). Available at http://www.health.gov/dietaryguidelines/2010.asp

Domestic violence statistics. (2012). Available at http://domesticviolencestatistics.org/domestic-violence-statistics/

Domestic violence: The facts. (2012). Available at http://staging.safehorizon.org/index/what-we-do-2/domestic-violence-abuse-147/domestic-violence-the-facts-195.html

Drake, B., Jolley, J., Lanier, P., Fluke, J., Barth, R., & Jonson-Reid, M. (2011). Racial bias in child protection? A comparison of competing explanations using national data. *Pediatrics, 127*(3), 471–478. Available at http://pediatrics.aappublications.org/content/127/3/471.abstract

Elder abuse statistics. (2012). Available at http://www.statisticbrain.com/elderly-abuse-statistics/

Elsawy, B., & Higgins, K. (2011). The geriatric assessment. *American Family Physician, 83*(1), 48–56. Available at http://www.aafp.org/afp/2011/0101/p48.html

Erikson, E. H. (1950). *Childhood and society.* New York, NY: W. W. Norton Company, Inc.

Erikson, E. (1963). *Childhood and society* (2nd ed.). New York, NY: W. W. Norton.

Erikson, E. H. (1968). *Identity: Youth and crisis.* New York, NY: W. W. Norton & Company, Inc.

Erikson, E. H. (1991). *Erikson's stages of personality development. Childhood and society.* New York, NY: W. W. Norton & Company.

Erikson, E. H., & Erikson, J. M. (1992). *The life cycle completed.* New York, NY: Norton.

Erikson, E. H., Erikson, J. M., & Kivnick, H. Q. (1986). *Vital involvement in old age.* New York, NY: W. W. Norton & Company.

Fitzpatrick, J., Fulmer, T., Wallace, M., & Flaherty, E. (Eds.). (2000). *Geriatric nursing research digest.* New York, NY: Springer.

Flaherty, E. (2008). Pain assessment for older adults. *American Journal of Nursing, 108*(6), 45–47.

Forgetfulness: It's not always what you think. (2012, November). Available at www.webmd.com/healthy…/forgetfulness-is-not-always-what-you-think

Forgetfulness: Knowing when to ask for help (September, 2012). Available at http://www.dementiacarecentral.com/node/726

Freud, S. (1930, reprinted in English 2002). *Civilizations and its discontents.* London, UK: Penguin.

Freud, S. (1949). *An outline of psychoanalysis* (authorized translation by James Strachey). New York, NY: W. W. Norton & Company, Inc.

From culture bound syndrome 'Susto' to a cultural impression of mental disorders. (2011, July 31). Available at http://jacquileigh.wordpress.com/2011/07/31/from-culture-bound-syndrome-%E2%80%98susto%E2%80%99-to-a-cultural-impression-of-mental-disorders/

Galanti, G. (2008). *Caring for patients from different cultures* (4th ed.). Philadelphia, PA: University of Pennsylvania Press.

Giger, J., & Davidhizar, R. (2012). *Transcultural nursing: Assessment and intervention* (6th ed.). St. Louis, MO: Elsevier.

Glasgow Coma Scale. (2012). Available at http://www.neuroskills.com/resources/glasgow-coma-scale.php

Gordon, M. (2010). *Manual of nursing diagnosis* (12th ed.). Sudbury, MA: Jones & Bartlett.

Guarnero, P. (2005). Mexicans. In J. Lipson & S. Dibble (Eds.), *Culture & nursing care* (pp. 330–342). San Francisco, CA: UCSF Nursing Press.

Hall, S. (2008). About the "Metropolitan Life" tables for height and weight. Available at www.halls.md/ideal-weight

Hamilton, B., & Ventura, S. (2012, April). Birth rates for U.S. teenagers reach historic lows for all ages and ethnic groups. NCHS Data Brief, no. 89. Available at http://www.cdc.gov/nchs/data/databriefs/db89.pdf

Hammer, R., Moynihan, B., & Pagliaro, E. (2013). *Forensic nursing: A handbook for practice* (2nd ed.). Burlington, MA: Jones & Bartlett.

HealthyPeople.gov. (2012). Sleep health. Available at http://healthypeople.gov/topicsobjectives2020/overview.aspx?topicid=38

Healthy People 2020. (2011). Health-related quality of life and well-being. Available at http://healthypeople.gov/2020/about/QoLWB-about.aspx

Healthy People 2020. (2012a). Maternal, infant, and child health. Available at http://www.healthypeople.gov/2020/topicsobjectives2020/objectiveslist.aspx?topicId=26

Healthy People 2020. (2012b). Nutrition and weight status. Available at http://www.healthypeople.gov/2020/topicsobjectives2020/overview.aspx?topicid=29

Healthy People 2020. (2012c). Substance abuse. Available at http://www.healthypeople.gov/2020/topicsobjectives2020/overview.aspx?topicid=40

Healthy People 2020. (2012d). Topics: Lesbian, gay, & transgender health. Available at www.healthypeople.gov/2020/topicsobjectives2020/default.aspx

Healthy People 2020. (2013a). Nutrition and weight status. Available at http://www.healthypeople.gov/2020/topicsobjectives2020/overview.aspx?topicid=29

Healthy People 2020. (2013b). Physical activity. Available at http://www.healthypeople.gov/2020/topicsobjectives2020/overview.aspx?topicid=33

Healthy People 2020. (2013c). Sexually transmitted diseases. Available at http://www.healthypeople.gov/2020/topicsobjectives2020/overview.aspx?topicid=37

Healthy People 2020. (2013d). Tobacco use. Available at http://www.healthypeople.gov/2020/topicsobjectives2020/overview.aspx?topicId=41

Hegar, A., Emans, S., & Muram, D. (2000). *Evaluation of the sexually abused child: A medical textbook and photographic atlas.* New York, NY: Oxford University Press.

Hockenberry, M. J., & Wilson, D. (2012). FACES Pain Rating Scale. *Wong's essentials of pediatric nursing* (9th ed.). St. Louis, MO: Elsevier.

Hummel, P, & Puchalski, M. (2000). N-Pass: Neonatal pain, agitation and sedation scale. In P. Hummel, M. Puchalski, S. Creech, & M. Weiss, (2004), N-PASS: Neonatal pain, agitation and sedation scale—

Reliability and validity. Available at http://www.anestesiarianimazione.com/2004/06c.asp

Humphreys, J., & Campbell, J. C. (2011). *Family violence and nursing practice* (2nd ed.). New York, NY: Springer.

Hutchinson, S. (2007). "Sinus headache" or migraine. Available at http://www.achenet.org/resources/sinus_headache_or_migraine/

Iannelli, V. (2012). Dental health guide for children: Caring for your child's teeth. Available at http://pediatrics.about.com/cs/pediatricadvice/a/dental_health.htm

Inside PA Training. (2011). The stethoscope and how to use it. Available at http://www.mypatraining.com/stethoscope-and-how-to-use-it

Institute of Medicine (IOM). (2010). The future of nursing: Leading change, advancing health. Available at http://www.iom.edu/Reports/2010/The-Future-of-Nursing-Leading-Change-Advancing-Health.aspx

International Association for the Study of Pain. (2011). Definition of pain. Available at http://www.iasp-pain.org

Is it forgetfulness or dementia? (May 19, 2009). Available at http://www.health.harvard.edu/healthbeat/HB_web/is-it-forgetfulness-or-dementia.htm

Jevon, P. (2008). Neurological assessment Part 4 - Glasgow Coma Scale 2. *Nursing Times, 104,* 30:24-25. Available at http://www.nursingtimes.net/neurological-assessment-part-4-glasgow-coma-scale-2/1768984. article

Joint Commission on Accreditation of Healthcare Organizations (JCAHO). (2012). Facts about pain management. Available at http://www.jointcommission.org/pain_management/

Kohlberg, L. (1978). The cognitive-developmental approach to moral education. In P. Scharf (Ed.), *Readings in moral education* (pp. 36-51). Minneapolis, MN: Winston Press.

Kohlberg, L. (1981). *The philosophy of moral development.* San Francisco, CA: Harper & Row.

Kohlberg, L. (1984). *The psychology of moral development: The nature and validity of moral stages.* San Francisco, CA: Harper & Row.

Kohlberg, L., & Gilligan, C. (1971). *The adolescent as a philosopher: The discovery of the self in a postconventional world.* Los Angeles, CA: Daedalus.

Kohlberg, L., & Ryncarz, R. (1990). Beyond justice reasoning: Moral development and consideration of a seventh stage. In C. Alexander & E. Langer (Eds.), *Higher stages of human development* (pp. 191-207). New York, NY: Oxford University Press.

Lee, M. (2008). *Race/ethnicity, socioeconomic status, and obesity across the transition from adolescence to adulthood.* Chapel Hill, NC: Melissa Sharon Lee. [Available on google books.com]

Lu, S., Leasure, A., & Dai, Y. (2010). A systematic review of body temperature variations in older people. *Journal of Clinical Nursing, 19*(1-2), 4-16. Abstract available at http://www.ncbi.nlm.nih.gov/pubmed/19868869

Manning, L. (2009). Preventing domestic, sexual violence and abuse can keep health care costs down. Available http://www.causes.com/causes/241644/updates/147606

McCaffrey, A., Eisenberg, D., Legedza, A., Davis, R., & Phillips, R. (2004). Prayer for health concerns: Results of a national survey on prevalence and patterns of use. *Archives of Internal Medicine, 164*, 858–862.

McCaffrey, M., & Pasero, C. (1999). Initial Pain Assessment Tool. *Pain: Clinical manual* (2nd ed., p. 60). St. Louis, MO: Mosby.

Medscape Nurses Education. (2008). Evaluation of acute abdominal pain reviewed. Available at http://www.medscape.org/viewarticle/573206

Memorial Sloan Kettering Cancer Center. (n.d.). Memorial Pain Assessment Card. Available at http://www.partnersagainstpain.com/printouts/A7012AS9.pdf

Micelli, D., & Mezey, M. (2007). Critical thinking related to complex care of older adults, Geriatric Nursing Education Consortium, The John A. Hartford Foundation Institute for Geriatric Nursing.

Miles, K. (2008–2011). Eye exams for older adults. Available at http://www.caring.com/articles/elderly-and-vision-care

Miller, S. (2010, September). Arterial disease. Lower extremity implications. *Lower Extremity Review.* Available at http://lowerextremityreview.com/article/arterial-disease-lower-extremity-implications

Morris, J. C. (1983). The Clinical Dementia Rating (CDR): Current version and scoring rules. *Neurology, 43*, 2412–2414. [May keep or delete but adding *Am Ac Neurol.* 2010]

NANDA International. (2012a). Glossary of terms. Available at http://www.nanda.org/DiagnosisDevelopment/DiagnosisSubmission/PreparingYourSubmission/GlossaryofTerms.aspx

NANDA International. (2012b). *Nursing diagnoses: Definitions and classification 2012–2014.* Oxford, UK: Wiley-Blackwell.

National Center for Hearing Assessment and Management, Utah State University. (2012). Newborn hearing screening. Available at http://www.infanthearing.org/screening/index.html

National Digestive Diseases Information Clearinghouse (NDDIC). (2012). Irritable bowel syndrome. Available at http://digestive.niddk.nih.gov/ddiseases/pubs/ibs/

National Heart, Lung, and Blood Institute (NHLBI). (2013, in development). Eighth report of the Joint National Committee on Prevention, Detection, Evaluation, and Treatment of High Blood Pressure (JNC 8). [in development]. Information and status available at http://www.nhlbi.nih.gov/guidelines/hypertension/jnc8/index.htm http://www.nhlbi.nih.gov/guidelines/indevelop.htm#status

National Institute of Deafness and Other Communication Disorders (NIDCD). (2011). Ten ways to recognize hearing loss. [Excerpt from NIH Publication No. 01 4913]. Available at http://www.nidcd.nih.gov/health/hearing/pages/10ways.aspx

National Institute of Dental and Craniofacial Research (NIDCR). (2013). Oral cancer. Available at http://www.nidcr.nih.gov/oralhealth/topics/oralcancer/

National Institutes of Health Osteoporosis and Related Bone Diseases National Research Center. (2012). The Surgeon General's report on bone health and osteoporosis: What it means to you. Available at http://www.niams.nih.gov/Health_Info/Bone/SCR/surgeon_generals_report.asp

National Institute of Neurological Disorders and Stroke (NINDS). (2012a). Traumatic brain injury: Hope through research. Available at http://www.ninds.nih.gov/disorders/tbi/detail_tbi.htm#193462321&com/bmi/bmicalc.htm

NIH Osteoporosis and Related Bone Diseases National Resource Center (2011a). Osteoporosis overview. Available at http://www.niams.nih.gov/Health_Info/Bone/Osteoporosis/overview.asp

National Pressure Ulcer Advisory Panel. (1998). Pressure Ulcer Scale for Healing (PUSH). PUSH Tool 3.0. Available at www.npuap.org

National Pressure Ulcer Advisory Panel. (2007). Pressure ulcer staging revised by NPUAP. Available at www.npuap.org

Nelson, H., Bougatsos, C., & Blazina, I. (2012). Screening women for intimate partner violence: A systematic review to update the U.S. Preventive Services Task Force recommendation. *Annals of Internal Medicine, 156*(11),796–808. Available at http://annals.org/article.aspx?articleid=1170891

Nursing Network on Violence Against Women International. (2012). Assessment tools. *Nutrition made incredibly easy* (2nd ed.). (2007). Philadelphia, PA: Wolters Kluwer/Lippincott Williams & Wilkins.

O'Brien, M. (2011). *Spirituality in nursing: Standing on holy ground* (4th ed.). Boston, MA: Jones and Bartlet.

Otto, S., Duncan, S., & Baker, L. (1996). Initial pain assessment for pediatric use only. Distributed by the City of Hope Pain/Palliative Care Resource Center. Available at http://www.cityofhope.org/prc/pain_assessment.asp

Overfield, T. (1995). *Biological variation in health and illness: Race, age and sex differences* (2nd ed.). Boca Raton, FL: CRC Press.

Parker, K. (n.d.). The boomerang generation: Feeling ok about living with mom and dad. Available at www.pewsocialtrends.org/2012/3/15

Piaget, J. (1952). *The origins of intelligence in children* (M. Cook, Trans.). New York, NY: International Universities Press.

Piaget, J. (1969). *The language and thought of the child* (M. Gabain, Trans.). New York, NY: Meridian Books.

Piaget, J. (1970). Piaget's theory. In P. H. Mussen (Ed.), *Carmichael's manual of child psychology* (3rd ed.). New York, NY: Wiley.

Piaget, J. (1981). *The psychology of intelligence* (M. Piercy & D. E. Berlyne, Trans.). Totowa, NJ: Littlefield & Adams.

Podsiadlo, D., & Richardson, R. (1991). Timed Get Up and Go Test: A test of basic functional mobility for frail elderly persons. *Journal of the American Geriatric Society, 39*(2), 142–148.

Purnell, L. D. (2012). *Transcultural health care: A culturally competent approach* (4th ed.). Philadelphia, PA: F. A. Davis.

Purnell, L. D. (2013). *Guide to culturally competent care* (4th ed.). Philadelphia, PA: F. A. Davis.

Schuster, C. S., & Ashburn, S. S. (1992). *The process of human development: A holistic life-span approach* (3rd ed.). Philadelphia, PA: J. B. Lippincott Company.

Screening older adults for symptoms of depression. (2008, January). *Chronicle of Nursing*. Available at http://www.asrn.org/journal-chronicle-nursing/265-screening-older-adults-for-symptoms-of-depression.html

Sheikh, J. I., & Yesavage, J. (1986). Geriatric Depression Scale (GDS): Recent evidence and development of a shorter version. In *Clinical gerontology: A guide to assessment and intervention* (pp. 165–173). New York, NY: The Haworth Press.

Silkman, C. (2008). Assessing the seven dimensions of pain: Pain dimensions: Sample assessment questions. *American Nurse Today, 3*(2), 13–15.

Skin Cancer Foundation. (2011). Skin cancer facts. Available at http://www.skincancer.org/skin-cancer-information/skin-cancer-facts#melanoma

SLUMS (The Saint Louis University Mental Status Examination for Detecting Mild Cognitive. Impairment and Dementia). (2002). Available at www.slu.edu

Smeltzer, S. (2008). Characteristics of arterial and venous insufficiency. In *Brunner & Suddarth's textbook of medical-surgical nursing* (11th ed., p. 979). Philadelphia, PA: Lippincott Williams & Wilkins.

Society of Pediatric Nurses. (2008). Position statement for measurement of temperature/fever in children. Available at http://www.pedsnurses.org/pdfs/downloads/gid,126/index.pdf

Soderstrom, C., Smith, G., Kufera, J., Dischinger, P., Hebel, R., McDuff, D., … Read K. M. (1997). The accuracy of the CAGE, the Brief Michigan Alcoholism Screening Test, and the Alcohol Use Disorders Identification Test in screening trauma center patients for alcoholism. *Journal of Trauma-Injury Infection & Critical Care, 43*(6), 962–969.

Spector, R. E. (2013). *Cultural diversity in health and illness* (8th ed.). Upper Saddle River, NJ: Prentice-Hall.

Stanford Sleepiness Scale. (2012). Available at http://chicagosleepapneasnoring.com/test-your-sleepiness/stanford-sleepiness-scale

Stephan, P. (2010). Inverted nipples, retracted nipples, and nipple changes. Available at http://breastcancer.about.com/od/whatisbreastcancer/tp/nipple-variations.htm

Stop Relationship Abuse Organization. (n.d.). Screening for intimate partner violence in the primary care setting. Available at http://stoprelationshipabuse.org/pdfs/Screening%20for%20IPV%20in%20the%20Primary%20Care,%20OBGYN,%20Pediatric,%20Mental%20Health%20Settings.pdf

Tanner, J. M. (1962). *Growth at adolescence* (2nd ed.). Oxford, UK: Blackwell Scientific Publications.

The Internet Stroke Center. (1997–2012). Stroke assessment scales. Available at http://www.strokecenter.org/professionals/stroke-diagnosis/stroke-assessment-scales/

The Skin Cancer Foundation. (2012). Early detection and self exams. Available at http://www.skincancer.org/skin-cancer-information/early-detection

Titus, M. O., Hulsey, T., Heckman, J., Losek, J. (2009). Temporal artery thermometry utilization in pediatric emergency care. *Clinical Pediatrics, 48*(2), 190–193.

Touhy, T. A., & Jett, K. (2012). *Ebersole and Hess' toward healthy aging: Human needs & nursing response* (8th ed.). St. Louis, MO: Elsevier Mosby.

Universal Pain Assessment Tool (UCLA). (2006). Available at http://www.anes.ucla.edu/pain

U.S. Department of Agriculture (USDA). (2011). USDA and HHS announce new dietary guidelines to help Americans make healthier food choices and confront obesity epidemic. Available at http://www.hhs.gov/news/press/2011pres/01/20110131a.html

U.S. Department of Agriculture (USDA), Center for Nutrition Policy and Promotion. (2010). MyPlate food guide. Available at http://www.choosemyplate.gov

U.S. Department of Agriculture (USDA), Center for Nutrition Policy and Promotion. (2012). Healthy eating index. Available at www.cnpp.usda.gov/HealthyEatingIndex.htm

U.S. Department of Agriculture (USDA) and Department of Health and Human Services (DHHS). (2010). Dietary guidelines for Americans. Available at http://health.gov/dietaryguidelines/dga2010/dietaryguidelines2010.pdf

U.S. Department of Health & Human Services (USDHHS). (2012). Osteoporosis and related bone diseases national resource center. Available at http://www.nutrition.gov/nutrition-and-health-issues/osteoporosis

U.S. Department of Health & Human Services (USDHHS). (n.d.). Understanding health information privacy. Available at http://www.hhs.gov/ocr/privacy/hipaa/understanding/index.html

U.S. Preventive Services Task Force (USPSTF). (2004b). Screening for family and intimate partner violence: Recommendation statement. Available at http://www.uspreventiveservicestaskforce.org/3rduspstf/famviolence/famviolrs.htm

U.S. Preventive Services Task Force (USPSTF). (2005). Screening for abdominal aortic aneurysm. Available at http://www.uspreventiveservicestaskforce.org/uspstf/uspsaneu.htm

U.S. Preventive Services Task Force (USPSTF). (2010). Screening for obesity in children and adolescents. Available at http://www.uspreventiveservicestaskforce.org/uspstf/uspsobes.htm

U.S. Preventive Services Task Force (USPSTF). (2012). Screening for prostate cancer. Available at http://www.uspreventiveservicestaskforce.org/prostatecancerscreening.htm

Verbal Descriptor Scale (VDS). (1992, February). *Acute Pain Management: Operative or Medical Procedures and Trauma, Clinical Practice Guideline No. 1.* AHCPR Publication No. 92–0032.

Violence wheel. (2009). Available at http://www.domesticviolence.org/violence-wheel/

VonBaeyer, C. (2007). Faces Pain Scale-Revised (FPS-R). Available at http://www.painsourcebook.ca

Wallace, M., & Shelkey, M. (2007). Katz index of independence in activities of daily living (ADL). *Annals of Long-Term Care, 11* (2). Available at www.annalsoflongtermcare.com

WebMD. (2010a). ABCDEs of skin cancer. Available at http://www.webmd.com/melanoma-skin-cancer/abcds-of-melanoma-skin-cancer

WebMD. (2011a). Eye exams and tests for children and teenagers. Available at http://www.webmd.com/eye-health/eye-exams-for-children-and-teenagers

WebMD. (2011b). High blood pressure in African-Americans. Available at http://www.webmd.com/hypertension-high-blood-pressure/hypertension-in-african-americans

World Health Organization (WHO). (2010). WHO pain guidelines. Available at http://www.whocancerpain.wisc.edu/?q=node/130

Zullo, N. (2012). Depression in elderly care recipients. Available at http://www.longtermcarelink.net/eldercare/depression_elderly_care_recipients.htm

Index

Note: Page number followed by b, f, or t indicates text in box, figure, or table.